VETERINARY ANESTHESIA AND PAIN MANAGEMENT SECRETS

VETERINARY ANESTHESIA AND PAIN MANAGEMENT SECRETS

STEPHEN A. GREENE, D.V.M., M.S., D.A.C.V.A.
Associate Professor of Veterinary Anesthesia
Department of Veterinary Clinical Medicine
University of Illinois College of Veterinary Medicine
Urbana, Illinois

HANLEY & BELFUS, INC./Philadelphia
An Imprint of Elsevier

Publisher: HANLEY & BELFUS, INC.
           Medical Publishers
           An Imprint of Elsevier
           210 South 13th Street
           Philadelphia, PA 19107
           (215) 546-7293; 800-962-1892
           FAX (215) 790-9330
           Web site: http://www.hanleyandbelfus.com

Note to the reader: Although the information in this book has been carefully reviewed for correctness of dosage and indications, neither the authors nor the editor nor the publisher can accept any legal responsibility for any errors or omissions that may be made. Neither the publisher nor the editor makes any warranty, expressed or implied, with respect to the material contained herein. Before prescribing any drug, the reader must review the manufacturer's correct product information (package inserts) for accepted indications, absolute dosage recommendations, and other information pertinent to the safe and effective use of the product described. This is especially important when drugs are given in combination or as an adjunct to other forms of therapy.

Library of Congress Cataloging-in-Publication Data

Veterinary anesthesia and pain management secrets / edited by Stephen A. Greene.
       p. cm. – (The Secrets Series®)
    Includes bibliographical references (p.).
    ISBN-13: 978-1-56053-442-6 ISBN-10: 1-56053-442-7 (alk. paper)

       1. Veterinary anesthesia—Examinations , questions, etc. 2. Pain in animals—
Treatment—Examinations, questions, etc. I. Greene, Stephen A., 1956-II. Series.

    SF914.V48 2002
    636.089'796'076—dc21   2001039966

ISBN-13: 978-1-56053-442-6
ISBN-10: 1-56053-442-7 (alk. paper)

**VETERINARY ANESTHESIA AND
PAIN MANAGEMENT SECRETS**

Permissions may be sought directly from Elsevier's Health Sciences Rights
Department in Philadelphia, PA, USA: phone: (+1) 215 239 3804, fax: (+1) 215 239 3805,
e-mail: healthpermissions@elsevier.com. You may also complete your request on-line
via the Elsevier homepage (http://www.elsevier.com), by selecting 'Customer Support'
and then 'Obtaining Permissions'.

Transferred to Digital Printing 2011.

CONTENTS

CONTRIBUTORS

G. John Benson, D.V.M., M.S., D.A.C.V.A.
Professor, Department of Veterinary Clinical Medicine, University of Illinois College of Veterinary Medicine, Urbana, Illinois

Nigel A. Caulkett, D.V.M., M.V.Sc., D.A.C.V.A.
Associate Professor, Department of Small Animal Clinical Sciences, University of Saskatchewan, Saskatoon, Saskatchewan, Canada

Sophie Cuvelliez, D.M.V., M.S., D.A.C.V.A., D.E.C.V.A.
Professor, Department of Clinical Sciences, Veterinary Medicine, Université de Montréal, Saint Hyacinthe, Québec, Canada

Thomas K. Day, D.V.M., M.S., D.A.C.V.A., D.A.C.V.E.C.C.
Emergency and Critical Care Veterinarian, Louisville Veterinary Specialty and Emergency Services, Louisville, Kentucky

Tom Doherty, M.V.B., M.Sc., D.A.C.V.A.
Associate Professor, Department of Large Animal Clinical Sciences, The University of Tennessee, College of Veterinary Medicine, Knoxville, Tennessee

Doris H. Dyson, D.V.M., D.V.Sc., D.A.C.V.A.
Associate Professor, Department of Clinical Studies, Ontario Veterinary College, University of Guelph, Guelph, Ontario, Canada

Jennifer Linda Fujimoto, D.V.M., D.A.C.V.A.
Senior Veterinarian, Animal Care Program, University of California at San Diego, La Jolla, California

David S. Galloway, D.V.M., M.M.A.S.
Major, U. S. Army Veterinary Corps; Resident of Small Animal Surgery, Department of Clinical Sciences, College of Veterinary Medicine, Oklahoma State University, Stillwater, Oklahoma

Stephen A. Greene, D.V.M., M.S., D.A.C.V.A.
Associate Professor of Veterinary Anesthesia, Department of Veterinary Clinical Medicine, University of Illinois College of Veterinary Medicine, Urbana, Illinois

Kurt A. Grimm, D.V.M., M.S., D.A.C.V.A., D.A.C.V.C.P.
Visiting Assistant Professor, Department of Veterinary Clinical Medicine, University of Illinois College of Veterinary Medicine, Urbana, Illinois

Tamara L. Grubb, D.V.M., M.S., D.A.C.V.A.
Assistant Professor, College of Veterinary Medicine, Oregon State University, Corvallis, Oregon

Ralph C. Harvey, D.V.M., M.S., D.A.C.V.A.
Associate Professor of Anesthesiology, Department of Small Animal Clinical Sciences, University of Tennessee College of Veterinary Medicine, Knoxville, Tennessee

Terrell G. Heaton-Jones, D.V.M.
Researcher, College of Veterinary Medicine, University of Florida, Gainesville, Florida

Jana L. Jones, D.V.M., D.A.C.V.A., D.A.C.V.E.C.C.
Assistant Professor, Department of Large Animal Clinical Sciences, College of Veterinary Medicine, University of Tennessee, Knoxville, Tennessee

Robert D. Keegan, D.V.M., D.A.C.V.A.
Associate Professor, Anesthesia Section Head, Department of Veterinary Clinical Sciences, Washington State University, Pullman, Washington

Lisa S. Klopp, D.V.M., M.S., D.A.C.V.I.M. (Neurology)
Assistant Professor, Department of Veterinary Clinical Medicine, University of Illinois College of Veterinary Medicine, Urbana, Illinois

Jeff C. H. Ko, D.V.M., M.S., D.A.C.V.A.
Associate Professor of Anesthesiology, Department of Veterinary Clinical Sciences, College of Veterinary Medicine, Oklahoma State University, Stillwater, Oklahoma

Kris T. Kruse-Elliott, D.V.M., Ph.D., D.A.C.V.A.
Associate Professor, Department of Surgical Sciences, University of Wisconsin, Madison, Wisconsin

Lynne I. Kushner, D.V.M., D.A.C.V.A.
Staff Anesthesiologist, Department of Clinical Sciences, Veterinary Hospital of the University of Pennsylvania; University of Pennsylvania School of Veterinary Medicine, Philadelphia, Pennsylvania

Leigh A. Lamont, D.V.M.
Resident in Anesthesiology, Department of Veterinary Clinical Medicine, University of Illinois College of Veterinary Medicine, Urbana, Illinois

Kip A. Lemke, D.V.M., M.S., D.A.C.V.A.
Associate Professor of Anesthesiology, Atlantic Veterinary College, University of Prince Edward Island, Charlottetown, Prince Edward Island, Canada

Khursheed Mama, D.V.M., D.A.C.V.A.
Assistant Professor, Department of Clinical Sciences, Colorado State University, Fort Collins, Colorado

Elizabeth A. Martinez, D.V.M., D.A.C.V.A.
Associate Professor, Department of Small Animal Medicine and Surgery, College of Veterinary Medicine, Texas A & M University, College Station, Texas

Sheila M. McCullough, D.V.M., M.S., D.A.C.V.I.M.
Clinical Assistant Professor, Department of Veterinary Clinical Medicine, University of Illinois College of Veterinary Medicine, Urbana, Illinois

Robert E. Meyer, D.V.M., D.A.C.V.A.
Associate Professor, Department of Anatomy, Physiological Sciences, and Radiology, North Carolina State University College of Veterinary Medicine, Raleigh, North Carolina

Luisito S. Pablo, D.V.M., M.S., D.A.C.V.A.
Associate Professor, Department of Large Animal Clinical Sciences, University of Florida, Gainesville, Florida

Jane Quandt, D.V.M., M.S., D.A.C.V.A.
Assistant Clinical Specialist in Anesthesiology, Department of Small Animal Clinical Sciences, College of Veterinary Medicine, Veterinary Teaching Hospital, University of Minnesota, St. Paul, Minnesota

David C. Rankin, D.V.M., M.S., D.A.C.V.A.
Staff Anesthesiologist, Wisconsin Veterinary Referral Center, Wankesha, Wisconsin

Thomas Riebold, D.V.M., D.A.C.V.A.
Professor, Department of Large Animal Clinical Sciences, College of Veterinary Medicine, Oregon State University, Corvallis, Oregon

Sheilah A. Robertson, B.V.M.S., Ph.D., D.A.C.V.A.
Associate Professor, Section of Anesthesia and Pain Management, University of Florida, Gainesville, Florida

Yves Rondenay, D.M.V.
Clinical Instructor, Veterinary Teaching Hospital, Université de Montréal, Québec, Canada

Julie A. Smith, D.V.M., D.A.C.V.A.
Hospital Director and Chief of Anesthesia, IAMS Pet Imaging, Vienna, Virginia

Lesley J. Smith, D.V.M., D.A.C.V.A.
Clinical Assistant Professor of Anesthesiology, Department of Surgical Sciences, School of Veterinary Medicine, University of Wisconsin, Madison, Wisconsin

William J. Tranquilli, D.V.M., M.S., D.A.C.V.A.
Professor of Clinical Medicine (Anesthesiology and Pain Management), Department of Clinical Medicine, University of Illinois College of Veterinary Medicine; University of Illinois Veterinary Medicine Teaching Hospital, Urbana, Illinois

Lois A. Wetmore, D.V.M., Sc.D., D.A.C.V.A.
Assistant Professor, Department of Clinical Sciences, Tufts University School of Veterinary Medicine, North Grafton, Massachusetts

Deborah V. Wilson, B.V.Sc., M.S., D.A.C.V.A.
Associate Professor, Department of Large Animal Clinical Sciences, Michigan State University, East Lansing, Michigan

PREFACE

It is my sincere hope that the reader will find the unique question-and-answer approach to be a breath of fresh air when compared with previously published texts on veterinary anesthesia and pain management. The contributing authors are noted experts in various veterinary medical specialties, including anesthesiology, clinical pharmacology, critical care, internal medicine, and neurology. Each has included subject matter that is of clinical relevance and interest. I am grateful for their diligent labors and will be forever in their debt.

As in other Secrets volumes, this book has been presented in an informative and easily understood style. It has been organized into nine sections: Patient Management, Patient Preparation, Pharmacology, Patient Monitoring, Perianesthetic Complications, Anesthesia and Systemic Disease, Special Anesthetic Considerations, Regional Anesthesia, and Pain Management for Small Animals. Each section contains salient information related to anesthetic management of small and large domestic species as well as amphibians, birds, camelids, laboratory animals, reptiles, and other wild animals. The inclusion of concepts and techniques related to pain management addresses the vital role of this increasingly emphasized aspect of veterinary medical care both in and out of the surgical theater.

I want to acknowledge William Lamsback and Mary Beth Murphy at Hanley & Belfus for offering their encouragement and inspiration to make this book more than a virtual reality.

Finally, I would like to dedicate this book to my colleagues, friends, and family (especially Erma, Kaitlin, and Jared) for their unwavering support of my professional efforts and to the memory of my father, Dr. Daryle E. Greene, who recognized the value of persistence in all worthwhile endeavors.

Stephen A. Greene, DVM, MS, DACVA

I. Patient Management

1. AIRWAY MAINTENANCE

Jane E. Quandt, D.V.M., M.S., D.A.C.V.A.

1. What are the advantages to endotracheal intubation versus a face mask for maintaining inhalant anesthesia?

- Maintenance of a patent airway.
- Improved efficiency of delivery of oxygen and anesthetic gases.
- Decreased exposure of waste gases to personnel.
- Intubation improves the efficiency of respiration by reducing the amount of dead space within the respiratory passages. The end of the endotracheal tube should be at the level of the animal's incisors to avoid endotracheal tube dead space.
- Respiratory support in the form of intermittent, positive-pressure ventilation is possible with intubation. This is required for animals undergoing thoracotomy or diaphragmatic hernia repair or receiving a neuromuscular blocking agent.
- An endotracheal tube with a cuff will reduce the risk of aspirating vomitus, blood, flush, or other material that may run into the oral cavity and breathing passages.

Animals undergoing general anesthesia should be endotracheally intubated.

2. What is the procedure for endotracheal intubation in the dog or cat?

- An endotracheal tube. Have more than one tube in varying sizes and in appropriate lengths. The tube cuffs should be checked to ensure there are no leaks. Note the amount of air required to fill the cuff.
- Sterile tube lubricant such as lidocaine gel or K-Y jelly. When lubricating a small endotracheal tube, be sure the lube does not obstruct the tube opening.
- Lidocaine spray (for cats) or 1% lidocaine solutiondrawn into a syringe. 0.1 ml is squirted onto the laryngeal area to decrease the risk of laryngospasm. A volume of 0.1 to 0.2 ml of lidocaine is sufficient, as excessive administration can be toxic.
- Gauze tie to hold the endotracheal tube in place.
- Laryngoscope or a good light source to visualize the laryngeal area.

3. What is the procedure for endotracheal intubation in the dog or cat?

When the animal, in sternal or lateral recumbency, reaches the appropriate plane of anesthesia and there are no signs of resistance such as gagging, swallowing, or chewing motion upon opening the mouth, the animal is ready to be intubated. Once the mouth is opened, the neck is extended so the head and neck are in a straight line. The upper jaw is held stationary, lips are pulled dorsally, and the lower jaw is pushed down with the tongue pulled forward and down. Use caution and do not cut the tongue on the teeth or pull the tongue excessively, which could damage the nerves.

The anesthetist using the laryngoscope or other light source should be able to see the epiglottis overlying the trachea. The laryngoscope blade or tip of the endotracheal tube is used to disengage the soft palate from the epiglottis. The blade can then be used on the back of the tongue, adjacent to the base of the epiglottis. When pushed downward, the blade pulls the epiglottis forward and down, allowing the entrance to the trachea to be visualized.

The endotracheal tube is inserted past the vocal folds and into the trachea. In cats, intubation is best done by advancing the tube when the vocal cords separate and the glottis opens. Don't

1

force the tube past the vocal cords if resistance is encountered; gently rotate the tube and advance. The curve of the tube should match the patient's neck when intubation is complete.

4. How can use of a stylet help in endotracheal intubation?
A small flexible endotracheal tube may bend during insertion. The use of a stylet, a thin metal rod or thick aluminum wire, inserted into the tube will prevent bending. The end of the stylet should not protrude beyond the end of the tube, as it may traumatize the laryngeal tissue. Once the tube is in the trachea, the stylet must be removed, as it will obstruct the airflow.

5. Describe correct placement of the endotracheal tube. How is the tube secured?
Once the tube is correctly placed the tube emerges from the glottis with the tip no further than the carina. The endotracheal tube connector should be at the level of the incisor teeth to avoid excessive dead space. Vocalization is impossible if the tube is properly placed. If the animal whines or makes vocal sounds, the tube is in the esophagus.

The tube is held in place with a snuggly tied piece of gauze. The tie should be snug to prevent slipping, which can occur when the tube becomes wet with saliva or other liquid, such as flush or blood. The tie ends are then passed behind the ears or behind the canine teeth and secured with a bow knot.

6. How much air should be put in the cuff of the endotracheal tube?
The reservoir bag is gently squeezed to 20 cm H_2O and the anesthetist listens for the sound of leaking air exiting the oral cavity. The cuff is inflated only until there is no longer a leak. The cuff should be inflated incrementally to prevent overinflation. If the leak is large, consider reintubation with a larger tube or check to make sure the tube is not in the esophagus. Excessive pressure in the cuff may cause ischemic injury and perhaps lead to tracheal stricture, tracheal ulceration, tracheitis, hemorrhage, tracheomalacia, fibrosis, or stenosis.

A surgery of long duration will require the endotracheal tube to be in place for lengthy times. To avoid constant pressure of the cuff on the same area of the trachea, the cuff should be deflated every 2 hours, the tube repositioned slightly, and the cuff reinflated. This will help prevent potential pressure necrosis of the tracheal mucosa.

7. What is the advantage of a cuffed versus a noncuffed tube?
The cuff helps to prevent leakage of waste gases. It will also reduce the risk of aspiration. Animals intubated with cuffed tubes are prevented from breathing room air, which may otherwise enter by flow from around the outside of the tube. If significant amounts of room air are breathed in, it is difficult to maintain the animal at an adequate anesthetic depth, as the air dilutes the anesthetic.

8. What precautions can be taken to avoid problems with endotracheal intubation?
Use a sterile or thoroughly disinfected endotracheal tube for each patient to prevent the spread of infectious disease.

The endotracheal tube should be lubricated with sterile xylocaine or K-Y jelly. Avoid using a lubricant containing benzocaine, as this can lead to a dose-dependent methemoglobinemia, which does not bind oxygen.

Intubation may stimulate the activity of the vagus nerve, increasing parasympathetic tone, especially in dogs. This may result in bradycardia, hypotension, and cardiac dysrhythmias. If the animal has an underlying cardiovascular disease, cardiac arrest may occur. Atropine or glycopyrrolate, an anticholinergic, given as part of the premedication can be helpful in preventing the parasympathetic stimulation.

Do not be forceful in the intubation, as this can damage the larynx, pharynx, or soft palate and lead to tissue edema. Ideally, the tip of the endotracheal tube should be past the larynx and not beyond the thoracic inlet. If the tube is advanced too far, it may enter one bronchus, resulting in ventilation to only one lung. Premeasure the length of the endotracheal tube and the distance between the nose and the thoracic inlet prior to anesthesia. The end of the tube should be at the level of the animal's incisors.

To avoid esophageal intubation, visualize the endotracheal tube going into the trachea. Esophageal intubation will lead to hypoxemia and an awakening patient.

Do not overinflate the cuff of the endotracheal tube, or pressure necrosis of the tracheal tissue may occur.

Watch that the endotracheal tube does not become obstructed with saliva, blood, or foreign material or become kinked.

9. Brachycephalic animals such as bulldogs, pugs, and Persian cats can be difficult to intubate. What special considerations are there for airway management in these breeds?

There are four common abnormalities with brachycephalic breeds:

- Elongated soft palate
- Everted laryngeal saccules
- Stenoic nares
- Hypoplastic trachea

These animals also have redundant pharyngeal tissue that makes visualizing the airway difficult. An array of endotracheal tubes in varying sizes should be readily available. The trachea may be smaller than the size of the animal would indicate. Preoxygenate to increase the safety margin for intubation. These breeds frequently have high vagal tone, and intubation stimulation may cause a vagal reflex and bradycardia. Preanesthetic administration of an anticholinergic can help prevent this from occurring.

In recovery, leave the endotracheal tube in for as long as possible. Once extubated, these animals need close monitoring to ensure that the airway stays patent. Keeping the animal's head and neck extended will help prevent the redundant tissue from obstructing the airway. Always keep the proper size of endotracheal tube near the animal's cage in case reintubation becomes necessary.

10. Are there any special considerations for the intubation of cats?

Cats have a narrow glottis that is easily traumatized; use care when intubating. If the laryngeal tissues are irritated during intubation, laryngospasm—reflex closure of the laryngeal cartilages—may occur. This can cause blockage of the airway. To prevent laryngospasm, use lidocaine spray on the larynx and lidocaine gel on the endotracheal tube to help desensitize the laryngeal tissue. Use a gentle intubation technique; advance the tube when the glottis is open.

The cat is more prone to laryngospasm with inadequate anesthetic depth. The laryngoscope is used to depress the tongue and not to pull the epiglottis forward and down. The blade should not touch the epiglottis, as this can cause trauma and edema.

A guide tube, such as a 5 to 8 French canine urinary catheter, that extends past the cuffed end of the endotracheal tube for a distance of 2 to 3 cm can be used to help make intubation easier. Pass the small catheter first and then thread the endotracheal over the catheter into the trachea.

11. What should you do if the cat has a laryngospasm?

Do not stimulate the larynx further; stop trying to intubate.

Supply oxygen by mask, so that any air that enters the trachea is oxygen-enriched.

Try one more dose of lidocaine spray on the larynx. If the spasm does not relax within 10 to 20 seconds, try deepening the anesthetic plane, or use a neuromuscular blocking agent. A neuromuscular blocking agent will cause relaxation of the tissues, but also apnea due to the paralysis, so intubation must be done immediately.

Do not force intubation, as this can damage the mucous membranes and larynx and lead to edema and then the danger of obstruction after extubation. It is also possible to penetrate the pharyngeal wall with forceful intubation.

You can secure a temporary airway by placing a 14-gauge needle or catheter in the trachea percutaneously. If all else fails, perform a tracheostomy.

12. When should the endotracheal tube be removed?

The endotracheal tube should be removed when the animal regains the ability to swallow and protect its airway. Do not allow the patient to chew the tube in half and aspirate the distal half.

This will necessitate reanesthetizing the animal to retrieve the tube, which is usually lodged at the carina. Care must also be taken that an animal with increased jaw tone does not bite down on the tube and create an obstruction.

Following a dental or other procedure in which blood or fluid is present in the oral cavity, be sure the oral cavity is wiped clean of any material the animal could aspirate, such as gauze, tissue fragments, and blood clots. Use a laryngoscope to fully visualize the mouth and upper tracheal area.

Extubation can be done with the tube cuff partially inflated to help act as a wedge and remove debris in the upper trachea. Do not leave the cuff fully inflated, as it can tear tracheal mucosa and damage the vocal cords. Once the animal is extubated, make sure it is breathing normally. It may help to extend the head and neck to maximize the integrity of the airway.

In the cat, don't delay extubation, as there can be the risk of hyper-responsive airway reflexes, laryngospasm, retching, or vomiting.

13. What are the indications for performing a tracheostomy?
- To relieve an upper respiratory tract obstruction
- To facilitate removal of respiratory secretions
- To decrease dead space
- To provide a route for inhalant anesthesia when oral or facial surgery is complex
- To reduce resistance to respiration
- When you are unable to orally intubate
- To reduce the risk of closed glottis pressure, or cough, following pulmonary or cranial surgery
- To facilitate artificial respiration

14. What is the technique for doing a tracheostomy?
Make a midline skin incision on the ventral neck equidistant from the larynx and the manubrium. Part the two sternohyoid muscles on the midline and continue blunt dissection down to the tracheal rings. Make an incision transverse between the rings; keep the incision small, only big enough for the tracheostomy tube. Alternatively, make a longitudinal incision to include two or three tracheal rings. Don't place the incision too close to the first tracheal ring, or it could potentially damage the cricoid cartilage and lead to subglottic laryngeal stenosis.

Place stay sutures around the tracheal ring adjacent to the incision on either side of the surgical opening. The sutures will aid in placement of the tube and are left in, labeled cranial and caudal, to help when the tube is routinely replaced or cleaned, or if it gets dislodged.

The tube ideally is two-thirds to three-fourths of the tracheal diameter, with a high-volume, low-pressure cuff. Inflate the cuff only as needed to prevent a leak with positive pressure ventilation and to help prevent aspiration. If a specifically designed tracheostomy tube is not available, an endotracheal tube can be used; it may need to be cut so it is short enough that it does not go into one bronchus.

Fasten the tube in place by tying it around the neck with umbilical tape or gauze. The soft tissue is loosely approximated with absorbable sutures and the skin is closed with nonabsorbable sutures. It is important to allow any air escaping around the tube to vent to the outside and not accumulate under the skin.

15. What is the postoperative care of the tracheostomy tube?
The lumen of the tracheostomy tube must be regularly cleaned to prevent obstruction with dried blood or mucus. The tube should be suctioned frequently, maybe as often as every 30 minutes after the initial placement, then decreasing to hourly and then to every 2 to 4 hours as the production of secretions lessens. Suctioning of the tube and airways is done using a soft sterile rubber or vinyl tube with an end-hole. The suction can be controlled using a thumb port or T-connector to allow application of intermittent suction. Suctioning must be intermittent, as continuous suction will lead to atelectasis and hypoxemia. Oxygenate the animal for 5 to 7 minutes with 100% oxygen prior to and after suctioning. After suctioning, give two to four positive pressure ventilations to help open the lower airways.

Humidification of the tube is important to prevent the drying of secretions that can block the tube. Humidification can be done with either a commercial humidifier or by injecting 1 to 5 ml of sterile water into the tube every hour. Many tracheostomy tubes come with an internal cannula that can be removed, cleaned, and resterilized, making for easier maintenance. The cannula is changed every 4 hours; the tracheostomy tube itself is changed every 24 to 48 hours if there is no inner cannula. Secretions and mucus can adhere to the inner cannula or tube and lead to obstruction of the airway, which necessitates the replacement of the tube or cannula with a clean one. The tube requires frequent monitoring, as obstruction can lead to death of the patient.

There is major risk for nosocomial infection when using tracheostomy tubes, therefore sterile technique must be used for suctioning and changing of the tube.

16. How should the tracheostomy tube be removed? When is this done?

Changing the tracheostomy tube can be dangerous if the new tube is not placed in a timely fashion. It is helpful to oxygenate the animal prior to tube removal and to use the sutures that were preplaced on the rings of the trachea cranial and caudal to the opening in the trachea. The sutures should be labeled as cranial and caudal and are used to gently retract the rings and to exteriorize the trachea to make the opening larger and easier to see. If the tracheostomy tube cannot be re-inserted, oral intubation can be done to establish an airway.

The tracheostomy tube can be removed when you believe that the animal is capable of returning to nasal or mouth breathing. To help determine whether the animal can breathe, deflate the cuff on the tube and occlude the tube opening. This technique is dangerous unless the tube allows sufficient air to flow around the tube. Alternatively, remove the tube and closely monitor the patient and re-intubate if necessary. If the animal cannot maintain normal breaths, the tube must be left in place.

Following tracheostomy tube removal, the animal must remain under close observation for several hours. A new tube must be ready for replacement if the animal's breathing becomes decompensated. Once it is safe for the animal to remain extubated, the site is allowed to heal in 7 to 10 days by second intention, as primary closure may predispose to subcutaneous emphysema.

17. What are armored endotracheal tubes?

Armored or reinforced endotracheal tubes are designed with helical wire or plastic implanted within the walls to prevent kinking of the tube and obstruction of the airway when the patient's head or neck is flexed. These tubes are used with ophthalmic surgery, head and neck surgery, cervical spinal taps, oral surgery, or any procedure in which the airway may become kinked.

The armored tubes have thicker walls than a standard tube with a smaller internal diameter, so there will be increased resistance to air flow. These tubes should be used only when necessary. They are very flexible and therefore more difficult to place. A stylet or guide tube will help facilitate insertion.

18. What special risk accompanies laser surgery? What is the best precaution?

Fire. Laser can cut through the endotracheal tube or ignite the tube, and the fire can become blowtorch-like in its effect. Heat, flame, and toxic products can be put down into the pulmonary parenchyma.

A red rubber endotracheal tube is more resistant to ignition and will produce less debris and inflammation.

19. How can the tube be protected against this risk?

When not using a red rubber endotracheal tube, protect the tube by wrapping with aluminum or copper adhesive-backed tape. The tape will reflect the laser, but make sure the adhesive is not flammable. One type of tape that can be used is self-adhesive 3M number 425 aluminum foil tape. Clean and dry the tube to be taped and wipe it with alcohol to remove residue so that the tape will stick. Cut the tape at angle of 60 degrees with the cut edge aligned with the proximal end of the cuff junction. Wrap the tube from the cuff up to the pilot tube in a spiral fashion with

30% overlap of the tape, so bending of the tube does not expose unprotected areas. Make sure there are no wrinkles in the tape that may abrade the tracheal mucosa.

The tube will be 1 to 2 mm larger than a normal tube after it has been wrapped. After wrapping, rewipe the tube with alcohol to provide a degree of cleanliness prior to intubation. Be aware that the tape itself can have rough edges that can damage the tissue. Also, pieces may break off to be aspirated, the tape may kink the tube, and the laser can reflect off the tube and damage the surrounding tissue. When the animal is extubated make sure the tape is intact on the tube.

20. What role does saline play in decreasing the risk?

The endotracheal tube cuff is filled with saline. The saline serves as a heat sink and absorbs the laser's energy, preventing combustion of the cuff. A small amount of methylene blue added to the saline will help signal when the cuff gets punctured by staining the tissue. If an air-filled cuff becomes perforated, oxygen will flow around the tube and enhance a fire, but if the cuff is filled with saline and breaks, there will be a fine spray to help decrease the fire. Pack the upper airway and oral cavity with saline-soaked sponges to decrease the risk of fire.

21. What other steps can be taken to reduce the risk?

The risk of fire can also be decreased by reducing the inspired oxygen to 30 to 50%.

Special laser tubes, Laser-Shield III by Xomed-Treace and Bivona "Fome-cuff" tube are available, but they are expensive. They are bulkier and more rigid than usual tubes and must be used carefully. They may cause mucosal abrasions.

In animals with a pre-existing tracheostomy tube, a metal tracheostomy tube can be used so laser entering the trachea would not cause ignition.

22. What do you do if there is a laser fire?

If there is a fire, remove the laser, turn off the oxygen (as oxygen will fuel the fire), and put the fire out. Then examine the airway. If possible, use a fiberoptic bronchoscope to evaluate the tracheal damage; the animal may need to reintubated. If there is severe damage with swelling and edema, a tracheostomy may be needed to establish an airway.

23. Are there any special requirements for endotracheal tubes in an animal undergoing MRI?

There can be no ferromagnetic object in the magnet, as this will degrade the image. There can be no wire in the endotracheal tube or the tube cuff. No wire spiral tubes or armored tubes can be used.

24. What is external pharyngotomy? When would it be used?

External pharyngotomy is a type of intubation that can be performed for oropharyngeal surgery or orthopedic procedures of the mandible or maxilla. This type of intubation aids in the visualization of the area and allows for normal dental occlusion so that proper reduction of jaw fractures can be achieved.

Initially place the endotracheal tube orally. Make a skin incision near the angle of the mandible. Pass hemostats bluntly through the incision into the caudal part of the pharynx. Remove the endotracheal tube adapter, grasp the tube, and pull it through from the pharynx through the subcutaneous tissue and skin incision. Replace the adapter and connect the tube to the breathing circuit. Secure with tape and suture.

Extubation is done with the cuff deflated and the tube pulled through the skin incision.

25. How is the equine patient intubated?

Flush the mouth prior to anesthesia to remove any grass or feedstuffs to prevent them from being carried into the airway during intubation. After the horse is anesthetized, the halter is removed, and the horse is placed in lateral recumbency with the head and neck extended. The airway should be in a straight line. Open the mouth and place a speculum. The speculum can be a metal one with teeth plates and a crank to open the mouth or polyvinyl chloride pipe wrapped with adhesive tape that can be placed between the upper and lower incisors. Pipe in varying diameters can be used for varying sizes of horses. Open the mouth gently to avoid trauma to the jaw. This is a "blind" intubation.

Introduce the lubricated tube into the mouth with the concave side of its curve directed toward the hard palate and advance it, keeping to midline until the tip is in the pharynx. This ensures it does not become impacted in the epiglottis. The tube may need to be rotated 0 to 90 degrees or more as it approaches the glottis. There should be no resistance as the tube enters the larynx and trachea. If the tube does not enter the trachea, the alignment of the animal's head and neck may be incorrect. Use caution when passing the tube, as the cuff can be damaged on the teeth.

Manipulation of the tube should be done in a gentle manner as edema or other injury can occur from excessive force. If there is resistance, retract the tube approximately 10 cm, rotate it 90 to 180 degrees, and readvance. Inflate the cuff only until there is no air leak at 20 to 30 cm H_2O. Overinflation of the cuff can cause collapse of the endotracheal tube.

26. Under what circumstances should the tube be removed?

Extubate the horse when it can swallow. Alternatively, the tube can be left in place until the horse is standing. The tube is probably best left in place if there is nasal turbinate edema that could lead to obstruction. Edema is more likely to occur in horses that have been anesthetized for a long time in dorsal recumbency with the head below heart level. Tape the endotracheal tube to the head, the helmet, or around the ear to prevent the horse from inhaling the tube.

27. What are the indications that upper airway obstruction has occurred in the horse following extubation?

With edema-obstruction there is a loud inspiratory snoring. It quickly disappears when the horse gets up and the head is higher than heart level. Phenylephrine, 10 to 20 mg in 12 ml of saline, sprayed into the nasal passages will decrease edema.

The soft palate can be displaced dorsally to the epiglottis, creating an obstruction. The soft palate enters the larynx during inspiration. This can be corrected by inducing swallowing. Manipulate the larynx by inserting a stomach tube to the area of the pharynx.

A nasotracheal tube or tracheostomy is needed if arytenoid paralysis occurs. There is a loud shrill noise with exaggerated inspiratory efforts.

28. What are the indications for nasal intubation in the equine?

Nasal intubation can be done for dental or mouth surgery to get the endotracheal tube out of the surgical field, as well as in the foal to allow an inhalant induction. Nasal intubation reduces pollution, as would occur with mask induction of the foal. The foal does not resent the inhalant when nasally intubated, as the animal cannot smell the gas.

29. What are the special considerations for nasal intubation in the equine?

Before considering nasal intubation, check both nostrils to make sure they are patent and there is no infection in the nose or sinuses. A tube passed through a contaminated area could then deposit contaminated particles in the lower airways. The nose must be cleaned of dirt and debris before the tube is passed. An extra long tube is needed for foals, 55 cm with a minimal curve, usually made of silicone rubber and having relatively thin walls for maximal internal diameter. In general, the nasal tracheal tube is one to two sizes smaller then an orotracheal tube for the patient.

30. How is nasal intubation performed in a foal?

In the awake foal, put lidocaine gel on the tip of the tube and inside the nostril. Keep the animal's head and neck extended and restrained to minimize jerking of the head and thus potential trauma to the meatus. Gently pass the tube through the external nares into the ventral meatus. If there is resistance to passage, the tube has probably gone into the middle meatus, or a smaller tube is needed. If there is continued resistance as the tube is passed into the pharyngeal area, the tube may be going esophageal, and the foal may swallow the tube. Do not rotate the tube, as this may lead to epistaxis. If the tube does not advance down one nostril, the other nostril can be tried.

Using gentle pressure, the tube is advanced into the pharynx and then to the larynx. If the foal coughs, the tube is close to the larynx and 3 ml 2% lidocaine can be injected down the tube to desensitize the epiglottis and arytenoid cartilages. There should be a loss of resistance as the tube advances into the trachea; the foal may cough and air flow can be felt coming from the end of the tube. Inability to palpate the tube in the trachea and lack of air movement through the tube is an indication of esophageal intubation.

After the tube has been properly placed, tape the tube to the muzzle to prevent the tube from being aspirated. The end of the tube should be at the nostrils and the cuff is distal to the larynx. When nasal intubation is only done to induce anesthesia, once the foal is anesthetized the nasal tube can be replaced with an oral tube so that there is less resistance to air flow.

31. How is nasal intubation performed in an adult horse?

In the adult, nasal intubation is usually done after induction of anesthesia. Keep the head and neck straight and gently advance the tube through the ventral meatus into the laryngeal area. There is lack of resistance as the tube passes into the trachea. The ventral nasal meatus will limit the size of tube that can be accommodated by the nostril. Extubate the nasal tube carefully, deflate the cuff, and withdraw in a slow and deliberate fashion. If the animal is conscious, restrain the head so that there is no jerking. Rapid rough extubation may cause nasal hemorrhage due to turbinate damage. The turbinates can also be damaged during intubation. Damaged turbinates can cause extensive hemorrhage. The horse can be recovered and allowed to stand with the tube in place.

Nasal intubation can be used if a horse recovering from anesthesia and extubated has developed nasal edema and needs an airway. Nasal intubation can be done without fully re-anesthetizing the horse, as would be necessary with oral intubation,

32. How is a large ruminant such as a cow intubated?

A large ruminant undergoing a lengthy general anesthesia procedure should be orally intubated to help prevent aspiration of rumen contents and saliva, of which there will be a copious flow. These animals have a high risk of regurgitation and aspiration. Flush the mouth clean of feed and debris prior to anesthesia. In adult cattle, the larynx cannot be visualized and intubation is done by palpation. Keep the anesthetized bovine in sternal recumbency until the endotracheal tube is in place to prevent aspiration. A speculum such as a Bayer dental wedge, Guenther mouth speculum, Weingart mouth speculum, or Drinkwater mouth gag is used to open the mouth. These are ruminant mouth gags that help protect the dental pad. A veterinarian with a small thin arm free of watches and rings, which may become lost into the cow, is the best candidate to perform the intubation technique. Pass the hand and arm through the speculum into the mouth and over the tongue and down to identify the epiglottis and arytenoid cartilages. Place the fingertips on the arytenoid cartilages and pass the lubricated tube between the dorsum of the tongue and arm. The tube is directed through the glottis by the fingertips and the hand is then withdrawn from the mouth as the tube is pushed on into the trachea. Rotating the tube 0 to 90 degrees as it approaches the arytenoid cartilages may help.

If the tube is too large to pass by the arm, pass a guide tube first and then pass the endotracheal tube over it. The guide tube is an equine stomach tube directed manually into the trachea as just described. The guide tube is removed once the endotracheal tube is in place. The intubation should be done as quickly as possible because the anesthetist's hand and arm will create an airway obstruction. Inflate the cuff immediately to help prevent aspiration. If the animal begins regurgitating before the tube is passed, apply external pressure over the esophagus to halt the flow of ruminal contents. When lubricating the tube, do not use lidocaine gel or a local anesthetic, as the mucous membranes of the trachea and larynx will be desensitized for some time after the tube is withdrawn, and the protective cough reflex will be absent and aspiration may be more likely to occur. Make sure the mouth is cleared of any ingesta before extubation.

33. Is intubation of the small ruminant different?

In small ruminants, direct visualization of the larynx is possible by use of a laryngoscope. Flush the mouth clean prior to anesthesia; a 60 cc syringe can be used. In the sheep and goat, once the animal is anesthetized, keep it in sternal recumbency until the endotracheal tube is in place. Extend the head and neck, keeping the airway straight. Use gauze loops around the upper and lower jaws to open the mouth. Pull the tongue forward and out of the mouth. Clean the mouth of saliva.

Place the blade of the laryngoscope behind the base of the tongue, in front of the epiglottis. Lift the blade horizontally to expose the larynx and vocal cords and pass the tube into the trachea. A guide tube can be used, such as a polyethylene catheter; do not use a metal rod because excessive force could damage the larynx or trachea. Pass the endotracheal tube over the guide tube into the trachea. Inflate the cuff as soon as possible and before the animal is placed in lateral recumbency.

In calves, the laryngoscope is used in the same manner. A guide tube can also be used; in bigger calves, a small equine stomach tube will be suitable as a guide tube.

As with adult cattle, small ruminants should not have the tube lubricateded with lidocaine gel, which would desensitize the mucous membranes of the trachea and larynx, making aspiration more likely. Make sure the mouth is free of ingesta prior to extubation.

34. Can nasal intubation be done in small ruminants?

Yes, the ventral nasal meatus is relatively large in sheep and goats, so a reasonably adequate tube size can be used. Make sure the nostrils are clean and patent. Pass a well-lubricated tube through the nostril into the ventral nasal meatus. Use a gentle, nonrotational movement when advancing the tube. If the tube does not pass, a laryngoscope can be used orally to expose the tip of the tube in the pharynx. A forceps can be used to assist the tube into the laryngeal opening as the tube is advanced through the nostril.

Nasal intubation can also be done in awake calves for an inhalant induction similar to that done in foals.

35. How is intubation performed in the llama?

Once the llama is anesthetized, extend the head and neck. Llamas also may regurgitate; this reflex is eliminated if there is adequate anesthetic depth. If there are rapid swallowing motions, the animal needs a deeper plane of anesthesia. Digital pressure on the esophagus can help prevent regurgitation. If there is regurgitation, lower the head to prevent aspiration. Clean the mouth before trying to intubate again.

Llamas need longer tubes, 40 to 55 cm for older animals, to go caudal to the larynx. The laryngoscope needs a long 250 to 350 mm blade. Gauze is used to hold open the jaws, because the mouth will not open widely. Depress the epiglottis to reveal the larynx. The base of the tongue has an elevation called torus linguae that blocks the view of the tracheal opening and impedes the tube. A stylet can be used to stiffen the tube and make it easier to pass; alternatively, a guide tube can be placed with the endotracheal tube threaded over it.

Keep the tube in until the llama is able to chew and cough to ensure that the animal can protect its airway. Watch the tube so that the animal does not bite it. If the llama is extubated too early, it may go back to sleep once stimulus of the tube is gone and may not be able to exchange air properly. Observe the animal following extubation for possible airway obstruction.

36. Can nasal intubation be performed in the llama?

To perform nasotracheal intubation, pass the tube between the ventral nasal concha and the nasal septum. The ventral nasal concha has a large smooth surface. Choanae, the caudal openings of the nasal cavities, lead to a large nasopharynx. Llamas depend on nasal breathing. Dorsal displacement of soft palate results in compromise of the airway. The tube lubricant should be water soluble with phenylephrine added to aid in vasoconstriction of nasal mucosa and help prevent hemorrhage. The tube is directed medially and ventrally through the nares into the ventral meatus. The bevel of the tube is directed laterally, so the tube tip courses along the nasal septum, minimizing the chance of traumatizing conchae. Slow, gentle pressure is used to advance the tube; twisting would abrade mucosa and cause epistaxis.

If the tube does not advance more than 10 cm in an adult llama, and the tube is of a proper size, it is probably in the middle meatus and contacting an ethmoid concha. If the tube continues to be manipulated, severe hemorrhage will result. Back the tube out and go into the ventral meatus. If the tube will not advance more than 25 cm in adult, the tube tip is probably in the pharyngeal diverticulum, a large diverticulum at the caudodorsal angle of the nasopharynx. Do not try to advance the tube as this will lead to injury. Withdraw the tube 3 cm, redirect it ventrally, and then advance the tube.

After the tube is in the nasopharynx, extend the head and neck to make the nasotracheal axis greater than or equal to 180 degrees; manipulate and rotate the tube as necessary to pass it into the larynx. Secure the nasal tube to the head so the animal will not aspirate it. The llama can be recovered with the tube in place.

37. What makes intubation difficult in the porcine?

Intubation of the pig is difficult to do but it improves oxygenation and ventilation and decreases the risk of aspiration. It is made difficult by the following factors:

- The mouth does not open widely.
- The larynx is rather loosely attached and mobile, is relatively small, and slopes ventrally, creating a sharp angle for passing the endotracheal tube.
- The laryngeal and tracheal diameters are small.
- Laryngeal spasm is easily provoked.

38. How can the pig be intubated?

With the pig anesthetized, it can be positioned in dorsal or sternal recumbency. The head and neck are slightly extended; use gauze loops around the upper and lower jaw to open the mouth. Pull the tongue out and forward; be careful not to cut it on the sharp incisor teeth. Use a laryngoscope to visualize the laryngeal area. Lidocaine spray and lubricant on the tube can decrease the risk of laryngospasm. To decrease the risk of laryngospasm, the pig needs to be fully anesthetized before any attempt can be made to pass the tube.

A guide tube (two 10 French canine urinary catheters connected lengthwise), can be passed first and the endotracheal tube then guided over the guide tube. Or, a stylet of malleable wire, such as copper or aluminum, placed inside the endotracheal tube but not protruding beyond the beveled end, will give stiffness to the tube and aid in its placement.

If the pig is in sternal recumbency, the endotracheal tube tip is kept ventral and advanced; it will meet resistance when the tip contacts the posterior floor of the larynx. When this occurs, rotate the tube 180 degrees, apply minimal pressure, and the tube will descend into the trachea; then rotate the tip back to the original position. The tube connector should be at the level of the snout and distal end of the endotracheal tube near the thoracic inlet.

Be gentle with the miniature pig. Traumatic intubation can lead to spasm, edema, and death.

39. How can you tell if the endotracheal tube is in the trachea in a large animal?

- Digital palpation in the adult bovine
- Observing or feeling the tube in the trachea
- Gas from the endotracheal tube on exhalation
- Absence of stertorous breathing sounds following intubation
- With a transparent endotracheal tube, seeing water vapor or condensation appear and then clear up with each breath
- When the animal is connected to an anesthesia machine, synchrony between the movement of the rebreathing bag and the thorax
- The end tidal carbon dioxide analyzer indicating the presence of carbon dioxide in the expired gas

40. What is retrograde intubation?

If direct visualization of the glottis or a portion of it is not possible, as in the case of a pharyngeal or an oral mass, one method to use is retrograde intubation.

A hypodermic needle is passed through the skin of the neck and into the trachea at the junction of the second and third tracheal rings. A guide wire, or canine urinary catheter that will pass easily through the needle, is maneuvered through the needle cranially into the larynx, pharynx, and oral cavity. It is then used as a guide for the passage of the endotracheal tube. After the tip of the tube is within the larynx, the needle and guide wire can be removed. The endotracheal tube is then advanced into the final position. The cuff of the tube should be caudal to the puncture site of the needle to avoid forcing gas subcutaneously or into the mediastinum during positive pressure ventilation.

Subcutaneous emphysema and pneumothorax are possible complications with this technique.

41. What is one-lung ventilation? Why would it be done?

One-lung ventilation, with collapse of the operative, nondependent, upper, nonventilated lung and ventilation to the lower, nonoperative, dependent lung is necessary for optimal safe thoracoscopy. Selective ventilation of the lower lung allows the upper, operative lung to collapse, and the tidal volume is delivered only to the lower lung. This will lead to significant ventilation-perfusion mismatching, which requires intensive support.

42. What are the techniques for establishing one-lung ventilation?

There are three techniques for establishing one-lung ventilation: bronchial blockade; endobronchial intubation; and use of a double-lumen endotracheal tube.

43. How does bronchial blockade work?

A balloon-tipped catheter, such as a Foley or Swan-Ganz, is inserted into the bifurcation of the trachea, and a single-lumen endotracheal tube is passd beside it. A fiberoptic bronchoscope is passed through the lumen of the endotracheal tube to guide the balloon-tipped catheter into the mainstem bronchus of the upper lung, then the cuff of the endotracheal tube is inflated. The bronchial blocker is not inflated until the upper lung has collapsed. The lumen of the bronchial blocker is used for aspiration and continuous positive airway pressure. These tubes are relatively easy to place but can become dislodged intraoperatively, possibly obstructing ventilation of one or both lungs.

44. How does endobronchial intubation work?

An endotracheal tube with a diameter smaller than the bronchus to be intubated is passed into the mainstem bronchus of the ventilated lower lung with bronchoscopic guidance. Care is needed to place and rotate to position the end-hole and the side-hole of the tube to prevent occlusion of early branching lobar bronchioles. Inaccurately positioning the bronchial cuff can lead to inadequate ventilation and accidental displacement of the tube. Endobronchial intubation does not provide a means for aspiration or intermittent ventilation of the upper lung. In some species, the right cranial lung lobe may not be ventilated when the right mainstem bronchus is selectively intubated.

45. How does intubation with a double-lumen endotracheal tube work?

Double-lumen tubes provide a means of controlling ventilation of either lung. A double-lumen tube is left- or right-sided. Essentially, it is two catheters bonded together side-by-side, each with a separate lumen to ventilate one of the lungs. A left-sided tube has a left side longer than right; with a right-sided tube, the right side is longer than the left. The shorter side ends in the trachea.

The proximal cuff is for the trachea, and the distal cuff is for the mainstem bronchus. This cuff causes separation and sealing off of the lungs from each other. The proximal cuff seals the lungs off from the environment. The right lung catheter on a right-sided tube must be slotted to allow ventilation of the right upper lobe because the right mainstem bronchus is too short to accommodate both right lumen tip and right endobronchial cuff.

Commercial tubes available are Carlens and Robertshaw tubes. Bear in mind these tubes are designed for use in humans.

A right- or left-oriented double-lumen endotracheal tube is passed the length of the trachea and rotated to seat in the appropriate mainstem bronchus. Blind intubation is inaccurate; a fiberoptic bronchoscope is passed through the lumen of the endotracheal tube to guide final positioning. Proper depth is when the cephalad surface of bronchial cuff is immediately below the carinal bifurcation.

Inflate the cuffs, ventilate, and auscultate both lungs. You should hear bilateral breath sounds; if not, back the tube out. Clamp one side, and there should be no breath sounds or chest movement. Unclamp the side, and sounds and movement should reappear. Do both sides to ensure adequate lung separation and cuff seal. Double-lumen tubes allow ventilation, aspiration, and insufflation of either lung, but they offer greater resistance because of their smaller diameter.

46. What are the potential complications of one-lung ventilation?

- Overinflation of the sealing balloon or cuff can cause the tube or catheter to be dislodged from position, this may impair ventilation and the cuff or balloon may partially or completely obstruct air flow to one or both lungs
- Overinflation of the cuff or balloon may displace the tracheal carina to the contralateral side and obstruct airflow, which can lead to inadequate ventilation or inappropriate collapse of the contralateral lung.
- Overinflation can lead to obstruction of cranial lobar bronchioles branching from the mainstem bronchus, causing inadequate ventilation.
- Overinflation of the endobronchial tube cuff may also lead to collapse of the tube lumen. Further overinflation can lead to bronchial or tracheal rupture
- With endobronchial intubation, passing the tube too far causes inadequate ventilation of the intubated lung

47. How is one-lung ventilation managed?

High concentrations (e.g., 100%) of oxygen must be used to prevent hypoxic pulmonary vasoconstriction in the ventilated lower lung. The ventilated lower lung will be responsible for all gas exchange and will need to have the normal tidal volume of 10 ml/kg by itself. However, high tidal volumes and high inspiratory pressures are not beneficial. Inspiratory pressures greater than 15 cm H_2O will increase pulmonary vascular resistance and blood flow will increase to the nonventilated upper lung.

Maintain eucapnia by increasing the respiratory rate by approximately 20%. Hypocapnia should be avoided, as it leads to increased pulmonary vascular resistance in the lower lung and inhibits hypoxic pulmonary vasoconstriction in the upper lung. Positive end-expiratory pressure (PEEP) can be applied to the ventilated lower lung to minimize atelectasis. Do not use pressures higher than 5 cm H_2O, as this will increase pulmonary vascular resistance in the lower lung and increase blood flow through the nonventilated upper lung. Continuous positive airway pressure (CPAP) can be applied to the upper lung by administering 100% oxygen at 5 to 10 cm H_2O to permit oxygen uptake in the upper lung. High levels of pressure will obstruct the surgeon's view. PEEP and CPAP can be combined.

BIBLIOGRAPHY

1. Bailey JE, Pablo LS: Anesthetic and physiologic considerations for veterinary endosurgery. In Freeman LJ (ed): Veterinary Endosurgery. St. Louis, Mosby, 1999, pp 24–43.
2. Benumof JL, Alfery DD: Anesthesia for thoracic surgery. In Miller RD (ed): Anesthesia. Philadelphia, Churchill Livingstone, 2000, pp 1665–1752.
3. Bistner SI, Ford RB, Raffe MR: Endotracheal intubation. In Bistner SI, Ford RB, Raffe MR (ed): Handbook of Veterinary Procedures and Emergency Treatment. Philadelphia, WB Saunders, 2000, pp 582–584.
4. Bistner SI, Ford RB, Raffe MR: Tracheotomy and tracheostomy. In Bistner SI, Ford RB, Raffe MR (ed): Handbook of Veterinary Procedures and Emergency Treatment. Philadelphia, WB Saunders, 2000, pp 622–625.
5. Gibbons G: Respiratory emergencies. In Murtaugh RJ, Kaplan PM (ed): Veterinary Emergency and Critical Care Medicine. St Louis, Mosby, 1992, pp 399–419.
6. Hall LW, Clarke KW: Anesthesia of the horse. In Hall LW, Clarke KW (ed): Veterinary Anesthesia. Philadelphia, Bailliere, 1991, pp 191–235.
7. Hall LW, Clarke KW: Anesthesia of the ox. In Hall LW, Clarke KW (ed): Veterinary Anesthesia. Philadelphia, Bailliere, 1991, pp 236–259.

8. Hall LW, Clarke KW: Anesthesia of the sheep, goat, and other herbivores. In Hall LW, Clarke KW (ed): Veterinary Anesthesia. Philadelphia, Bailliere, 1991, pp 260–274.
9. Hall LW, Clarke KW: Anesthesia of the pig. In Hall LW, Clarke KW (ed): Veterinary Anesthesia. Philadelphia, Bailliere, 1991, pp 275–289.
10. Hartsfield SM: Airway management and ventilation. In Thurmon JC, Tranquilli WJ, Benson GJ (ed): Veterinary Anesthesia. Baltimore, Williams & Wilkins, 1996, pp 515–556.
11. Harvey RC: Anesthesia for severe upper airway obstruction. In Haskins SC, Klide AM (ed): The Veterinary Clinics of North America Small Animal Practice Opinions in Small Animal Anesthesia. Philadelphia, WB Saunders, 1992, pp 452–453.
12. McKelvey D, Hollingshead KW: General anesthesia. In McKelvey D, Hollingshead KW (ed): Small Animal Anesthesia Canine and Feline Practice. St. Louis, Mosby, 1994, pp 55–118.
13. McKelvey D, Hollingshead KW: Anesthetic equipment. I: McKelvey D, Hollingshead KW (ed): Small Animal Anesthesia Canine and Feline Practice. St . Louis, Mosby, 1994, pp 163–213.
14. McKelvey D, Hollingshead KW: Anesthetic problems and emergencies. In McKelvey D, Hollingshead KW (ed): Small Animal Anesthesia Canine and Feline Practice. St. Louis, Mosby, 1994, pp 235–282.
15. Quandt JE: Anesthetic considerations for laser, laparoscopy, and thoracoscopy procedures. Clin Techn Small Animal Pract 14:50–55,1999.
16. Rampil IJ: Anesthesia for laser surgery. In Miller RD (ed): Anesthesia. Philadelphia, Churchill Livingstone, 2000, pp 2199–2212.
17. Riebold TW, Geiser DR, Goble DO: Large Animal Anesthesia Principles and Techniques. Ames, Iowa State University Press, 1995.
18. Riebold TW, Engel HN, Grubb TL, et al: Orotracheal and nasotracheal intubation in llamas. J Am Vet Med Assoc 204:779–783, 1994.
19. Shawley RV, Bednarski RM: Endotracheal intubation in the horse. In Muir WW, Hubbell JAE (ed): Equine Anesthesia Monitoring and Emergency Therapy. St Louis, Mosby, 1991, pp 310–324.
20. Steffey EP: Inhalation anesthesia. In Hall LW, Taylor PM (ed): Anaesthesia of the Cat. Philadelphia, Bailliere, 1994, pp 157–193.
21. Taylor PM: Accidents and emergencies. In Hall LW, Taylor PM (ed): Anaesthesia of the Cat. Philadelphia, Bailliere, 1994, pp 249–273.
22. Thurmon JC, Tranquilli WJ, Benson GJ: Airway management and ventilation. In Thurmon JC, Tranquilli WJ, Benson GJ (ed): Essentials of Small Animal Anesthesia and Analgesia. Philadelphia, Williams & Wilkins, 1999, pp 292–325.

2. OXYGENATION AND VENTILATION

Sheilah A. Robertson, B.V.M.S., Ph.D., D.A.C.V.A., D.E.C.V.A., M.R.C.V.S.

1. What are the normal values for an arterial blood sample collected from an awake patient breathing room air?

A blood gas machine measures three things from a sample of arterial blood: pH, partial pressure of CO_2 ($PaCO_2$), and partial pressure of oxygen (PaO_2); all other values are calculated and derived from nomograms.

Variable	Normal Range
pH	7.35–7.45
$PaCO_2$	35–45 mm Hg
PaO_2	80–110 mm Hg

2. What differences would be seen if the patient were breathing 100% oxygen?

The only factor that will show a significant change is the PaO_2. The predicted "ideal" PaO_2 in a patient breathing 100% oxygen is approximately 500 mm Hg. PaO_2 can be predicted if the percentage of inspired oxygen (FIO_2) is known; see question 3.

3. How can you predict what the PaO_2 should be for each patient?

In a healthy animal with no shunts, V/Q inequality, or diffusion impairment, the predicted PaO_2 is approximately four to five times the percentage of inspired oxygen, or fraction of inspired oxygen (FIO_2). For example, if the patient is breathing 50% oxygen ($FIO_2 = 0.5$), its PaO_2 should be 4 or $5 \times 50 = 200$–250 mm Hg. If the animal is breathing 100% oxygen ($FIO_2 = 1.0$), its PaO_2 should be 400–500 mm Hg.

4. What are the definitions of hypoxemia and hypoxia?

Sometimes the words *hypoxemia* and *hypoxia* are used interchangeably, and there is no universal agreement on the definition of these terms. A distinction can be made, however.

Hypoxemia refers only to the situation in blood and means "low oxygen content in the blood." It can be a result of reduced PaO_2, reduced hemoglobin saturation (SaO_2), or low hemoglobin content. The severity can be assessed by calculating the total amount of oxygen in the blood (oxygen content). Normal PaO_2 values are in the range of 85–110 mm Hg for most animals and hypoxemia is often defined as a PaO_2 of less than 60 mm Hg.

Hypoxia is a broader term that refers to impaired oxygen delivery and also takes into account cardiac output, perfusion, and oxygen extraction by tissues. If these definitions are used, a patient could have normal blood oxygen content, yet be hypoxic secondary to a low cardiac output. This highlights the fact that the clinician must look at the whole picture, not just a blood gas result.

5. How do you calculate the oxygen content of blood?

The oxygen content of blood (CaO_2) is measured in ml O_2/dl and is calculated by the following equation:

$$CaO_2 = \text{amount of } O_2 \text{ bound to hemoglobin} + \text{amount dissolved in plasma}$$

The amount of oxygen bound to hemoglobin is calculated by:

SaO_2 (arterial hemoglobin saturation expressed as a decimal fraction) $\times$ hemoglobin content (g/dl) $\times$ 1.34 (the O_2 binding capacity of hemoglobin).

The amount of dissolved oxygen is calculated by multiplying the PaO_2 by 0.003, the solubility constant for dissolved oxygen in plasma. For example, a dog with an Hb of 15 g/dl, a PaO_2 of 95 mmHg, and a SaO_2 of 98% will have a blood oxygen content of:

$$0.98 \times 15 \times 1.34 + 95 \times 0.003 = 19.98 \text{ ml/dL}$$

6. Which of the following patients is more hypoxemic?

PATIENT	PaO$_2$ (MM HG)	SaO$_2$ (%)	HB (G/DL)
A	90	97	6
B	55	85	15

Using the oxygen content equation:

$$CaO_2 = SaO_2 \times Hb \times 1.34 + 0.003 \times PaO_2,$$

the CaO$_2$ of patient A is 8.06 ml/dl and that of patient B is 17.25 ml/dl. This emphasizes the importance of looking at the overall picture, not isolated results.

7. How much oxygen do animals need to meet their metabolic demands?
An animal's oxygen consumption is correlated with its metabolic rate. The latter is influenced by the ratio of body weight to surface area (small animals have a higher metabolic rate than large animals), body temperature (metabolic rate falls as temperature decreases), and level of consciousness (awake versus anesthetized). To meet their basal metabolic needs, dogs consume 4–7 ml/kg/min of oxygen, and values of 3–14 ml/kg/min have been reported for anesthetized dogs. Oxygen consumption rates are lower with barbiturate and inhalant anesthetics and higher with ketamine.

8. Does cyanosis always occur if an animal becomes hypoxemic?
No, absence of cyanosis does not always equate with normal arterial oxygen values. Reduced or *un*oxygenated hemoglobin is purple, and when a sufficient amount is present it gives the skin and mucous membranes a blue-purple or cyanotic color. Cyanosis can develop when hypoxemia is present (for example, reduced oxygen uptake in the lungs secondary to a right-to-left shunt), if hemoglobin is unable to carry oxygen (methemoglobinemia), or when blood stagnates in peripheral capillary beds (for example, when cardiac output is low or there is arteriolar constriction). Approximately 5 g/dl of unoxygenated hemoglobin has to be present in capillaries for cyanosis to be clinically detected; therefore, a severely anemic animal may never be cyanotic even if it is severely hypoxemic. The color of mucous membranes and skin are also influenced by pigmentation and lighting conditions, making cyanosis an unreliable clinical indicator of oxygenation problems in animals.

9. Can you measure oxygen delivery to tissues?
There is no simple way to measure the oxygen delivery to individual organs and tissue beds. The total amount of oxygen transferred or delivered per minute can be calculated by multiplying the cardiac output by the oxygen content of blood (CaO$_2$). Note that delivery of oxygen to tissues can be increased two different ways.

10. What are the causes of hypoxemia in animals?
There are four primary causes:
• Shunt
• Ventilation-perfusion inequality (V/Q mismatch)
• Hypoventilation
• Diffusion impairment
A fifth, less common cause is a low inspired oxygen concentration, which could occur if a hypoxic gas mixture was accidentally used; for example, if the oxygen supply ran out while nitrous oxide was being used.

11. What does it mean when an animal with a low PaO$_2$ does not respond to supplemental oxygen?
This means the patient has a shunt and that some blood reaches the arterial system without first passing through ventilated areas of the lung. Unlike the other causes of hypoxemia (V/Q

mismatch, hypoventilation, and diffusion impairment), hypoxemia caused by a shunt cannot be abolished by administering 100% oxygen.

12. How is the adequacy of ventilation assessed in patients?

This can be assessed by using the alveolar ventilation equation:

$$V_A = V_{CO_2} \times K / PA_{CO_2}$$

V_A is the volume of alveolar gas in the tidal volume. Alveolar gas is the component of the tidal volume that is important for gas exchange; the remainder is dead space ventilation. V_{CO2} is the volume of expired CO_2 per unit time and K is a constant (0.863). In most normal patients, PA_{CO_2} is similar to $PaCO_2$. The relationship between alveolar ventilation and CO_2 is important to understand; if an animal's alveolar ventilation decreases by 50%, but CO_2 production remains the same, the alveolar (and arterial) CO_2 doubles. Therefore, a rise in $PaCO_2$ is always present in the face of hypoventilation. If an animal is breathing room air (21% oxygen), hypoventilation will also cause a decrease in alveolar and arterial oxygen, but if it is breathing an enriched oxygen mixture, the arterial oxygen may be normal or increased.

13. Can a capnograph be reliably used to substitute for repeated blood gas analysis of carbon dioxide in all situations?

No. A capnograph continuously measures exhaled (and inhaled) carbon dioxide concentrations that under ideal conditions reflect alveolar concentrations. It is usually presumed that alveolar and capillary CO_2 are equilibrated; therefore, the end-tidal CO_2 concentration ($ETCO_2$) can be used to monitor $PaCO_2$. The $ETCO_2$ often underestimates actual $PaCO_2$; this alveolar to arterial difference is due to dead space ventilation but is minor in many clinical situations. However, there are some situations, such as during thoracotomy in dogs, in which the $ETCO_2$ is a very unreliable indicator of adequacy of ventilation. It is important to measure the $PaCO_2$ in a patient and to determine the end-tidal:alveolar gradient before relying on a capnograph to guide decisions.

14. What is an acceptable $PaCO_2$ in an anesthetized patient?

If the patient has no intracranial pathology, an upper limit of 60 mm Hg is usually acceptable. Mild hypercapnia may be beneficial because it stimulates the sympathetic nervous system and supports cardiovascular function. Hyperventilation to values below 20–25 mm Hg should be avoided, as this may result in decreased cerebral blood flow and oxygen delivery to the brain.

15. Why is it important to maintain normocapnia or mild hypocapnia in animals with increased intracranial pressure?

Determinants of cerebral blood flow (CBF) include $PaCO_2$, PaO_2, cerebral perfusion pressure, and autoregulation. The $PaCO_2$ is the most important of these factors. Increases and decreases in CO_2 cause pH-mediated dilation or constriction of cerebral vessels, respectively. The relationship is linear with an increase or decrease in CBF of 1 ml per 100 g of brain tissue per minute for every 1 mm Hg increase or decrease in $PaCO_2$.

16. What are the possible causes of an increase in $PaCO_2$ during anesthesia?

$PaCO_2$ may rise because of:

- Decreased elimination
  - Hypoventilation secondary to central nervous system depression caused by anesthetic drugs
  - Respiratory muscle weakness secondary to use of neuromuscular blocking agents or hypokalemia
  - Intrinsic pulmonary disease that may be severe enough to interfere with diffusion of CO_2 across the alveolar membrane. This is an unusual cause because CO_2 is 30 times more diffusible than oxygen.
- Rebreathing
  - Exhausted soda-lime

- Excessive dead space, which can be due to an incompetent or missing one-way valve in the anesthetic circuit, excessive endotracheal tube length, or an inappropriately large capnograph adaptor between the patient and the breathing circuit
- Increased production
    - Although rare in animals, malignant hyperthermia has been reported and leads to excessive CO_2 production

17. If I use a pulse oximeter on anesthetized patients and the hemoglobin saturation (SaO_2) remains greater than 95%, can I be assured that ventilation is adequate?

No! A pulse oximeter measures only hemoglobin saturation. Even if an animal is severely hypoventilating and has a greatly elevated $PaCO_2$, hemoglobin saturation will often be normal if the animal is breathing 100% oxygen. An example of this is shown in the following blood gas analysis from an animal during anesthesia. The cause of the severe hypoventilation was an excessively deep plane of anesthesia. Normal values are shown in parenthesis.

Pulse oximeter reading 98% (95–98%)

Arterial blood gas results:

pH	6.944 (7.400)
PaO_2	454 mm Hg (4–5 $\times$ inspired concentration)
$PaCO_2$	114 mm Hg (40–45)
Base Excess	12.2 mEq/l (–4 to + 4)

18. When the $PaCO_2$ is very high in an anesthetized patient, why doesn't the animal hyperventilate to blow off the excess carbon dioxide?

In conscious animals, the relationship between $PaCO_2$ and minute ventilation is linear. Under anesthesia, there is a decrease in ventilation and a rise in $PaCO_2$ and a marked change in the CO_2/ventilation response curve. These changes become greater as the level of anesthesia deepens. They are caused by central nervous system depression and a decrease in sensitivity of the central chemoreceptors. At high levels, CO_2 alone can cause unconsciousness (CO_2 narcosis); in dogs, a CO_2 of 245 mm Hg produces anesthesia. Ketamine is the one anesthetic agent that has minimal effect on the CO_2/ventilation response curve.

19. I've heard that if you give a low dose of a neuromuscular blocking agent you can preferentially relax the skeletal muscles but preserve the respiratory muscles so that you don't need to manually or mechanically ventilate the patient. Is this true?

No. The extent and duration of neuromuscular blockade is highly variable between individuals. The practice of using a "low" dose of a neuromuscular blocking agent such as pancuronium to paralyze the ocular muscle but "spare" the respiratory muscles has been shown to be dangerous. It is essential to monitor adequacy of ventilation by measuring the $PaCO_2$ and/or $ETCO_2$ in all animals that receive neuromuscular blocking agents.

20. When you decide to use a mechanical ventilator how do you choose the various settings such as tidal volume, respiratory rate, and peak inspiratory pressure?

As a general guide, the tidal volume (TV) of most animals is 10–15 ml/kg body weight. Adequate inflation of the lungs of a normal animal can usually be achieved with inflation pressures of 15–20 cm H_2O. The respiratory rate (RR) will differ between species and sizes of animal. An animal's minute ventilation can be calculated by multiplying the TV by RR, but the only way to check the *adequacy* of ventilation is to measure the $PaCO_2$.

21. What is the I:E ratio? Why is it important during intermittent positive pressure ventilation (IPPV)?

This is the ratio between the inspiratory (I) and expiratory (E) phases of the respiratory cycle. During spontaneous ventilation, the intrathoracic pressure becomes negative and the volume of blood returning to the heart is increased. During IPPV, the reverse is true; positive pressure is created in the thorax, resulting in collapse of large vessels and a decrease in the volume of blood returning to the heart. If the inspiratory phase is prolonged, or the I:E ratio is small, there may not be sufficient time during expiration for adequate filling of the heart, resulting in a decreased cardiac output. To avoid this, the inspiratory time should be less than 2 seconds and the I:E ratio 1:2 to 1:4.

22. Should you avoid potent opioids in animals after thoracic surgery because of the danger of respiratory depression?

Opioids are known to cause respiratory depression, but this is less common in animals than in humans, and is unusual at clinical doses and in animals that are in pain. The shallow respiration that is a feature of thoracic pain is likely to cause a decreased PaO_2 and elevated CO_2, and good pain management will usually improve respiratory gas exchange in these patients.

23. Why are pregnant animals more likely to become hypoxic if they become apneic?

During pregnancy, there is a decrease in the functional residual capacity (FRC) of the lung. The FRC is the lung's oxygen "reservoir," and a decrease in FRC plus an increase in oxygen consumption in pregnant animals results in a rapid drop in PaO_2 during apnea.

24. What does the term "preoxygenation" mean and what are the advantages of this technique?

Preoxygenation is a technique that can be used prior to induction of general anesthesia to delay the onset of hypoxemia. 100% oxygen is administered by facemask for 5 minutes, during which time the air occupying the functional residual capacity (FRC), or "reservoir," in the lungs is replaced by 100% oxygen. In the event of a complete airway obstruction or apnea, it takes about 3–4 minutes for a patient that has been preoxygenated to become hypoxemic, compared with only 90 seconds after breathing room air. This is a valuable technique to use if the patient's FRC is reduced (as in pregnancy), the patient has an airway obstruction, or difficult intubation is predicted after induction of anesthesia.

25. If oxygen is essential for survival, what does the term "oxygen toxicity" mean?

Exposure of animals to high concentrations of oxygen over prolonged periods causes lung damage. Increased free radical formation is thought to be the mechanism that causes membrane damage, and reported changes include interstitial and alveolar edema, atelectasis, intra-alveolar hemorrhage, decreased lung compliance, and arterial hypoxemia. There is considerable variation in susceptibility to toxicity, but an FIO_2 of greater than 60% for 12 to 24 hours is likely to cause problems.

BIBLIOGRAPHY

1. Hartsfield S: Anesthetic machines and breathing systems. In Thurmon JC, Tranquilli WJ, Benson GJ (eds): Lumb and Jones' Veterinary Anesthesia, 3rd ed. Baltimore, Williams & Wilkins, 1996, pp 394–395.
2. Lee DD, Meyer RE, Sullivan TC et al: Respiratory depressant and skeletal muscle relaxant effects of low-dose pancuronium bromide in spontaneously breathing isoflurane anesthetized dogs. Veterinary Surgery 27: 473-479, 1998.
3. Wagner AE, Gaynor JS, Dunlop CI, et al: Monitoring adequacy of ventilation by capnography during thoracotomy in dogs. J Am Vet Med Assoc 212:377–379, 1998.
4. West JB: Pulmonary Pathophysiology: The Essentials, 5th ed. Baltimore, Lippincott, Williams & Wilkins, 1998.
5. West JB: Respiratory Physiology: The Essentials, 5th ed. Baltimore, Lippincott, Williams & Wilkins, 1998.

3. ELECTROLYTES

Lois A. Wetmore, D.V.M., Sc.D., D.A.C.V.A.

1. What pre-existing disease processes or conditions typically have associated electrolyte abnormalities?

Acid/base abnormalities
- Acidosis: hyperkalemia, hypercalcemia (ionized), hyperchloremia
- Alkalosis: hypokalemia, hypocalcemia (ionized), hypochloremia

Cardiac disease
- Congestive heart failure: hyponatremia (with hypervolemia)

Endocrine disease
- Hypoadrenocorticism: hyponatremia, hyperkalemia, hypercalcemia
- Hyperadrenocorticism: hypernatremia
- Hypoparathyroidism: hypocalcemia
- Hyperparathyroidism (primary or secondary): hypercalcemia
- Hyperaldosteronism: hypernatremia, hypokalemia
- Diabetes insipidus: hypernatremia

Gastrointestinal disease
- Vomiting: hypochloremia, hyponatremia or hypernatremia, hypokalemia
- Diarrhea: hyponatremia or hypernatremia, hyperchloremia, hypomagnesemia, hypokalemia
- Anorexia: hypokalemia, hypomagnesemia
- Protein-losing enteropathy: hypocalcemia, with or without hypomagnesemia
- Gastric dilation volvulus: hypochloremia
- Equine colic: hypocalcemia, hypomagnesemia

Pancreatic disease
- Pancreatitis: hypocalcemia, hypomagnesemia, hyponatremia

Pregnancy/lactation
- Eclampsia: hypocalcemia
- Parturient paresis: hypocalcemia

Renal/urinary disease
- Acute renal failure: hypocalcemia
  - Oliguric phase: hypernatremia, hyperkalemia, hypermagnesemia
  - Diuretic phase: hyponatremia, hypokalemia, hypomagnesemia
- Chronic renal failure:
  - With polyuria: hypermagnesemia, hypokalemia (cats), hypocalcemia (dogs and cats), hypercalcemia (horses, dogs, and cats)
  - With oliguria: hyperkalemia
- Renal tubular acidosis: hypokalemia
- Nephrotic syndrome: hyponatremia (with hypervolemia)
- Urinary tract obstruction: hyperkalemia
- Ruptured bladder and uroabdomen: hyperkalemia, hyponatremia (foals)
- Ethylene glycol poisoning: hypocalcemia
- Peritoneal dialysis: hypomagnesemia, hypokalemia

Skin/musculoskeletal disease
- Myositis: hyperkalemia
- Tissue destruction: hyperkalemia
- Burns: hyperkalemia
- Hyperkalemic periodic paralysis in quarter horses (HYPP): hyperkalemia

Tumors
  • Anal sac apocrine gland adenocarcinoma: hypercalcemia
  • Lymphoma: hypercalcemia
  • Multiple myeloma: hypercalcemia
  • Other endocrine neoplasias: hypercalcemia
Other
  • Dehydration: hypernatremia, hyperchloremia, hypercalcemia
  • Hypoalbuminemia: hypocalcemia
  • Blood transfusion (citrate): hypocalcemia, hypomagnesemia
  • Excessive dietary supplementation (large animals): hypercalcemia
  • Excessive dietary supplementation (small animals): hypernatremia, hyperkalemia, hypercalcemia
  • Hypervitaminosis D: hypercalcemia
  • Hypertonic fluid administration: hypernatremia
  • Hypokalemic periodic paralysis (Burmese cats): hypokalemia
  • Age:
    • Young animals: hypercalcemia, hyperphosphatemia
  • Idiopathic:
    • Cats: hypercalcemia
  • Iatrogenic:
    • Thyroidectomy: hypocalcemia
    • Parathyroid gland tumor removal: hypocalcemia

2. What medications predispose to electrolyte abnormalities?

Diuretics
  • Potassium-sparing (spironolactone, triamterene, amiloride): hyperkalemia
  • Loop diuretics: hypochloremia, hypocalcemia, hypokalemia, hypomagnesemia
Dietary supplements
  • Salt substitute: hyperkalemia
  • Laxatives/ antacids: hypermagnesemia
Positive inotropes:
  • Digitalis: relative hypomagnesemia (shift magnesium into the cell); magnesium deficiency will magnify the effect of digitalis cardiotoxicity
  • Catecholamines: hypomagnesemia, hypokalemia
Antibiotics
  • Aminoglycosides: hypomagnesemia
  • Cyclosporine: hyperkalemia
  • Penicillins: hypokalemia
Other
  • Angiotensin-converting enzyme inhibitors: hyperkalemia
  • Insulin: hypokalemia
  • Steroids: hypocalcemia
  • Sodium bicarbonate: hypernatremia, hypocalcemia, hypokalemia
  • Mannitol: hypernatremia

3. What clinical changes can be seen in anesthetized patients that are associated with electrolyte abnormalities ?

Cardiac Arrhythmias: This is the most significant change associated with electrolyte abnormalities in anesthetized animals. The arrhythmias frequently develop during anesthesia in previously asymptomatic animals.

Hypotension: Anesthetized patients can be hypotensive for many reasons, but typically the hypotension resolves with fluid administration or lightening of the patient's anesthetic depth. Patients with pre-existing electrolyte disorders more commonly have hypotension that is unresponsive to fluid administration, and lightening the anesthetic depth results in patient movement with minimal improvement in mean arterial blood pressure.

Delayed Recovery: Electrolyte abnormalities that result in muscle weakness will potentially contribute to a delay in recovery from general anesthesia. This includes hyperkalemia, hypokalemia, hypercalcemia, hypocalcemia (majority of cases present with muscle fasciculations and tetany), hypermagnesemia, and hypomagnesemia.

4. Describe the cardiac changes associated with different electrolyte abnormalities.

Hypocalcemia: Occurrence of electrocardiographic changes (tachycardia and prolonged QT interval) not consistent in hypocalcemic patients.

Hypercalcemia: Rarely causes clinically significant cardiac problems in awake animals. During anesthesia, changes in cardiac electrical activity may occur, including prolongation of the PR interval, shortening of the QT interval bradycardia, atrioventricular block, and cardiac arrest.

Hypokalemia: Bradycardia, supraventricular and ventricular arrhythmias, prolonged QT interval, ST segment deviations, decreased amplitude of T waves, development of U waves, delayed ventricular repolarization, and increased duration of the action potential. Patients with hypokalemia are unresponsive to the effects of class I antiarrhythmics (e.g., lidocaine, procainamide, quinidine).

Hyperkalemia: Peaked T waves, decrease in size of P waves and R waves, prolonged P-R interval, and widened QRS complexes. Bradycardia is typically present with higher potassium concentrations (>7.0), although some patients present with ventricular tachycardia.

Hypomagnesemia: Peaked T waves, mild ST segment depression, prolonged P-R interval, widened QRS complexes, atrial fibrillation, ventricular tachycardia, supraventricular tachycardia, torsades de pointes, ventricular bigeminy, premature ventricular contractions, and ventricular fibrillation may occur with one or more of these arrhythmias occurring at different times in a single anesthetized patient. The arrhythmias should resolve once the inhalant anesthetic is turned off and the patient recovers from anesthesia. If rate control is necessary in the presence of atrial fibrillation or ventricular arrhythmias, magnesium sulfate (0.15–0.3 mEq/kg, dilute to <20% solution with 5% dextrose in water) can be administered intravenously over 5 to 15 minutes. Concurrent use of calcium may negate the effects of magnesium administration. Magnesium may increase neuromuscular blockade when used concurrently with nondepolarizing neuromuscular blocking agents.

Hypermagnesemia: Bradycardia, third-degree atrioventricular block, asystole, widening of QRS complexes.

5. Describe the blood pressure changes associated with different electrolyte abnormalities.

Hypocalcemia: Effect not determined, although both hypotension due to vasodilation and hypertension have been reported in human patients with hypocalcemia.

Hypercalcemia: Causes vasoconstriction. Patients with vasoconstriction may have an extreme response to anesthetic agents that cause vasodilation, resulting in profound hypotension due to a relative hypovolemia under anesthesia.

Hypokalemia: Hypotension due to a decrease in systemic vascular resistance.

Hypomagnesemia: Causes hypertension. Patients with vasoconstriction may have an extreme response to drugs that cause vasodilation, resulting in profound hypotension under anesthesia.

Hypermagnesemia: Causes a decrease in peripheral vascular resistance. Myocardial contractility is probably not affected by elevated magnesium concentrations.

6. When is treatment for electrolyte abnormalities indicated in anesthetized patients?

With few exceptions, most electrolyte abnormalities should be diagnosed and corrected prior to anesthesia. When this is not possible, anesthetic agents that potentiate cardiac arrhythmias, such as α_2-agonists, halothane, and barbiturates should be avoided.

Every effort should also be made to prevent changes in electrolytes that may be caused by general anesthesia. As an example, in an animal with mild hyperkalemia and a urinary tract obstruction, it is advantageous to use intermittent positive-pressure ventilation to maintain awake

$PaCO_2$ levels and prevent the worsening of the hyperkalemia that could result from respiratory acidosis because of general anesthesia. Acidosis also increases the ionized serum calcium level and should be prevented in anesthetized patients with hypercalcemia. Conversely, acidosis may be preferred in a hypocalcemic patient because it causes a relative increase in available ionized calcium.

Monitoring electrolyte changes under anesthesia is usually unnecessary unless specific changes are anticipated (e.g., potassium levels in a horse susceptible to hyperkalemic periodic paralysis).

Any time a patient under anesthesia has cardiac arrhythmias because of electrolyte abnormalities, the electrolyte abnormality should be corrected or the procedure stopped and the animal recovered from anesthesia. Only when the procedure is required to correct the electrolyte abnormality (e.g., placement of a dialysis catheter in a patient with renal failure) should the anesthesia be continued until the procedure is completed, despite the presence of cardiac arrhythmias.

7. What fluids should be administered to patients with sodium abnormalities and how fast can they be administered?

Hypernatremia: Fluid administration to a hypernatremic patient, especially one with concurrent dehydration, can result in cerebral edema if a change in serum sodium occurs too rapidly. Dehydrated patients requiring anesthesia should receive an isotonic fluid with a sodium concentration similar to that of normal plasma. Typically, hypernatremia resolves with correction of dehydration. If hypernatremia persists, 0.45% NaCl with 2.5% dextrose, or 5% dextrose in water can be given slowly, while the serum sodium concentration is serially measured to ensure a decrease no faster than 0.5–1 mEq/hr. This typically can be achieved using a fluid rate of 3–6 ml/kg/hr, depending on the sodium concentration in the administered fluid.

Hyponatremia: Correction of serum sodium in hyponatremic patients should occur slowly (0.5–1 mEq/hr) using an isotonic crystalloid solution such as lactated Ringer's solution. The use of more concentrated (up to 3%) NaCl solutions is controversial. It is especially important to treat this electrolyte abnormality during or after anesthesia when signs of cerebral edema are present (absence of palpebral reflex, papillary edema, hypertension). Aggressive treatment of hyponatremia, especially chronic hyponatremia, may result in an irreversible, fatal condition known as osmotic myelinosis. Clinical signs associated with this condition do not develop for 1 to 3 days.

8. How fast can potassium be administered to a hypokalemic anesthetized patient?

Potassium chloride should be infused at a rate no faster than 0.5–1 mEq/kg/hr to correct significant hypokalemia. Patients with more severe potassium deficits will tolerate potassium administration rates at the upper end of the dose range. The concentration of potassium in the administered fluid should not exceed 60 mEq/L unless administered through a central line. In anesthetized patients it is important to concurrently administer a fluid with normal potassium (e.g., lactated Ringer's solution) so that in the event of acute blood loss, fluids may be bolused without exceeding the maximum safe rate for potassium administration. Patients receiving potassium supplementation under anesthesia must be closely monitored for development of cardiac arrhythmias.

9. How can you rapidly and safely decrease potassium levels in an anesthetized hyperkalemic patient?

Elevated blood potassium can be successfully reduced by either increasing the elimination of potassium in the urine or by shifting extracellular potassium into the intracellular compartment. Although the latter method is not a permanent solution to the problem, it is an acceptable temporary solution in anesthetized patients. Since cardiac arrhythmias may develop in anesthetized hyperkalemic patients with relatively small increases in serum potassium (6–7 mEq/L), treatment to reduce the potassium concentration is more frequently required in these patients.

10. What agents can be used to decrease potassium levels?

Potassium free fluids: Many options are available. Typically 0.9% NaCl is used at 10–40 ml/kg/hr (higher rates if dehydration or hypovolemia is present).

Sodium bicarbonate: When possible, this drug should be administered based on the patient's blood gas analysis. When this is unavailable, sodium bicarbonate at 0.5–1 mEq/kg IV may be given if the patient is unlikely to have pre-existing metabolic alkalosis.

Insulin and glucose: A dose of 0.5–1.0 U regular insulin per kilogram body weight with 2 g dextrose per unit insulin can be given intravenously to dogs to shift potassium intracellularly. The low end of the insulin range should be used for cats. Foals and horses require an even lower dose of insulin (0.05–0.15 U/kg IV) followed by an infusion of 5% dextrose 4.4–6.6 ml/kg with an initial rate of 0.1–0.2 ml/kg/min. Administration of 5% dextrose without insulin is slower but may also be effective in correcting hyperkalemia in small animals and horses with hyperkalemic periodic paralysis. This technique is effective at decreasing serum potassium within 15 to 30 minutes of administration and lasts up to several hours.

Calcium: A dose of 10% calcium chloride (0.5 ml/kg IV slowly) or 10% calcium gluconate (0.5–1 ml/kg/over 15 minutes) can be used to block the adverse cardiovascular effects caused by hyperkalemia. This treatment does not decrease serum potassium. Hyperkalemia raises (makes less negative) the resting membrane potential (RMP) of cell membranes. As the RMP gets closer to the threshold potential, cells depolarize more easily (hyperexcitability). As the RMP continues to rise, it approaches the threshold potential and cells then take longer to repolarize, resulting in bradycardia. Calcium administration increases the threshold potential, moving it further above the RMP, therefore normalizing the relationship between the RMP and the threshold potential.

11. How can anesthesia increase blood potassium levels in an anesthetized patient?

All anesthetic agents decrease the sensitivity of the brain to elevated carbon dioxide partial pressure. This decrease is dose-related and more severe with some anesthetic agents (opioids, barbiturates, isoflurane, sevoflurane) than others (ether, halothane, ketamine). In addition to closely monitoring patients under anesthesia and avoiding excessive anesthetic depth, you should ventilate patients with some pre-existing electrolyte abnormalities to avoid respiratory acidosis. This is important in patients with hyperkalemia and hypercalcemia, since acidosis increases the serum concentrations of these electrolytes.

Depolarizing muscle relaxants (e.g., succinylcholine) can cause a release of potassium from muscle cells, especially when repeatedly administered. Prior administration of diazepam can prevent this increase and should be used in hyperkalemic patients when succinylcholine must be given.

12. What is the difference between total serum calcium and ionized calcium values?

Total calcium consists of protein-bound calcium (35%), ionized calcium (55%), and complexed calcium (10%). The percentage of serum calcium in the ionized and protein-bound states is influenced by the pH of the blood, with alkalosis causing a decrease in the ionized calcium and acidosis causing an increase in the proportion of calcium that is in the ionized form. Total serum calcium concentration is usually used to assess the calcium status of an animal, despite the fact that ionized calcium is the biologically active form. Ionized calcium should be measured when clinical signs of hypocalcemia or disease states causing hypocalcemia are present (e.g., equine colic, lactation), even when total calcium concentrations are normal since ionized calcium can be abnormal in the face of a normal total serum calcium level. When this occurs, calcium should be administered, despite a normal total calcium concentration. Normal values for total and ionized calcium are given in the table.

Normal and Abnormal Perioperative Electrolyte Values in Dogs and Cats

ELECTROLYTE	SERUM ELECTROLYTE CONCENTRATION	
	NORMAL RANGE	LEVEL REQUIRING CORRECTION
Sodium(mEq/L)	145–154, dog 151–158, cat	>165 or < 135, dog >165 or <145, cat
Chloride (mEq/L)	107–113, dog 117–123, cat	Treatment is required only when acid/base changes are excessive Hyperchloremia with pH <7.20 Hypochloremia with pH ≥7.48

(continued on next page)

Normal and Abnormal Perioperative Electrolyte Values in Dogs and Cats (continued)

ELECTROLYTE	SERUM ELECTROLYTE CONCENTRATION	
	NORMAL RANGE	LEVEL REQUIRING CORRECTION
Potassium (mEq/L)	3.5–5.3, dog and cat	>6.5 or < 2.5
Ionized calcium		
(mmol/L)	1.2–1.5, dog	
	1.1–1.4, cat	
(mg/dL)	5.0–6.0, dog	>7.0 or <5.0, dog
	4.5–5.5, cat	>6.5 or <4.5, cat
Total calcium		
(mg/dL)	9.0–11.5, dog	>14.5 or < 6.5, dog
	8.0–10.5, cat	>13.5 or <7.0, cat
(mmol/L)	2.2–3.8, dog	
	2.0–2.6, cat	
Ionized magnesium		
(mg/dL)	1.04–1.36, dog	<0.8, dog
Total magnesium		
(mg/dL)	1.7–2.4, dog	<1.2, dog
	1.7–2.7, cat	

13. How does albumin affect the total calcium level measured in serum?

Albumin is the predominant protein bound to calcium (80–90%), and changes in serum albumin will change the measured total serum calcium. Adjusting the total serum calcium level to account for this variation is particularly important when the serum albumin level is outside of the normal range. The formula used to adjust the total serum calcium is as follows:

$$\text{Adjusted Ca (mg/dL)} = \text{Measured Ca (mg/dL)} - \text{albumin (g/dL)} + 3.5$$

This formula should not be used to adjust for changes in albumin in young dogs or cats. It is true in these patients that decreases in albumin are associated with decreases in serum calcium, but a linear relationship does not exist, precluding the use of this formula. The adjusted total serum calcium is relevant only because it is used to reflect the ionized calcium value. If albumin values are not available or there is a question regarding the adjusted value, the ionized calcium should be measured.

14. How fast can calcium be administered to a hypocalcemic anesthetized patient?

If cardiac signs of hypocalcemia appear, hypocalcemic dogs and cats should be treated with a bolus of 10% calcium gluconate (100 mg/ml) 0.5–1.0 ml/kg slowly over a 10- to 20-minute period, while monitoring the electrocardiogram (ECG) for signs of bradycardia. Additional calcium gluconate at 0.05–0.15 mg/kg/hr may be given slowly with concurrent ECG monitoring if repeated measurements of ionized calcium remain below normal, although correction of the cardiac arrhythmias is all that is required during anesthesia.

In hypocalcemic horses, 23% calcium gluconate can be administered slowly at 0.25–0.5 ml/kg/hr while monitoring the ECG for evidence of bradycardia. Concurrent administration of dobutamine through the same catheter is acceptable in hypotensive horses if calcium and dobutamine are not added to the same bag of fluids.

Administration of calcium to patients without pre-existing hypocalcemia is indicated under certain circumstances (e.g., as treatment for hyperkalemia). When calcium (2–10 ml of a 10% calcium gluconate solution) is used in these patients, it should be administered slowly and the ECG should be monitored to ensure that cardiac arrhythmias do not worsen.

15. How often should a patient's blood calcium concentration be measured after a parathyroidectomy?

Since parathyroid hormone (PTH) is responsible for minute-to-minute adjustments in the serum ionized calcium concentration in the body, and the half-life of PTH in the serum is only 3 to 5 minutes, removal of the parathyroid glands potentially has an acute effect on blood calcium levels. Surgical thyroidectomy may result in partial or complete removal of the parathyroid glands in the dog, since both the cranial and the caudal parathyroid glands are embedded in the body of each thyroid lobe. In cats, the cranial parathyroid glands are external to the thyroid parenchyma and can be dissected free of the thyroid gland prior to its removal.

Patients that have a parathyroid tumor removed also risk extreme postoperative fluctuations in serum ionized calcium levels because of presurgical suppression of the normal gland's PTH production by excessive PTH production by the tumor. In these cases, hypocalcemia is frequently noted within 12 to 120 hours after surgery. A baseline calcium level should be established immediately postoperatively and then reassessed at regular intervals (every 6 hours) for up to 5 days or until the calcium fluctuations have stabilized. Treatment of postoperative hypocalcemia should be acutely done using intravenous calcium preparations administered slowly while the patient is carefully monitored (as described above).

Once clinical signs of hypocalcemia (muscle tremors, tetany, seizures, cardiac arrhythmias) disappear, 10 ml of 10% calcium gluconate can be added to 250 ml lactated Ringer's solution and administered at a rate of 60 ml/24 hours (cats) or 1.25 ml/kg/hr (dogs). After the patient is alert and stable enough to accept oral medication, calcium lactate or carbonate tablets (25 mg/kg/day elemental calcium) and vitamin D can be administered until there is adequate time for ectopic parathyroid tissue to hypertrophy (2–3 weeks) or damaged parathyroid glands to revascularize.

16. Since serum magnesium values reflect less than 1% of the total body magnesium, how significant is an abnormal magnesium value?

Like calcium, serum magnesium exists in three distinct fractions: magnesium bound to protein (33%), that complexed with anions (12%), and ionized magnesium (55%). The ionized fraction is considered to be the only fraction that is biologically active. Like potassium, the vast majority of the body's magnesium exists intracellularly, and measurement of serum magnesium is thought to be a poor reflection of the magnesium stores in the body. Although there are many more accurate estimates of the total body magnesium value, the serum magnesium concentration obtained from commercial laboratory analysis of serum is the most readily available sample for determination of magnesium concentration. It is important to recognize that serum magnesium levels can be normal in the face of low total body magnesium. When abnormal serum magnesium levels are identified, their significance must be determined on a case-by-case basis using patient history and clinical signs.

It is very common for critically ill anorexic dogs and cats, especially those on magnesium-free fluids, to have hypomagnesemia. Magnesium levels should be regularly monitored and magnesium supplemented in the intravenous fluids of these patients. Any sick patient that has been repeatedly shown to have abnormal magnesium values should be evaluated immediately prior to anesthesia, and elective procedures should not be performed until the serum magnesium value has returned to within the normal range.

17. How does the administration of hypertonic saline affect the blood sodium level?

Hypertonic saline is administered to patients in various types of shock (noncardiogenic) to rapidly increase blood volume. It is available alone (7% NaCl) or in combination with 6% dextran 70 and is dosed at 4–6 ml/kg, although there are reports of safe administration of up to 10 ml/kg to animals in hemorrhagic shock. The combination of 7% NaCl with dextran appears to have a longer duration of action than 7% NaCl alone. When 7% NaCl is administered at the recommended dose to patients with normal blood electrolytes, the serum sodium concentration rises above normal to a value usually below 165 mEq/L, and the serum osmolality increases to near 360 mOsm/kg. These changes are generally well tolerated. Ventricular premature contractions are commonly observed but are usually transient. Administering 7% NaCl above 6 ml/kg should be done cautiously with repeated measurements of serum sodium concentration to avoid concentrations greater than 165 mEq/L.

Patients with pre-existing hypernatremia, dehydration, or hyperosmolality should not receive hypertonic saline solutions. Administration of 7% NaCl faster that 1 ml/kg/min usually results in a vagally mediated bradycardia, hypotension, rapid shallow breathing, and bronchoconstriction. These signs will disappear once the infusion rate has been slowed.

18. What electrolyte monitoring regimen should you use when anesthetizing horses that are carriers of heterozygous or homozygous for the gene causing hyperkalemic periodic paralysis? What other clinical signs can be observed in these horses under anesthesia?

Hyperkalemic periodic paralysis (HYPP) is an autosomal dominant genetic disease of quarter horses and cross-breeds. Clinical signs associated with this disease include muscle fasciculations, weakness, prolapse of the third eyelid, tachypnea, inspiratory stridor, laryngospasm, dysphagia, recumbency, and death. Compared with heterozygous horses, homozygous animals tend to show more extreme clinical signs that usually appear earlier in life. Serum potassium concentrations are typically elevated when clinical signs are present. The elevations can be slight or high enough to cause cardiac arrhythmias.

Anesthesia can precipitate the onset of clinical signs associated with HYPP. Horses under anesthesia may have bradycardia or tachycardia, tachypnea, hypercapnia, muscle fasciculations, and hyperthermia. Recovery can be prolonged from hours to several days or can occur normally, but clinical signs develop shortly after recovery. Horses known to be carriers of the HYPP gene should be maintained on preventative medication such as acetazolamide and have serum potassium levels measured the day before and the day of surgery prior to induction of anesthesia. If normal, induction of anesthesia can be done using a standard equine induction technique. Halothane should be avoided as an anesthetic maintenance agent because of its arrhythmogenic effects. During anesthesia, the patient should be positive-pressure ventilated, and isotonic maintenance fluids, with or without a low concentration of potassium, should be administered at a standard infusion rate. Also, serum potassium concentration should be repeatedly measured (every 30 minutes to 1 hour) and the patient closely monitored for clinical signs of HYPP, including evaluation of the ECG for changes consistent with the presence of hyperkalemia.

If the patient does develop hyperkalemia and bradycardia, in addition to standard treatments for hyperkalemia listed in question 10, small doses (1 ml to a 465 kg horse) of 1:1000 epinephrine can be given to increase the heart rate and facilitate intracellular potassium movement. It is important to remember that patients can have clinical signs and not have elevations in the serum potassium concentration. Horses that do develop clinical signs should be treated symptomatically, and you should serially monitor electrolytes, especially potassium, calcium, and magnesium, for deviations from normal that would contribute to worsening the severity of signs.

19. How does gastrointestinal disease in horses affect electrolyte levels? How significant are these changes in an anesthetized horse?

Perioperative hypomagnesemia and hypocalcemia have been reported in horses with surgical intestinal colic. These changes in serum electrolyte concentrations are believed to be due to the ileus, endotoxemia, and sepsis commonly present with intestinal displacement and obstruction. Intravenous administration of fluids low in magnesium and calcium also contributes to the severity of these electrolyte abnormalities. Measured ionized magnesium and calcium values are more likely to reflect the deficiency than are total serum values.

Hypocalcemia and hypomagnesemia are believed to contribute to the presence of intraoperative hypotension and cardiac arrhythmias. Administering dobutamine in these cases before correcting electrolyte abnormalities frequently results in tachyarrhythmias with minimal improvement of blood pressure. To effectively treat the hypotension without raising the heart rate over 60 beats/minute, you should supplement calcium before or during dobutamine administration.

Generally, ionized calcium and magnesium concentrations should be measured prior to or immediately after the onset of anesthesia for surgical correction of intestinal displacement or obstruction. If the ionized calcium level is abnormal, administer 23% calcium gluconate slowly while monitoring the ECG for evidence of bradycardia. Low ionized magnesium levels can be corrected more slowly by administration of a magnesium-containing maintenance fluid (e.g.,

Plasma-Lyte A, Baxter Healthcare Corporation, Round Lake, Illinois). There are currently no specific guidelines for magnesium replacement therapy in awake or anesthetized horses.

20. What is the composition of electrolytes in various fluids?

FLUID	SODIUM	CHLORIDE	POTASSIUM	CALCIUM	MAGNESIUM	OTHER	OSMOLARITY (MOSMOL/L)
	ELECTROLYTE CONCENTRATION (MEQ/L)						
Lactated Ringer's solution	130	109	4	2.7	—	Lactate, 28	273
Lactated Ringer's + 5% dextrose	130	109	4	2.7	—	Dextrose (50 g/l), Lactate, 28	525
0.9% sodium chloride	154	154	—	—	—	—	308
0.45% saline, 2.5% dextrose	77	77	—	—	—	Dextrose (25 g/L)	280
5% dextrose and water	—	—	—	—	—	Dextrose (50 g/L)	252
Plasma-Lyte 56	40	40	13	—	3	Acetate, 16	111
Plasma-Lyte A or Normosol-R	140	98	5	—	3	Acetate, 27, Gluconate, 23	295
Normosol-M + 5% Dextrose	40	40	13	—	3	Acetate, 16 Dextrose (50 g/L)	364
6% hetastarch in 0.9% NaCl	154	154	—	—	—	Hetastarch (60 g/L)	308
Hypertonic saline	1232	1232	—	—	—	—	2464
Sodium bicarbonate (8.4%)	1000	—	—	—	—	Bicarbonate, 1000	2000
Potassium chloride	—	2000	2000	—	—	—	4000
10% calcium chloride	—	1360	—	1360	—	—	2040
10% calcium gluconate	—	—	—	465	—	Gluconate, 465	680
Cal-Dextro C	87	—	—	1099	—	Gluconate, 1099, Dextrose (44.9 g/L), Boric acid, 571 Bromine, 87	Un-available
Cal-Dextro #2	87	—	—	841	316	Gluconate, 841 Dextrose (165g/l) Phosphorous, 949 Boric acid, 517 Bromine, 87	Unavailable
Cal-Nate 1069 (23% calcium borogluconate)	—	—	—	1069	—	Gluconate, 1069	6,782
50% magnesium sulfate	—	—	—	—	4065	Sulfate, 4065	4060
50% magnesium chloride	—	4624	—	—	4624	—	Unavailable

BIBLIOGRAPHY

1. Aldrich J, Haskins SC: Monitoring the critically ill patient. In Bonagura JD (ed): Kirk's Current Veterinary Therapy XII. Philadelphia, W.B. Saunders, 1995 pp 98–105.
2. Caywood DD: The larynx, trachea, and thyroid and parathyroid glands. In Harvey CE, Newton CD, Schwartz A (eds): Small Animal Surgery. Philadelphia, Lippincott, 1990, pp 189–210.
3. Chew DJ, Carothers M: Hypercalcemia. Vet Clin North Am Small Anim Pract 19:265–287, 1989.
4. Cornick JL, Seahorn TL, Hartsfield SM: Hyperthermia during isoflurane anaesthesia in a horse with suspected hyperkalemic periodic paralysis. Equine Vet J 26:511–514, 1994.
5. Dhupa N: Magnesium therapy. In Bonagura JD (ed): Kirk's Current Veterinary Therapy XII. Philadelphia, W.B. Saunders, 1995 pp 132–133.
6. DiBartola, SP: Hyponatremia. Vet Clin North Am Small Anim Pract 19:215–230, 1989.

7. DiBartola SP, de Morais HA: Disorders of potassium: Hyperkalemia and hypokalemia. In DiBartola SP (ed): Fluid Therapy in Small Animal Practice, 2nd ed. Philadelphia, W.B. Saunders, 2000, pp 83–107.

8. Flanders JA: Parathyroid glands. In Slatter D (ed): Textbook of Small Animal Surgery 2nd ed. Philadelphia, W.B. Saunders, 1993, pp 1523–1536.

9. Garcia-Lopez JM, Provost PJ, Rush JE, et al: Prevalence and prognostic importance of hypomagnesemia and hypocalcemia in horses that have colic surgery. Am J Vet Res 62:7–12, 2001.

10. Hardy RM: Hypernatremia. Vet Clin North Am Small Anim Pract 19:231–240, 1989.

11. Johnson PJ: Physiology of body fluids in the horse. Vet Clin North Am Equine 14:1–22, 1998.

12. Kadar E, Rush JE, Wetmore LA, et al: Hypomagnesemia and cardiac arrhythmias in a dog following pamidronate, calcitonin and furosemide administration for hypercalcemia of malignancy. Manuscript in preparation.

13. Kimmel SE, Waddell LS, Michel KE: Hypomagnesemia and hypocalcemia associated with protein-losing enteropathy in Yorkshire Terriers: Five cases (1992–1998) J Am Vet Med Assoc 217:703–706, 2000.

14. Martin LG, Van Pelt DR, Wingfield WE: Magnesium and the critically ill patient. In Bonagura JD (ed): Kirk's Current Veterinary Therapy XII. Philadelphia, W.B. Saunders, 1995, pp 128–131.

15. Naylor JM: Equine hyperkalemic periodic paralysis: Review and implications. Can Vet J 35:279–285, 1994.

16. Naylor JM: Hyperkalemic periodic paralysis. Vet Clin North Am Equine 13:129-144, 1997.

17. Pascoe PJ: Perioperative management of fluid therapy. In DiBartola SP (ed): Fluid Therapy in Small Animal Practice, 2nd ed. Philadelphia, W.B. Saunders, 2000, pp 307–329.

18. Plumb DC: Veterinary Drug Handbook, 3rd ed. Ames, Iowa State University Press, 1999, pp 699–700.

19. Robertson SA, Green SL, Carter SW, et al: Postanesthetic recumbency associated with hyperkalemic periodic paralysis in a quarter horse. J Am Vet Med Assoc 201:1209–1212, 1992.

20. Rosol TJ, Chew DJ, Nagode LA, et al: Disorders of calcium: Hypercalcemia and hypocalcemia. In DiBartola SP (ed): Fluid Therapy in Small Animal Practice, 2nd ed. Philadelphia, W.B. Saunders, 2000, pp 108–162.

21. Russell LC, Rush JE: Cardiac arrhythmias in systemic disease. In Bonagura JD (ed): Kirk's Current Veterinary Therapy XII. Philadelphia, W.B. Saunders, 1995, pp 161-166.

22. Scavelli TD, Peterson ME: The thyroid. In Slatter D (ed): Textbook of Small Animal Surgery 2nd ed. Philadelphia, W.B. Saunders, 1993, pp 1514-1523.

23. Schertel ER, Tobias TA: Hypertonic fluid therapy. In DiBartola SP (ed): Fluid Therapy in Small Animal Practice, 2nd ed. Philadelphia, W.B. Saunders, 2000, pp 496–506.

24. Sealer D: Fluid and electrolyte therapy. In Thurmon JC, Tranquilli WJ, Benson GJ (eds): Lumb and Jones' Veterinary Anesthesia, 3rd ed. Philadelphia, Williams & Wilkins, 1996, pp 585–589.

25. Spier SJ, Carlson GP, Holliday TA, et al: Hyperkalemic periodic paralysis in horses. J Am Vet Med Assoc 197:1009–1017, 1990.

26. Willard MD: Disorders of potassium homeostasis. Vet Clin North Am Small Anim Pract 19:241–263, 1989.

4. FLUID THERAPY

Khursheed Mama, D.V.M., D.A.C.V.A.

1. When is fluid therapy indicated?

Fluid therapy is indicated in a multitude of circumstances in which an animal is unable to compensate for changes in its fluid and electrolyte balance. The nature of therapy is specific to each circumstance and should be based on the individual patient's needs.

2. What is the preferred route of administration for fluids? Why?

Intravenous. This allows for more precise and controlled delivery to the patient.

3. What are common sites for intravenous catheterization in dogs and cats?

The cephalic, medial (cat), or lateral (dog) saphenous and jugular veins are most commonly used.

4. Are there other routes of administration that can be used for fluid administration?

Yes, many other routes, including intraosseous, intraperitoneal, oral, and subcutaneous can be used to administer fluids. The intraosseous route, while more invasive, is useful in small patients when intravenous catheterization is challenging. Fluids can be delivered at similar rates via this route. Other routes have limitations, such as slower or unreliable absorption, the potential to cause peritonitis, and the possibility of infection.

5. What terminology is used to classify types of fluids?

Fluids can be classified under the broad categories of crystalloids and colloids. Crystalloid solutions are those containing ions or solutes that redistribute to all fluid compartments within the body. Colloid solutions contain large molecular weight substances that remain predominantly within the vascular compartment.

6. What defines a balanced or unbalanced crystalloid solution?

Crystalloid solutions can be termed *balanced* if their components are similar to those contained in extracellular fluid and *unbalanced* if this is not the case.

7. Crystalloid solutions are also classified based on tonicity. What is the basis of this classification?

Solutions are classified as hypertonic, hypotonic, or isotonic based on their osmolality relative to that of blood and extracellular fluid.

8. Some crystalloid solutions are considered acidifying. What is an example of such a solution? Why is this term used?

Sodium chloride is an acidifying crystalloid solution. It is an unbalanced solution in that it contains no bicarbonate precursor. Hence, when large volumes are administered rapidly, it may result in a dilutional acidemia (by virtue of diluting plasma bicarbonate).

9. Despite this acidifying effect there are circumstances in which normal saline is the replacement solution of choice. What are some examples?

Saline is the fluid of choice in a patient with metabolic alkalosis (e.g., pyloric obstruction) or in a patient that is hyperkalemic as a result of its primary disease (e.g., Addison's disease, ruptured bladder).

10. In hyperkalemic patients, although normal saline is useful because it does not contain potassium, an acidifying solution may actually be undesirable. Is there a way to modify saline to decrease this acidifying effect?

Yes, sodium bicarbonate can be added to the saline solution. Since plasma normally contains 18 to 24 mEq/L of bicarbonate, this amount can be added to a liter of saline to minimize the acidifying effect of saline alone.

11. When administering fluids, it is helpful to think of replacement, maintenance, and ongoing losses. What does each of these terms represent?

When a patient is first presented, its hydration status will determine initial replacement fluid therapy. Hence, replacement therapy addresses the deficit fluid volume. If the patient weighs 10 kg and is 10% dehydrated, 1 L of balanced electrolyte solution will constitute the replacement component of fluid to be administered (10% × 10 kg = 1 L).

Maintenance fluid therapy is directed at maintaining normal sensible losses (e.g., urinary production 1–2 ml/kg/hr for a small animal patient) and insensible losses (e.g., respiratory, cutaneous). Note that this may sometimes be termed normal ongoing losses. This is estimated based on the patient's body weight and maintenance energy requirements (approximately 70–80 kcal/kg/day for the dog and 50–60 kcal/kg/day for the cat) that are commonly used to arrive at the daily fluid requirement (approximately 25–50 ml/kg/day).

Abnormal ongoing losses may also occur during the patient's stay in the medical facility. Examples of this include fluid loss due to vomiting, diuresis, etc. These losses can be quantitated (by weighing the animal as needed during the day) and then replaced on a volume per weight basis (500 ml for 0.5 kg loss).

12. Ideally, what types of fluids should be used to replace losses?

Isotonic solutions containing a composition similar to that of extracellular fluid are generally used for replacement of losses. Maintenance solutions contain lower sodium and higher potassium levels that better match the composition of sensible and insensible losses. Solutions to replace abnormal ongoing losses should be selected based on the presumed or measured composition of the loss.

13. What are some examples of commercially available solutions used for replacement and/or maintenance?

Lactated Ringer's solution, Normosol-R, Plasma-Lyte 148 (or R), and normal saline (0.9%) are examples of replacement solutions. Normosol-M, Plasma-Lyte 56 (or M), and half-strength saline (0.45%) are examples of maintenance solutions.

14. What are the main components in these solutions?

Replacement solutions: These solutions are generally isotonic and contain electrolytes in a similar composition to that of plasma: Na^+, 130–154 mEq/L; K^+, 4–5 mEq/L; Cl^-, 98–154 mEq/L. Additionally, some solutions contain other ions such as Ca^{++} and Mg^{++} and an alkalinizing substance or bicarbonate precursor in the form of acetate, lactate, or gluconate.

Maintenance solutions: These solutions are generally hypotonic: Na^+, 40–55 mEq/L; K^+, 13–20 mEq/L; Cl^-, 40–55 mEq/L. These solutions may also contain bicarbonate precursors, other ions, and dextrose.

Detailed information about the composition of different fluids can be found in the references listed at the end of this chapter.

Ongoing loss solutions: No commercially available solutions specifically meet this requirement. Often a replacement solution supplemented with potassium is used to meet this need.

15. What are the guidelines for speed of administration for these two types of fluid?

Replacement solutions can be rapidly administered as determined by the needs of the patient. Frequently half the calculated deficit is administered in 10 to 20 minutes and the patient's hydration and demeanor reassessed and the administration rate adjusted. In general, maintenance solutions should be administered slowly in keeping with the normal sensible and insensible losses. Ongoing losses are generally replaced over a few hours; rate of administration is limited by the maximal rate of administration of potassium and type of fluid administered.

16. What is the recommended maximal rate for intravenous administration of potassium?
In general, a rate of 0.5 mEq/kg/hour should not be exceeded.

17. What are signs that potassium administration may be too rapid?
Electrocardiographic changes such as tall-tented T waves, widened QRS complexes, prolonged P-R interval, absence of P-waves, and bradycardia are associated with hyperkalemia. Cardiac arrest will result if hyperkalemia is not treated.

18. What is the treatment for hyperkalemia?
Intravenous administration of 10 mg/kg calcium chloride, administration of 0.5–1 mEq/kg sodium bicarbonate, administration of potassium-free fluids (e.g., NaCl), potassium-wasting diuretics, insulin and glucose (dextrose), and gastrointestinal exchange resins.

19. Although 5% dextrose in water is commercially available and could be considered an isotonic solution (osmolality, 250 mOsm/L), rapid administration and or large doses may result in patient compromise. Can you explain this?
While isotonic in the fluid preparation, when given to the patient, the dextrose is utilized by cells, leaving behind only free water that is hypotonic and may lead to cellular edema and lysis.

20. How would you administer dextrose to a patient that needed it?
If the fluids are to be administered rapidly, dextrose may be added to a commercial replacement solution such as lactated Ringer's to achieve the desired concentration of dextrose. For example, to get a 5% dextrose solution, 100 ml of 50% dextrose is added to 1 L of lactated Ringer's solution (i.e., 50 mg/ml ÷ 500 mg/ml × 1000 ml). Maintenance solutions containing dextrose are also available for patients in whom slower administration is appropriate.

21. What is the recommended 'maintenance' fluid administration rate for the anesthetized patient?
5–10 ml/kg/hour, IV.

22. Why does this maintenance rate exceed the rate suggested previously as adequate to replace normal sensible and insensible losses?
Although the terminology used is the same, anesthetic maintenance differs from traditional maintenance and is a source of confusion to many. The fluid administration rate during anesthesia is higher because, in addition to compensating for normal sensible and insensible losses, maintenance of vascular volume is crucial to ensure adequate tissue perfusion in the anesthetized patient. This is especially important because normal compensatory homeostatic mechanisms may be altered in these patients. Hence, fluids may be administered to counteract the hemodynamic changes that occur with anesthetic drugs (e.g., vasodilation) and/or to compensate for volume losses (e.g., hemorrhage) related to the primary disease or the procedure.

23. Are there patients in whom a lower anesthetic maintenance administration rate should be considered?
There are many patients in whom lower fluid administration rates should be used. Examples include patients in congestive heart failure, patients with regurgitant murmurs, pulmonary edema, etc, or patients with clinically significant reductions in hematocrit or total protein values.

24. What is the recommended fluid administration rate to replace blood loss in a patient with a normal packed cell volume and total protein? What is the basis for this guideline?
Three times the volume lost if crystalloid solutions are used. Approximately two-thirds of the crystalloid solution administered will redistribute to the interstitial and intracellular fluid spaces

within 20 to 30 minutes. Hence, only about one-third of the amount of crystalloid given will remain in the vascular space.

25. What is the role of anions such as lactate, acetate, and gluconate in crystalloid solutions?

These anions, when metabolized (largely by oxidation), utilize a hydrogen ion and generate bicarbonate equivalent to that contained in the extracellular fluid compartment. Hence, they help maintain normal blood pH and may be referred to as alkalinizing solutions.

26. Are there circumstances under which a specific anion may be preferred?

Lactate and acetate predominate as the anions present in commercially available fluids, and, although both result in an equivalent alkalinizing effect, there are circumstances under which one may be preferred. Concern has been expressed about the administration of lactate to patients with severe hepatic disease, as enzyme systems responsible for the clearance of lactate may become saturated. Similarly, in patients with cancer, lactate metabolism may be impaired or be associated with a high-energy expenditure. Acetate, which is metabolized at sites throughout the body, may be preferred in these patients. The disadvantage of acetate-containing solutions is that rapid administration may result in significant hypotension mediated via vasodilation.

27. What are some of the fluid incompatibilities one should be aware of?

Fluids containing calcium should not be mixed with bicarbonate-containing solutions or citrated blood products, as these may precipitate. Inotropes (e.g., dobutamine) should not be administered with bicarbonate-containing solutions, as the latter may reduce the efficacy of the former.

28. What are the indications for the use of colloids?

Colloids may be used in patients in whom rapid intravenous volume expansion (e.g., hypovolemia, hemorrhage) is desired or in the patient that needs oncotic support (e.g., hypoproteinemia, hypoalbuminemia).

29. How do colloids work?

Colloidal solutions contain large molecular weight particles that remain within the vascular space and help maintain oncotic pressure by holding or drawing water into the vascular space. Unlike crystalloid solutions, colloids help maintain vascular volume for hours to days.

30. What determines the duration of effect of different colloid solutions?

The molecular weight of the compound: the larger the particles, the longer the compound will remain within the vascular space to generate its effect. The number of particles is also significant, as this will determine the osmotic capacity of the fluid.

31. Are these values (for molecular weight and number) readily available?

Yes. Average molecular weight is designated M_w and number molecular weight (i.e., total weight of all molecules, divided by the number of molecules) is designated M_n. See the references listed at the end of the chapter for more information regarding the specific values for the commercially available synthetic colloid solutions.

32. What are some of the commercially available synthetic colloid solutions?

Dextran 70, Dextran 40, Hetastarch, Pentastarch, Gelatin

33. How and at what rate should colloids be administered? Is there a maximal limit?

Colloids are given intravenously. Hetastarch and Dextran 70 can be administered at rates of 1–2 ml/kg/hour if used for ongoing oncotic support. Alternatively, rapid administration up to 20 ml/kg is used in a patient in an acute hypotensive, hypovolemic crisis.

34. What are some concerns when administering colloids?

The primary concern has been the influence of colloidal solutions on coagulation. Both direct effects (interfere with platelet function) and indirect effects (by virtue of dilution of coagulation factors, etc) may contribute. Similarly, hemodilution and a reduced hematocrit may be clinically significant with sustained or large volume colloid use. Inappropriate administration may also lead to hypervolemia. Anaphylactic reactions have been reported in humans but have not been documented in dogs and cats.

35. Are there other solutions that may be considered colloids?

Yes, blood and its components are considered colloids. Refer to the appropriate chapter in this book for information on this subject.

BIBLIOGRAPHY

1. DiBartola SP: Introduction to fluid therapy. In DiBartola SP (ed): Fluid Therapy in Small Animal Practice, 2nd ed. W.B. Saunders, 2000, pp 265–280.
2. Pascoe PJ: Perioperative management of fluid therapy. In DiBartola SP (ed): Fluid Therapy in Small Animal Practice, 2nd ed. W.B. Saunders, 2000, pp 307–329.
3. Greco DS: The distribution of body water and general approach to the patient. Adv Fluid Electrolyte Disorders 28(3): 473–482, 1998.
4. Mathews KA: The various types of parenteral fluids and their indications. Adv Fluid Electrolyte Disorders 28(3), 483–513, 1998.

5. BLOOD AND BLOOD PRODUCTS

Luisito S. Pablo, D.V.M., M.S., D.A.C.V.A.

1. What is blood component therapy?

Blood component therapy involves the administration of a specific blood product according to the need of the clinical condition of the patient.

2. What are the advantages of blood component therapy in the field of anesthesia?

The main advantage of blood component therapy during anesthesia is the minimal volume needed for administration, preventing circulatory overload. For example, in anemic patients with normal blood volume, the administration of packed red blood cells is preferable over whole blood. The colloid component of whole blood can result in volume overload when attempting to increase the oxygen-carrying capacity of the patient. The use of specific blood components may also lead to fewer complications associated with transfusion because unnecessary components are not administered. There are other advantages, which may not have direct impact on anesthesia. They include longer storage time for some components (plasma and plasma derivatives), a better use of blood resources, and a better therapeutic approach to the patient's problem.

3. What are the available blood products that can be used in small animals before, during, and after anesthesia?

- Packed red blood cells
- Fresh frozen plasma
- Cryoprecipitate
- Cryoprecipitate-poor plasma
- Platelet-rich plasma

4. How can practitioners acquire these products if they do not have the capability to process the whole blood?

Veterinary blood banks can supply most of the blood components. One way to find veterinary blood bank is to search the Internet. References are also available listing the different blood banks.

5. What are the common indications of blood component therapy during the perioperative period?

- Severe hemorrhage during surgery
- Acute and chronic anemia due to a variety of causes (trauma, neoplasia, chronic inflammation)
- Hypoproteinemia
- von Willebrand's disease
- Coagulopathies (disseminated intravascular coagulation and liver disease)
- Thrombocytopenia

6. List the contents of the different blood and blood products used clinically.

- Whole blood: red blood cells, clotting factors, proteins, von Willebrand's factor (vWf), and platelets
- Packed red blood cells: red blood cells only
- Fresh frozen plasma (FFP): all clotting factors, including albumin and vitamin K-dependent proteins
- Stored frozen plasma (SFP): similar to FFP with reduced concentration of cofactors V and VIII
- Cryoprecipitate: high concentration of factor VIII, fibrinogen, vWF, and fibronectin

- Cryoprecipitate-free plasma: similar to FFP or SFP with decreased factor VIII, fibrinogen, vWF, and fibronectin

7. Give specific indications for the different blood products.
- Whole blood: massive blood loss (>20% of blood volume) before and during anesthesia, coagulopathy resulting in massive blood loss, and some patients with disseminated intravascular coagulation
- Packed red blood cells: less severe blood loss during surgery and normovolemic anemia
- Fresh frozen plasma (FFP): von Willebrand's disease, hemophilia A and B, liver disease, coagulopathy, disseminated intravascular coagulation, rodenticide intoxication, and hypoproteinemia
- Stored-frozen plasma (SFP): similar indications as for FFP except in patients with hemophilia A or wVf deficiency
- Cryoprecipitate: disseminated intravascular coagulation, vWF deficiency, hemophilia A, and generalized sepsis (fibronectin enhances mononuclear phagocytic activity)
- Cryoprecipitate-free plasma: similar indications to FFP or SFP except in conditions that require factor VIII, fibrinogen, vWF, and fibronectin

8. What is the best approach to correcting hypoalbuminemia?
In hypoalbuminemia, fresh frozen plasma should be not used as the only source of albumin. To increase the albumin concentration by 1 g/dl, plasma should be given at 45 ml/kg and can be expensive. Without concurrent administration of other colloids, albumin from the transfused plasma equilibrates rapidly with the extravascular space. The best approach is to administer synthetic colloids (e.g., hetastarch and dextrans) in addition to plasma.

9. Do blood and blood products require special administration sets?
Blood and blood products should be administered through a 170 μm filter because they have microagglutinates.

10. Is there any specific temperature requirement for the blood products before their administration to the patient?
Blood and blood products, except platelet-rich plasma, should be warmed before transfusion, especially in small patients. However, the temperature should not be more than 37°C. Higher temperature will result in hemolysis and precipitation of numerous proteins. Platelet-rich plasma can be kept at 22°C during transfusion.

11. How do you determine the dose for blood and blood products? What are the typical infusion rates for the different blood products?
The dose for whole blood and packed red blood cells is based on the patient's packed cell volume (PCV) and the desired increase in PCV. The formula used is:

$$\text{ml of blood required} = \text{Blood volume} \times \frac{(\text{desired PCV} - \text{recipient PCV})}{\text{Donor PCV}}$$

The volume is administered slowly for the first 5 to 15 minutes at a rate of 5.0 ml/kg/hour. The animal is closely observed at this time for adverse reactions. The rate is increased to 10.0–22.0 ml/kg/hour if no complications are observed. If the patient is hypovolemic, the rate of infusion can be increased up to 66 ml/kg/hour.

Fresh frozen plasma, frozen plasma, and cryoprecipitate-poor plasma are administered at 10.0 ml/kg and repeated until the bleeding is controlled. Cryoprecipitate is administered to effect at 1 U/10 kg and repeated 12 hours after, if bleeding continues. The dose for platelet-rich plasma is 1 U/10 kg.

The recommended rate of infusion for plasma products is 22 ml/kg per 24 hours in a normovolemic patient. In hypovolemic patients, the rate of infusion should not be more than 22.0 ml/kg/hour. The rate is further reduced to 4.0 ml/kg/hour in patients with compromised cardiac function.

12. Which crystalloid solution can be mixed with blood during administration?

Normal saline (0.9%) can be mixed with blood. Crystalloid solutions that contain calcium will activate the coagulation system. Some preparations are either hypotonic or hypertonic, resulting in hemolysis.

13. How would you detect acute transfusion reaction during anesthesia?

Hypotension is the most common sign associated with transfusion reaction in anesthetized patients. Both acute hemolytic reactions and acute hypersensitivity reactions will be manifested as hypotension. Tachycardia may be manifested if the acute hemolysis results in shock. Anesthesia will mask the early signs of hemolytic transfusion reaction, which include pyrexia, tremors, vomiting, dyspnea, and salivation. The presence of hypotension and tachycardia due to the ongoing blood loss will complicate the detection of an acute hemolytic transfusion reaction. It is important to remember that acute hemolytic reaction can occur within minutes of the start of the transfusion. If hypotension persists despite blood transfusion and other therapeutic modalities (positive inotrope and lowered anesthetic concentration), it is prudent to stop the transfusion and check the blood for hemolysis.

With acute hypersensitivity, vasoactive substances (histamine, serotonin, kallikreins, and proteases) are released. In this case, there will be no hemolysis. The onset of a reaction is usually 1 to 45 minutes from the start of infusion. In dogs, in addition to hypotension, urticaria can be seen with acute hypersensitivity reaction. Acute hypersensitivity reaction can also result in severe shock.

14. What steps should be taken to minimize reaction to the blood and blood products?

Transfusion reaction can be minimized by cross-matching in dogs. Incompatibilities occur as a result of earlier sensitization of the recipient or the presence of naturally occurring isoantibodies in either the donor or recipient. It is important to remember that compatible cross-match does not stop the patient from being sensitized against donor cells. Incompatibility reaction can occur as early as 4 days following transfusion. Based on this, previously transfused patients should always be cross-matched, even if blood from the same donor is used. A dog that has never received donor blood can be safely given a blood transfusion without cross-match.

If the animal will receive plasma product repeatedly, a minor cross-match is advisable. Minor cross-match will detect antibodies in donor plasma against the cells of the recipient.

In cats, blood-typing or cross-matching should be done before transfusion. Cats have naturally occurring alloantibodies. Untyped or uncross-matched blood given to a cat that has never received a transfusion can be fatal.

15. When are blood or blood products needed when hemorrhage occurs during anesthesia? Which blood products can be administered in this situation?

Whole blood is generally required when massive blood loss occurs during anesthesia. Blood loss is considered massive if more than 20% of the blood volume is lost. Whole blood is also indicated if there is blood loss and the patient is hypoproteinemic. If whole blood is not available, a combination of fresh frozen plasma and packed red blood cells can be used. If the blood loss is less than 20% of the blood volume and the packed cell volume of the patient is approaching 20%, packed red blood cells can be administered. The volume of blood products administered should equal the blood loss and it must be administered at a rate that should replace the loss as rapidly as possible.

16. A dog or a cat is under general anesthesia and severe bleeding occurs unexpectedly. No cross-match was made before anesthesia, and hemoglobin-based oxygen carrying solution is not available. How do you approach this situation?

If the patient is a dog that has not been transfused before, whole blood or packed red blood cells from any donor can be infused. If the dog has had a previous blood transfusion, synthetic colloid may have to be used until a cross-match is performed.

In cats, the breed may play a role in the decision making. If the cat belongs to a breed with type B frequency of 0%, blood from a type A donor can be used without cross-match. If the patient belongs to one of the breeds with known type B blood, the patient has to be typed before transfusion. Blood typing using a card is quicker than cross-matching. Cross-matching is not necessary in this case.

17. The patient has low oxygen carrying capacity, and no blood or blood products are available. What is an alternative therapy?

Hemoglobin-based oxygen-carrying solutions.

18. What is Oxyglobin? What are its main indications during perioperative period?

Oxyglobin is an ultrapurified, polymerized hemoglobin solution (13.0 mg/dl) of bovine origin in a modified Ringer's lactated solution. It has a pH of 7.8 and an osmolality of 300 mOsm/kg. It is less viscous than blood.

It is mainly indicated in relieving the signs associated with anemia. It has also been used to improve and maintain perfusion. It can be used in patients that develop severe hemorrhage during anesthesia or any shock state in which volume loading is necessary.

19. How is Oxyglobin administered to dogs and cats?

A standard intravenous set is all that is needed to administer Oxyglobin to dogs and cats. In very small patients, an infusion pump will aid in accurate dosing. In cats, Oxyglobin is given at 10.0 ml/kg at an infusion rate not to exceed 5.0 ml/kg/hour. The dose range in dogs is 15.0–30.0 ml/kg with the rate of administration limited to 10.0 ml/kg/hour. In cases of hemorrhagic and hypovolemic shock, bolus administration can be used.

20. Are there any reported complications associated with Oxyglobin?

Oxyglobin has been reported to increase pulmonary resistance. Patients with pulmonary thromboembolism or pulmonary contusion developed pulmonary edema and died. As a result of this, it is best to avoid Oxyglobin in patients with pulmonary disease. Other significant complications associated with Oxyglobin include volume overload and interference with some blood tests.

21. What are the indicators of improvement following transfusion therapy during anesthesia?

Laboratory data are needed to accurately determine the improvement brought about by the transfusion therapy. The administration of whole blood and packed red blood cells should result in higher hematocrit and plasma hemoglobin level. When using Oxyglobin, the plasma hemoglobin level should be checked because the hematocrit will stay low. The administration of plasma to increase colloid oncotic pressure will lead to increased plasma protein levels. Improvement due to synthetic colloid cannot be measured by a refractometer and will need an oncometer to determine colloid oncotic pressure. The administration of cryoprecipitate should normalize buccal mucosa bleeding time (2–4 minutes).

The more practical approach in von Willebrand's disease is to observe the presence of uncontrolled bleeding during surgery. Uncontrolled bleeding indicates the need for more cryoprecipitate. With the other blood products, improvement in clinical signs will be more important indicator of effective therapy. An important end point of therapy when treating coagulopathies will be when active bleeding ceases. Coagulation tests using prothrombin time (PT) and activated partial thromboplastin time (aPTT) can assist in determining the success of therapy.

In case of hemorrhage, hypovolemia, and shock during anesthesia, effective transfusion therapy should result in normal heart rate, improved systemic blood pressure, normal central venous pressure, increased urine output, and pink mucous membranes. The respiratory rate may not change because of the blunting effect of anesthetics. If capnography is being used for monitoring, increased expired CO_2 without any change in the ventilatory status indicates an improving perfusion state.

22. The patient has a clinical condition that necessitates blood products before anesthesia. When is the best time to administer these blood products?

The time to administer the blood products is determined by the severity of the problem and the need to perform surgery immediately in life-threatening conditions. If there is bleeding associated with coagulopathies, administration of plasma components before anesthesia should be timed such that the patient should have received the initial dose before surgery. With von Willebrand's disease, cryoprecipitate is started about 1 to 2 hours before surgery and usually continues through surgery until the required dose is given. More units of cryoprecipitate will be needed if there is bleeding during surgery. With anemic patients (PCV < 20%), the whole blood or packed red blood cells are administered until the desired PCV is reached. A desired PCV may be set at 25%. In invasive procedures during which blood loss is expected, infusion of packed red blood cells continues through surgery at a rate of 5.0 ml/kg/hour. In hypoproteinemic patients, plasma is administered before anesthesia until a plasma protein concentration of ≥ 4.0 g/dl is reached.

23. What are the signs of volume overload during anesthesia?

Volume overload during anesthesia may be manifested as serous nasal discharge, chemosis, and pulmonary crackles and edema. With severe pulmonary edema, frothy fluid may be found in the endotracheal tube and breathing circuit. If central venous pressure (CVP) is being monitored during anesthesia, there will be sudden elevation in CVP. Tachypnea, dyspnea, and tachycardia are commonly associated with circulatory overload in conscious patients. These signs may not even be manifested during anesthesia, however, because anesthetics tend to blunt these responses.

BIBLIOGRAPHY

1. Feldman BF: Blood transfusion guidelines. In Bonagura JE (ed): Kirk's Current Veterinary Therapy XIII Small Animal Practice. Philadelphia, WB Saunders Co, 2000, pp 400–403.
2. Giger U: Blood typing and crossmatching to ensure compatible transfusions. In Bonagura JE (ed): Kirk's Current Veterinary Therapy XIII Small Animal Practice. Philadelphia, WB Saunders Co, 2000, pp 396–399.
3. Harrell KA, Kristensen AT: Canine transfusion reactions and their management. Vet Clin North Am (Small Animal Pract) 25:1333–1364, 1995.
4. Hohenhaus AE: Blood transfusions and blood substitutes. In DiBartola SP (ed): Fluid Therapy in Small Animal Practice, 2nd ed. Philadelphia, WB Saunders Co, 2000, pp 451–464.
5. Kerl ME, Hohenhaus AE: Packed red blood cell transfusions in dogs: 131 cases. J Am Vet Med Assoc 202:1495–1499, 1989.
6. Kristensen AT, Feldman BF: General principles of small animal blood component administration. Vet Clin North Am (Small Animal Pract) 25:1277–1290, 1995.
7. Wardrop KJ: Transfusion medicine. In August JR (ed): Consultations in Feline Internal Medicine. Philadelphia, WB Saunders Co, 2001, pp 461–467.

6. THE AUTONOMIC NERVOUS SYSTEM (ANS)

Lisa S. Klopp, D.V.M., M.S., D.A.C.V.I.M. (Neurology)

1. What is the autonomic nervous system?

The autonomic nervous system (ANS) is an involuntary system that controls physiologic homeostasis. It is involved in control of various vegetative and protective functions. Although the system is involuntary, it integrates to subserve voluntary function. For example, if an animal is threatened and needs to flee, somatic systems will be modulated by the ANS: cardiac output, blood supply, and respiratory rate increase to supply nutrients and oxygen to working somatic muscles.

2. What is the basic anatomy of the autonomic nervous system?

The autonomic nervous is a two-neuron system. The first neuron, termed the preganglionic neuron, originates in the central nervous system (CNS) and the second, termed the postganglionic neuron, arises in a ganglion (collection of nerve cell bodies outside the central nervous system). The postganglionic axon terminates on the effector organ.

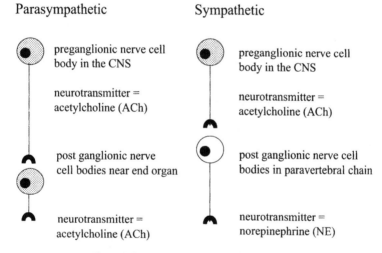

Figure 1. The two neuron organization of the ANS

3. What are the two divisions of the autonomic nervous system?

The autonomic nervous system is divided functionally and anatomically into the parasympathetic and sympathetic nervous systems. These divisions tend to have opposing functions (eg. parasympathetic innervation to the heart decreases heart rate, whereas sympathetic innervation increases it). When one division is activated, the influence from the other is decreased. The balance of input from the two systems depends on the requirements of the animal at that time. Some organs receive only sympathetic innervation and the activity is regulated by changes in the amount of discharge in sympathetic pre- and postganglionic fibers.

4. What is the specific anatomy of the parasympathetic division of the autonomic nervous systems?

Preganglionic nerve cell bodies originate in the brain stem and sacral spinal cord (see figures).

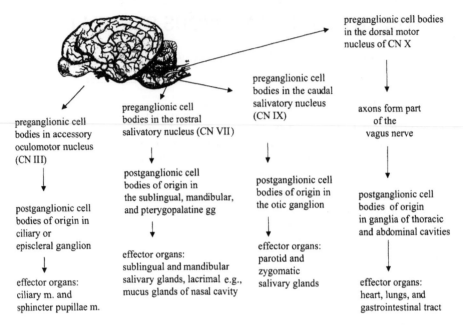

preganglionic cell bodies in the dorsal motor nucleus of CN X

↓

preganglionic cell bodies in the caudal salivatory nucleus (CN IX)

axons form part of the vagus nerve

preganglionic cell bodies in the rostral salivatory nucleus (CN VII)

preganglionic cell bodies in accessory oculomotor nucleus (CN III)

↓

postganglionic cell bodies of origin in the sublingual, mandibular, and pterygopalatine gg

↓

postganglionic cell bodies of origin in the otic ganglion

↓

postganglionic cell bodies of origin in ganglia of thoracic and abdominal cavities

↓

postganglionic cell bodies of origin in ciliary or episcleral ganglion

↓

effector organs: ciliary m. and sphincter pupillae m.

effector organs: sublingual and mandibular salivary glands, lacrimal e.g., mucus glands of nasal cavity

effector organs: parotid and zygomatic salivary glands

effector organs: heart, lungs, and gastrointestinal tract

Figure 2. Brain stem origins of the parasympathetic nervous system

    In the brain stem, parasympathetic preganglionic cell bodies are found in some of the cranial nerve nuclei. These include cranial nerve (CN) III (accessory oculomotor nuclei or Edinger-Westphal nucleus), CN VII (rostral salivatory nucleus), CN IX (caudal salivatory nucleus), and CN X (dorsal motor nucleus of CN X). These nuclei are the origin of the preganglionic neurons providing parasympathetic innervation to the eye (CN III), the salivary and lacrimal glands (CN VII and IX), and thoracic and abdominal organs (CN X).

    Preganglionic neuronal cell bodies in the sacral region (S1-3) originate in the intermediate lateral gray matter. These preganglionic neurons give rise to parasympathetic innervation of structures in the pelvic canal (see figure).

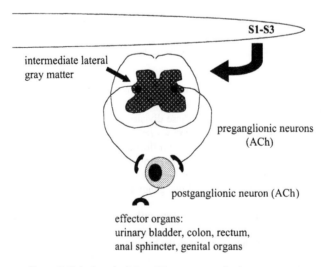

S1-S3

intermediate lateral gray matter

preganglionic neurons (ACh)

postganglionic neuron (ACh)

effector organs: urinary bladder, colon, rectum, anal sphincter, genital organs

Figure 3. Spinal cord origins of the parasympathetic nervous system

5. What is the specific anatomy of the sympathetic division of the autonomic nervous system?

Preganglionic neuronal cell bodies originate in the intermediate lateral gray matter of the spinal cord from (C_8) T1–L_{4-5}. The preganglionic axonal fibers exit the spinal canal with the ventral nerve roots and join spinal nerves for a short distance. They then enter communicating branches that course to the sympathetic (or paravertebral) chain. The sympathetic chain is a bilateral collection of pre- and postganglionic sympathetic axonal fibers and general visceral afferent sensory axonal fibers. The preganglionic fibers course to the chain (paravertebral) ganglia which are located in the thoracic and abdominal cavities ventrolateral to the vertebral bodies. These ganglia are located along the sympathetic chain and are associated and numbered according to the spinal nerves. The pre- and postganglionic axons are of variable length, depending on the spinal cord segments from which they arise (preganglionic), the location of the ganglion, and the final destination of the postganglionic fiber. The adrenal gland is considered a "postganglionic neuron." It is innervated directly by a preganglionic axon.

The sympathetic nervous system is topographically arranged. The rostral thoracic sympathetic cell bodies are responsible for sympathetic innervation of the head and neck (i.e. eyes, blood vessels, salivary glands). The midthoracic sympathetic cell bodies result in innervation of the organs of the thoracic and abdominal cavity (i.e., heart, lungs, spleen). The preganglionic cell bodies that originate in the lumbar region give rise to innervation of the caudal abdominal cavity and pelvic cavity (i.e. bladder, rectum, genital organs).

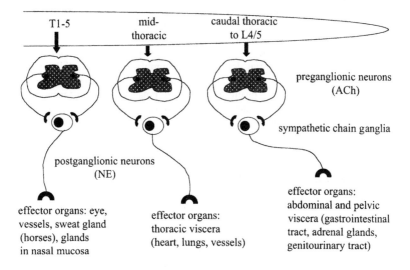

Figure 4. Spinal cord origins and topographic organization of the sympathetic nervous system

6. Describe the differences in neurochemistry between the parasympathetic and sympathetic divisions of the autonomic nervous system.

In both divisions, the neurotransmitter released from the preganglionic neuron is acetylcholine (see figure at question 2). The postganglionic neurons of the parasympathetic nervous system also release acetylcholine. The postganglionic neurons in the sympathetic division release norepinephrine. Some sympathetic cholinergic postganglionic neurons have been identified, however. These neurons may innervate vessels in skeletal muscles, the nictitating membrane in the cat, and some sweat glands.

7. Describe the synthesis and metabolism of acetylcholine.

Acteylcholine is synthesized from choline and acetyl coenzyme A via the enzyme choline acetyltransferase (ChAT):

$$\text{choline + acetyl coenzyme A} \xrightarrow{[ChAT]} \text{acetylcholine + coenzyme A.}$$

Following its synthesis in the nerve terminal, acetylcholine is transported into synaptic vesicles via the vesicular acetylcholine transporter protein. The precursor choline is provided to the nerve for acetylcholine synthesis by two mechanisms. Once released, acetylcholine in the synaptic cleft is hydrolyzed to acetate and choline via acetylcholinesterase (AchE). In addition, choline is derived from membrane phosphatidylcholine. Both sources of choline are available in the extracellular space (synaptic cleft) and a high-affinity uptake system brings choline back into the nerve terminal.

$$\text{acetylcholine} \xrightarrow{[AchE]} \text{acetate + choline}$$

8. Describe the receptors for acetylcholine.

Originally, subtyping of acetylcholine receptors was based on the actions of two alkaloids, nicotine and muscarine. Both types of receptors are located on the dendritic zone of the postganglionic neuron, but the nicotinic effects tend to predominate. Muscarinic receptors are present on the effector organs that respond to parasympathetic stimulation.

9. How do the nicotinic receptors function?

Nicotinic receptors are found primarily on the postsynaptic ganglionic membranes and the skeletal muscle. In the autonomic ganglia, the primary electrophysiologic event following stimulation is rapid depolarization of the postganglionic membrane mediated by ACh acting on the receptors. This results in an excitatory postsynaptic potential by opening of a cation channel. Secondary events following the initial depolarization amplify or suppress this signal and are mediated by actions on postganglionic muscarinic receptors and intracellular peptides (substance P, angiotensin, enkalphins), which result in decreased potassium conductance. In addition, inhibitory postsynaptic potentials mediated by catecholamines (dopamine and/or norepinephrine) play a role. Acetylcholine may facilitate cation-conductance in adrenergic interneurons to stimulate the release of norepinephrine or dopamine. In general, these secondary events regulate the sensitivity of the postsynaptic ganglia to repetitive depolarization.

10. How do the muscarinic receptors function?

There are four subtypes of muscarinic receptors (M_1, M_2, M_3, and M_4). Muscarinic receptors are found on visceral smooth muscle, cardiac muscle, secretory glands, and endothelium of the vasculature. With the exception of the endothelial cell, these sites receive primary cholinergic innervation and excite or inhibit function in a tissue-dependent manner. Responses within an individual tissue can vary. Smooth muscle in many organs exhibits intrinsic electrical or mechanical activity. Therefore, acetylcholine modifies, rather than initiates, muscle activity in these organs. Exogenously administered acetylcholine results primarily in stimulation of effector organs rather than the nicotinic receptors of the postganglionic membranes. This is believed to be due both to a large abundance of muscarinic receptors on effector organs and poor blood flow to ganglia.

Responses of Effector Organs to Acetylcholine via Muscarinic Receptors

EFFECTOR ORGAN	ORGAN RESPONSES
Vascular endothelium	Vasodilation mediated by release of endothelium-derived relaxation factor (nitric oxide)
Eye	
Iris (constrictor pupillae muscle)	Miosis
Ciliary muscle	Accommodation of the lens to near vision
Bronchi	Bronchoconstriction
	Increased secretions

Continued on next page

Responses of Effector Organs to Acetylcholine via Muscarinic Receptors (continued)

EFFECTOR ORGAN	ORGAN RESPONSES
Heart	Bradycardia
Sinoatrial node	Decreased conduction velocity
Atrioventricular node	(atrioventricular block at high doses)
Atria	Decreased contraction (negative inotropy)
Ventricles	
Gastrointestinal tract	Increased smooth muscle tone
	Increased secretions
	Sphincter relaxation
Urinary bladder	Detrusor muscle contraction
	Sphincter relaxation
Penis	Erection
Uterus	Varies depending on hormonal influences
Salivary gland	Increased secretion

11. Describe the synthesis of catecholamines.

Norepinephrine (NE), epinephrine (E), and dopamine (DA) are endogenous catecholamines. Norepinephrine is found in postsynaptic ganglia and epinephrine is a hormone released from the adrenal medulla. The adrenal medulla is innervated by a preganglionic neuron, thus the adrenal medulla behaves like a postganglionic neuron. Dopamine, an important CNS neurotransmitter, has biological activity in the periphery, primarily influencing renal blood flow. The initial precursor for catecholamine synthesis is tyrosine. L-tyrosine is found free in the cytosol of adrenergic neurons and is converted to L-dopa by tyrosine hydroxylase. Tyrosine hydroxylase is found in all cells that synthesize catecholamines. Tyrosine hydroxylase is the rate-limiting enzyme in catecholamine synthesis and requires tetrahydrobiopterin and oxygen as cofactors.

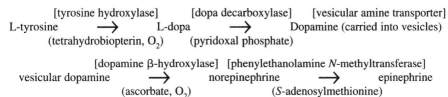

L-dopa in the cytosol is converted to dopamine by dopa decarboxylase, which requires pyridoxal phosphate as a cofactor. Dopamine is taken into storage vesicles, where it is converted to norepinephrine by the action of dopamine β-hydroxylase. Dopamine β-hydroxylase uses ascorbate (vitamin C) and oxygen as its cofactors. In tissues that produce epinephrine (e.g., adrenal gland), norepinephrine is converted to epinephrine by phenyethanolamine *N*-methyltransferase. This enzyme requires *S*-adenosylmethionine as a cofactor.

12. How is the supply of catecholamines regulated?

Catecholamines are found in low concentration in the cytosol. Storage vesicles maintain a ready supply of catecholamines for release in the nerve terminal. Effective regulation of synthesis maintains a steady supply of catecholamines by altering the rate of synthesis of tyrosine hydroxylase and dopamine β-hydroxylase. Tyrosine hydroxylase is subject to end-product feedback inhibition. Therefore, increased intracytosolic catecholamine concentrations will decrease tyrosine hydroxylase activity.

13. How are the actions of catecholamines terminated?

The actions of catecholamines are terminated by three methods: (1) re-uptake into nerve terminals; (2) diffusion out of synaptic clefts with metabolism by extraneuronal tissues; and (3) metabolic transformation. Catecholamines diffuse into the synaptic cleft and are taken up or transported back into the terminal axon. The carrier or transporter protein is located on the outer membrane of the axon terminal. This transporter is saturable and couples energy-dependent transport with the Na^+ gradient across neuronal membranes. A transporter specific for norepinephrine is found only on noradrenergic neurons, whereas a transporter with a specific affinity for dopamine is found on dopaminergic neurons.

14. Describe the metabolism of catecholamines.

Catecholamines are metabolized by two enzyme pathways, monoamine oxidase (MAO) and catechol-O-methyltransferase (COMT). Both MAO and COMT are found in effector tissues and MAO is also found in catecholamine-producing neurons.

Monoamine oxidase is a flavin-containing enzyme located on the outer mitochondrial membrane, and it inactivates cytosolic catecholamines. In neurons, it inactivates catecholamines not protected within storage vesicles. MAO oxidatively converts catecholamines to aldehydes. The aldehydes are then converted either to acids by aldehyde hydrogenase or to glycols by aldehyde reductase. There are two isomers of monoamine oxidase, MAO-1 and MAO-2. It is MAO-1 that is responsible for metabolism of norepinephrine and serotonin.

Catechol-O-methyltransferase, a cytosolic enzyme, is found in all cells in the body, including erythrocytes. COMT in the liver and kidney is probably the most important method of inactivating circulating catecholamines. COMT requires magnesium and inactivates catecholamines by transferring a methyl group from the co-substrate S-adenosylmethionine to the 3-hydroxy group of the catecholamine ring.

15. Describe the receptors for catecholamines.

Adrenergic receptors can be divided into four subsets: α_1, α_2, β_1, and β_2. A β_3 receptor has been identified but plays little role in the functions of the ANS. Each subtype can be inhibited or facilitated by various pharmacologic agents. The actions mediated by the receptors tend to be very different. Therefore, the effects of norepinephrine on any organ may vary.

Responses of Effector Organs to Catecholamines

EFFECTOR ORGAN	RECEPTOR	ORGAN RESPONSES
Arterioles		
Coronary and pulmonary	α_1	Vasoconstriction
	β_2	Vasodilation
Mesenteric and renal	α_1	Vasoconstriction
	β_2	Vasodilation
Skin	α_1	Vasoconstriction
Skeletal muscle	α_1	Vasoconstriction
	β_2	Vasodilation
Cerebral	α	Mild vasoconstriction
Veins	α_1	Vasoconstriction
	β_2	Vasodilation
Eye		
Radial muscle	α_1	Contraction, mydriasis
Ciliary muscle	β	Relaxation for far vision
Lungs		
Bronchi	β_2	Bronchodilation
Glands	α_1	Decreased secretion
	β_2	Increased secretion
Heart	all β_1	Increased heart rate
Sinoatrial node		Increased atrial and ventricular contractility (positive
Atrioventricular node		inotropy)

Continued on next page

Responses of Effector Organs to Catecholamines (continued)

EFFECTOR ORGAN	RECEPTOR	ORGAN RESPONSES
His-Purkinje system Atria Ventricles		Increased atrial and ventricular conduction velocity (postive chronotropy) Increased automaticity
Gastrointestinal tract	$\alpha_1, \beta_{1,2}$ α	Smooth muscle relaxation (decreased motility and tone) Increased sphincter contraction
Spleen	α	Splenic contraction, increased erythrocyte levels (especially dogs)
	β_2	Relaxation
Urinary bladder Trigone and internal sphincter Detrusor muscle	 α_1 β_2	Retention: Contraction Fundus relaxes
Uterus	α β	Contraction $\Big\}$ depends on hormonal status Relaxation
Salivary gland	α_1	Increased secretion
Metabolism	β α_2 β_2	Activated adrenoreceptors on liver, skeletal muscle, adipose tissue result in increased blood glucose, free fatty acids, and lactic acid Inhibited insulin secretion Glucagon release
Skin	α	Erector pili muscle contraction results in piloerection

Dopamine receptors DA_1 and DA_2 are located on coronary, renal, and splanchnic arterioles. Stimulation of these receptors by dopamine results in vasodilation of these vessels.

16. How are the effects of sympathomimetic agents mediated?

Sympathomimetic agents mediate their effects by direct, indirect, or mixed direct and indirect mechanisms. Direct mechanisms are mediated by binding and stimulation of adrenergic receptors. Indirect mechanisms are associated with a release of endogenous catecholamines. Agents that mediate their effects by mixed or indirect mechanisms tend to lose efficacy with repeated dosages or when catecholamine stores are depleted.

17. What are the effects on the autonomic nervous system of drugs commonly used during anesthesia?

Effects of Drugs Commonly Used During Anesthesia on the Autonomic Nervous System

AGENT	MECHANISM OR RECEPTOR SITE OF ACTION	USES IN ANESTHESIA	EFFECTS ON THE AUTONOMIC NERVOUS SYSTEM (ANS)
Anticholinergics Atropine Glycopyrrolate	Muscarinic receptors	Inhibit vagal- induced bradycardia Decrease salivation Decrease gastric acid secretion	Arrhythmias: Sinus tachycardia Second-degree atrioventricular block Ventricular premature contraction Ventricular bigeminy Mydriasis Decreased intestinal motility Bronchodilation Decreased urinary bladder and urethral tone

Continued on next page

Effects of Drugs Commonly Used During Anesthesia on the Autonomic Nervous System (continued)

AGENT	MECHANISM OR RECEPTOR SITE OF ACTION	USES IN ANESTHESIA	EFFECTS ON THE AUTONOMIC NERVOUS SYSTEM (ANS)
Dissociative agents Ketamine Tiletamine	Interruption of ascending transmission from unconscious to conscious parts of the brain via depression of the thalamocortical region	Induction or maintenance of short anesthesia in dogs and cats Analgesia (relatively poor visceral analgesia with some unique analgesic effects through NMDA-receptor antagonism) Superficial sleep	Increased cerebral blood flow and intracranial pressure Decreased cardiovascular function but increased sympathetic tone results in overall stimulation of cardiovascular function: Increased cardiac output Tachycardia Increased arterial blood pressure Myocardial sensitization to catecholamine-induced arrhythmias Profuse salivation (ketamine)
Benzodiazepines Midazolam Diazepam	Enhanced effect of the inhibitory neurotransmitter, gamma-amino butyric acid (GABA) by binding to benzodiazepine portion of the GABA receptor activates chloride channels resulting in neuronal hyperpolarization	Tranquilization Muscle relaxation Anticonvulsant	Minimal cardiovascular effects Decreased cerebral blood flow
α_2 agonists Medetomidine Xylazine	α_2 receptors in the dorsal horn of the spinal cord inhibit release of nociceptive neurotransmitters (substance P, calcitonin gene-related peptide) α_2 receptors in the locus ceruleus mediate sedation Stimulation of presynaptic α_2 receptors in the ANS indirectly result in decreased norepinephrine release both centrally and peripherally	Analgesia Sedation Muscle relaxation	Arrhythmias: Bradycardia (responsive to atropine) First- and second-degree atrioventricular block Sinus arrest Atrioventricular dissociation Decreased cardiac output Variable effects on peripheral vascular resistance Decreased gastrointestinal motility and secretion
Phenothiazines Acepromazine	Affects the basal ganglia, hypothalamus, limbic system, reticular activating system Blocks dopamine (5-HT) receptors and dopaminergic actions	Tranquilization Premedication Sedative Antiemetic Antihistamine	Decreased vasomotor reflexes (blocks α_1-mediated vasoconstriction) and stimulation of β_2 receptors by circulating endogenous epinephrine: Hypotension Hypothermia Reflex sinus tachycardia Antiarrhythmic (local blockade of α_1 effects on myocardium) Cardiac contractility usually normal, may be mildly decreased Decreased gastrointestinal motility

Continued on next page

Effects of Drugs Commonly Used During Anesthesia on the Autonomic Nervous System (continued)

AGENT	MECHANISM OR RECEPTOR SITE OF ACTION	USES IN ANESTHESIA	EFFECTS ON THE AUTONOMIC NERVOUS SYSTEM (ANS)

Opioids
  Morphine
  Oxymorphone
  Fentanyl
  Meperidine
  Hydromorphone
  Buprenorphine
  Butorphanol
	Classified as angonists, antagonists, or mixed
	Four classes of opioid receptors $(\mu, \kappa, \Delta, \sigma)$
	The most important receptors for opioids used clinically are the μ and κ receptors
	μ (mu receptor)
	Two subtypes (μ_1, μ_2)
	Supraspinal and spinal analgesia, euphoria
	Sedation
	κ (kappa receptor)
	Three subtypes (κ_{1-3})
	Spinal analgesia
	Dysphoria
	Sedation
		Analgesia
		Sedation
			Cardiovascular depression:
			  Atropine-sensitive bradycardia
			  Hypotension induced by histamine release after rapid intravenous administration (morphine, meperidine)
			  Tachycardia (meperidine)
			  Transient decrease in cardiac output, mean arterial pressure, systemic vascular resistence (oxymorphone)
			Salivation (fentanyl, morphine)
			Delayed gastric emptying
			Decreased small intestinal propulsion
			Urinary retention
			Diarrhea or constipation
			Miosis in dogs, mydriasis in cats

Barbiturates
  Thiopental
  Pentobarbital
	Prevent passage of impulse to the cerebral cortex
	Bind the GABA receptor and decrease the rate of dissociation of inhibitory neurotransmitters from the receptor
	Inhibit the effects of glutamate (excitatory neurotransmitter)
	Alters synaptic transmission by inhibition of sodium and calcium channels and potentiation of potassium channels
		Rapid parenteral induction or maintenance of anesthesia	Dose-dependent cardiovascular depression:
			  Transient hypotension
			  Secondary transient tachycardia
			  Cardiac output decreased
			Arrhythmias:
			  Ventricular premature contraction
			  Ventricular extrasystole
			  Ventricular bigeminy
			Decreased cerebral blood flow and metabolic rate
			Anticonvulsant (pentobarbital)

Propofol		Hypnotic agent Parenteral induction or maintenance of anesthesia	Direct myocardial depression Peripheral vasodilation, venodilation Decreased arterial blood pressure and cardiac output (dose-dependent) Heart rate increased or unchanged

Gas inhalants
  Methoxyflurane
  Halothane
  Isoflurane
  Sevoflurane
	Not completely understood; various theories proposed	General anesthesia (loss of consciousness, muscle relaxation, analgesia)	Dose-dependent decrease in cardiac contractility, cardiac output, arterial blood pressure, stroke volume
			Peripheral vasodilation
			Myocardial sensitization to catecholamine-induced arrhythmias (especially halothane)

Continued on next page

Effects of Drugs Commonly Used During Anesthesia on the Autonomic Nervous System (continued)

AGENT	MECHANISM OR RECEPTOR SITE OF ACTION	USES IN ANESTHESIA	EFFECTS ON THE AUTONOMIC NERVOUS SYSTEM (ANS)
			Decreased renal blood flow Increased cerebral blood flow (dilation of cerebral vessels)
Sympathomimetic agents Dopamine Dobutamine Epinephrine	β_1 receptors— positive inotropy D_1 and D_2 receptors —vasodilation of renal and mesenteric vasculature α_1 receptors— vasoconstriction β_1 receptors- positive inotropy See table 2 at question 15	Inotropic support Maintain splanchnic (renal) blood flow Treat shock Hypotension Restore cardiac activity after cardiac arrest Treat bradycardia that is unresponsive to anticholinergics	Low doses of dopamine vasodilate renal, mesenteric, coronary, and cerebral vessels High doses of dopamine stimulate α and β receptors Rapidly metabolized, adverse effects are short-lived High doses of epinephrine stimulate α receptors See table at question 15. Typically, adverse effects manifest as fear, anxiety, cardiac arrhythmias, and cerebral hemorrhage
Ephedrine (non-catecholamine adrenergic agonist)	Indirect and direct-acting adrenergic effects Most effects due to release of norepinephrine from the adrenergic nerve terminal	Increase blood pressure Positive inotrope	Hypertension Cardiac arrhythmias

BIBLIOGRAPHY

1. Siegel GJ, Agranoff BW, Albers RW, et al (eds): Basic Neurochemistry. Molecular , Cellular, and Medical Aspects, 6th ed. Philadelphia, Lippincott-Raven Publishers, 1999.
2. Boothe DM (ed): Small Animal Clinical Pharmacology and Therapeutics. Philadelphia, W.B. Saunders, 2001.
3. Mathews CK, van Holde KE: Information processing and expression in multicellular organisms. In Mathews CK, van Holde KE (eds): Biochemistry. Redwood City, CA, The Benjamin/Cummings Publishing Co, Inc., 1990, pp 1046–1047.
4. Weiner N, Taylor P: Drugs acting at synaptic and neuroeffector junctional sites. In Gilman AG, Goodman LS, Rall TW, Murad F (eds): The Pharmacologic Basis of Therapeutics. New York, Macmillan Publishing Co, 1980, pp 66–180.
5. Aherns FA: Pharmacology. Baltimore, Williams & Wilkins, 1996.

II. Patient Preparation

7. PREANESTHETIC EVALUATION

Leigh A. Lamont, D.V.M.

1. What is the purpose of preanesthetic patient evaluation?

The purpose of the preanesthetic evaluation is to determine the patient's physical status. The anesthetist can then use this information to make a variety of decisions regarding anesthetic management of the case, including the choice, dose, and route of administration of anesthetic drugs, indications for specific types of intraoperative and postoperative monitoring, and the development of a pain management strategy. A thorough preanesthetic evaluation may facilitate anticipation of unexpected events and prevent an emergency situation. Remember the old adage, "For every mistake that is made for not knowing, a hundred are made for not looking."

2. What factors determine a patient's physical status?

Determination of physical status always begins with assessment of the patient's signalment, a thorough history and a complete physical examination. Based on this information, suitable laboratory tests can be chosen to further evaluate the patient. Remember, extensive laboratory testing is not a substitute for a thorough physical examination. The need for further work-up, such as radiography, ultrasonography, and electrocardiography, may be indicated by abnormalities noted in the initial evaluation and, in most cases, these procedures should be completed prior to contemplating anesthesia.

3. What factors must be considered when assessing a patient's signalment and history?
• Signalment: species, age, breed, sex
• Body weight
• Presenting complaint, duration and severity
• Symptoms of organ system disease: diarrhea, vomiting, polyuria/polydypsia, seizures, behavior change, exercise intolerance, coughing, dyspnea, weight loss, poor body condition
• Concurrent medications: organophosphates, H_2-blockers, antibiotics (e.g., aminoglycosides), cardiac glycosides, phenobarbital, nonsteroidal anti-inflammatories, calcium channel blockers, β-blockers, catecholamine-depleting drugs
• Previous anesthesia
• Allergies
• Recent feeding

4. What factors must be considered when performing a physical examination?
• General body condition: obesity, cachexia, pregnancy, hydration, temperature, attitude, temperament
• Cardiovascular: heart rate and rhythm, auscultation (murmurs), arterial blood pressure, pressure quality and regularity, capillary refill time
• Pulmonary: respiratory rate, depth and effort, mucous membrane color, auscultation (wheezes, crackles), upper airway obstruction, percussion
• Nervous system, special senses: seizure, coma, or stupor, syncope, vision, hearing
• Gastrointestinal: diarrhea, vomiting, abdominal distension, auscultation (gut sounds), rectal palpation if indicated
• Hepatic: icterus, bleeding abnormalities, altered mentation

- Renal: kidney palpation, urinary bladder palpation, oliguria/anuria, polyuria/polydypsia
- Integument: neoplasia, trauma, parasite infestation, hair loss
- Musculoskeletal: weakness, lameness, ataxia, fractures, muscle mass

5. Which laboratory tests must be run as part of a preanesthetic evaluation?

This depends on the patient's signalment and presenting complaint, the physical examination findings, and the planned surgical procedure. Minimum evaluation should include a packed cell volume and total plasma protein concentration, even in young healthy animals. Additional laboratory tests are often indicated, including complete hematologic evaluation, serum chemistry evaluation, urinalysis, blood gas assessment, and coagulation profiles. For normal values for routine laboratory tests in domestic animals, the reader is referred to the publications cited at the end of the chapter.

6. What is the ASA classification of patient physical status?

This refers to the American Society of Anesthesiologists (ASA) system of classification. Based on the integration of information obtained from signalment, history, and physical examination findings, patients can be placed into one of five potential categories. Classification of overall health is an essential part of any anesthetic record system and should be done for every patient undergoing anesthesia.

7. Describe the categories in the ASA classification system:

Category	Physical Status	Examples
I	Normal, healthy patient	Routine ovariohysterectomy, prophylactic dental cleaning
II	Patient with mild systemic disease	Cruciate rupture repair, equine arthroscopy
III	Patient with severe systemic disease	Femur fracture repair with myocardial contusions, feline urethral obstruction
IV	Patient with severe systemic disease that is a constant threat to life	Equine large bowel torsion, hemorrhaging splenic hemangiosarcoma
V	Moribund patient not expected to survive 24 hours with or without surgery	Any of the above in extreme shock, with massive tissue damage, severe metabolic derangement, etc.

8. What is meant by operative risk?

Operative risk refers to the uncertainty and potential for an adverse outcome associated with anesthesia and surgery in any patient, whether classified as an ASA I or ASA IV level patient. It should be noted that physical status, anesthetic risk, and operative risk are not synonymous.

9. How does all of this information affect how I perform anesthesia?

After determining the patient's physical status and the operative risk, and communicating these to the animal's owner, you can formulate an anesthetic plan. Additional considerations for the anesthetic plan include the type and duration of surgical procedure, body positioning, drug selection (to provide anesthesia and analgesia), airway management, fluid management, body temperature management, intraoperative monitoring, anticipation of potential complications, and availability of emergency drugs and equipment.

REFERENCES

1. Muir WW, Hubbell JAE, Skarda RT, Bednarski RM: Patient evaluation and preparation. In Handbook of Veterinary Anesthesia, 3rd ed. St. Louis, Mosby, 2000, pp 8–18.
2. Thurmon JC, Tranquilli WJ, Benson GJ: General considerations for anesthesia. In Essentials of Small Animal Anesthesia and Analgesia. Philadelphia, Lippincott Williams & Wilkins, 1999, pp 1–9.

8. PREMEDICATION

Doris H. Dyson, D.V.M., D.V.Sc., D.A.C.V.A.

1. How is the dose of premedication chosen when the quoted range is often so large?

Doses should be selected according to the patient's individual needs and the desired effect. Select a higher dose if the desired effect is greater (more pain expected). Reduced doses are usually chosen for sick or depressed animals (reduce sedative drug doses or eliminate, but rarely reduce analgesic drug dose unless used for sedation).

Combinations have additive or even synergistic effects; therefore, a lower dose of a drug is chosen when it is used in a combination (sedative drug dose is reduced rather than analgesic drug dose, since the sedative is considered to have more adverse effects).

Smaller animals have a higher dose requirement than larger animals (e.g., cats and little dogs compared with German Shepherd size) based on metabolic scaling.

Personal preference is often involved in decisions. Doses are selected based on what the anesthetist is prepared to deal with. A lower dose of acepromazine (or none) is combined with an opioid in geriatric patients when the advantages are not worth the potential hypotension. Another anesthetist may feel that the added sedation of a higher dose is worthwhile in certain cases, since he or she is prepared to monitor for and treat hypotension if it occurs.

2. How do you select between the profound (full agonist) opioids that are available for premedication in advance of a surgery associated with significant pain?

Selection of morphine, hydromorphone, or oxymorphone is based primarily on availability and personal preference. All three provide long-duration, profound analgesia, and their use is associated with a similar degree of respiratory depression (under general anesthesia), bradycardia (vagal induced), and panting.

Sometimes morphine or hydromorphone are rejected because of the higher incidence of vomiting associated with them. Sometimes they may be selected over oxymorphone because of cost benefit.

Full-agonist opioid use in large animals is primarily morphine for postoperative analgesia following more painful orthopedic procedures.

3. When would the vomiting associated with opioids be a contraindication to their use?

This adverse effect could be a concern in animals with stomach or esophageal obstruction, and in those at greater risk for aspiration. Morphine and hydromorphone show a higher incidence of vomiting than oxymorphone in dogs. Other less profound (partial agonist or mixed agonist/antagonist) opioids (butorphanol, buprenorphine, meperidine) rarely cause vomiting.

Intravenous administration of hydromorphone in depressed dogs (most gastric torsion cases) as part of an induction regimen appears to produce sedative effects before the vomiting center effect can occur. I have not seen any vomiting in these cases.

If vomiting occurs repeatedly with prolonged administration of opioids for analgesia (pre- or postoperatively), a different opioid should be selected, if possible, for the comfort of the animal.

4. When would you choose midazolam or diazepam as part of the premedication?

Benzodiazepines produce no adverse cardiovascular or respiratory effects and thus are preferred to acepromazine or α_2 agonists in sick, depressed, or geriatric animals and small ruminants. In such cases involving small animals, opioids alone produce enough sedation that a benzodiazepine is chosen only when extra restraint is required or if ketamine is selected.

Midazolam is preferred over diazepam if an intramuscular or subcutaneous route is chosen (water solubility allows use in mixtures and allows better absorption).

Small ruminants are very susceptible to pulmonary edema from xylazine administration (secondary to pulmonary inflammatory macrophage reaction); therefore, intravenous diazepam is the preferred premedication.

Diazepam is used in horses, but because of the concern for ataxia it is limited to premedication of excitable foals. In adult horses, it is included with induction rather than premedication.

5. What premedication is suitable when a fentanyl patch has been in place preoperatively?

Fentanyl is a μ agonist and should not be combined with an agonist-antagonist opioid (butorphanol) capable of reducing the sedative and analgesic effects. Other sedatives and opioids are suitable. The effect from a fentanyl patch is usually mild to moderate and not sufficient for significant surgical pain. Premedication for very painful procedures can include one of the profound opioids (no or minimal reduction of dose). If mild or no pain is involved, premedication can be a sedative or meperidine (alone or combined).

If a patch is placed preoperatively for the postoperative analgesic effects, use of butorphanol would not be contraindicated as a premedication due to its relatively short effect, but there is no rationale behind such a selection.

6. If an animal is premedicated with butorphanol, does this mean that epidural morphine will be ineffective?

No. Epidural morphine takes 60 minutes for effect and although low morphine doses are used, the drug is placed directly at the site of action (spinal receptors). This will likely outweigh any butorphanol effects from systemic administration (especially considering butorphanol was given much earlier than epidural effect is expected to occur).

7. Does the use of ketamine in the premedication of cats result in any analgesic effects?

Possibly. Ketamine has been effective for analgesia in burn patients, although good analgesic doses and their expected duration are not established in small animals. Ketamine is a good somatic analgesic and may provide effective analgesia for abscess lancing, laceration repair, and possibly postoperative castration pain. Degree of pain and doses used, along with duration achieved, require assessment of patients postoperatively to guarantee that the expected effect occurred.

Anesthetic demands may be higher during the castration procedure in cats (visceral stimulus) if other analgesics are not given as part of the premedication.

Visceral analgesia is ineffective for peri- and postoperative pain from ovariohysterectomy. Orthopedic procedures would also require use of more profound opioids, and/or nonsteroidal anti-inflammatory drugs.

8. If pain is not expected during a procedure and propofol is chosen as an induction agent, is there any reason to premedicate the animal?

Yes. The main advantage of premedication is reduction in the dose of induction and maintenance drugs with expected reduction in negative effects. Although smooth induction and recovery occur with propofol, it produces vasodilation and cardiac output depression that could be reduced by the lower doses needed in the premedicated animal.

Premedication will also reduce the cost of anesthesia considering the expense of propofol. This savings is not significant, however, unless opening a second vial of propofol can be avoided. The remaining propofol should not be kept beyond the day it is opened and therefore may end up being discarded anyway.

9. Is there a role for meperidine as a premedicant?

Yes and no. It can be useful but is not a necessity. Meperidine can be used for a short duration opioid effect, with lesser adverse effects. It may be selected for cerebrospinal fluid taps, as an antitussive (alternative to butorphanol), and for short procedures with mild associated pain, given alone in older animals, or given with acepromazine in healthy small animals.

Butorphanol can also be selected for such procedures, although its MAC reduction effect has not been as clearly noted as shown with μ agonists (such as meperidine).

10. Do premade mixtures for premedication (e.g., butorphanol/acepromazine/anticholinergic combinations) provide the analgesia required in all cases?

No. You need to assess the dose (mg/kg) of the opioid in the mixture to determine whether it would be suitable for that procedure. Often the dose is very low and suitable only for mild pain. Butorphanol in these mixtures may be effective in a healthy animal undergoing ovariohysterectomy if a fast, uncomplicated surgery is done.

All animals must be considered with respect to their individual needs for analgesia. They then must be monitored postoperatively to determine whether expectations were correct.

Typical mixtures contain approximately 0.3 mg/kg butorphanol for cats and 0.1–0.15 mg/kg butorphanol for dogs. The analgesic dose recommendation when using butorphanol for ovariohysterectomy in the cat is 0.2–0.4 mg/kg and in the dog is 0.2 mg/kg. Clearly, this dose will not achieve good analgesia in all circumstances.

You should make yourself familiar with the mixture used by doing a few calculations. Variations can exist. Do not assume its effectiveness, even in elective cases. The meperidine mixture found in some clinics is suitable only for mild postoperative pain (e.g., after castration).

11. Are premade mixtures for premedication (e.g., butorphanol/acepromazine/anticholinergic combinations) suitable for surgeries other than elective cases?

Yes and no. All the drugs included and their doses must be determined to be safe and appropriate for the case. The premade mixtures usually have a dose of acepromazine that is appropriate for healthy animals (0.04–0.05 mg/kg for dogs and 0.1–0.15 mg/kg for cats). This should be taken into consideration as well as the drug and dose included for analgesia (see question 10). It may also be better to avoid an anticholinergic in some patients (e.g., cardiac compromised patients), unless there is a clear need for it.

12. Is an anticholinergic required if an opioid is part of the premedication?

No, although inclusion for healthy animals is common, safe, and reasonable. Some clinicians choose to make their premedication mixture without an anticholinergic. Often, if separate drugs are mixed at the time of premedication, the anticholinergic is not included. Smaller volumes for premedication are possible. An anticholinergic can always be given intravenously at the time bradycardia is noted. The antisialogogue effect is rarely required.

13. Should bradycardia following opioid analgesic administration be treated?

Yes, if the level of bradycardia is significant (with respect to patient size) and the animal is under general anesthesia. Evidence exists to indicate improved cardiac output and thus better perfusion when vagal-induced bradycardia (as a result of opioid administration) is treated during inhalant anesthesia. Otherwise, the depressive inhalant effects may add to the negative effect of low heart rate. Evidence exists from unpublished data that cardiac output benefit does not exist if significant hypovolemia is present.

A heart rate of 80–120 bpm in cats and 60–80 bpm in dogs (related to patient size) is worth treating. Bradycardia is considered to be less detrimental in the awake animal following opioid administration.

14. Should bradycardia following α_2 administration be treated?

Controversy exists, but evidence points to a detrimental effect of anticholinergic medication in sedated animals (increased myocardial work). In the anesthetized animal under isoflurane (with associated vasodilation effects), treatment with an anticholinergic is advised to improve cardiac output.

15. If an animal was premedicated with an analgesic, how do you judge when to give more or how much more to give at the end of the surgery?

A very rough guideline can calculate dose on board:

[dose given / duration expected × time from injection]

Add further drug to achieve the desired dose. For example, after 2 hours, a dose of oxymorphone of 0.05 mg/kg may have the effect of 0.025 mg/kg (4-hour expected duration). Therefore, if a full dose is desired for recovery, another 0.025 mg/kg can be given as the anesthetic is about to be turned off.

You must carefully consider what dose is required for the pain involved when you supplement an analgesic dose, to avoid long recoveries or dysphoria (overestimated dose) or pain awareness at recovery (fear of giving more drug or underestimated dose).

16. What is the advantage of providing analgesia in the premedication of an animal going for surgery (when no pain exists before the surgery)?

Preemptive analgesia reduces "wind-up" of pain receptors during a surgery and therefore reduces the amount of drug required to control pain. This is a well-accepted theory that may be difficult to prove in clinical studies because of the inherent limitations associated with measuring pain in animals. Most anesthesiologists in veterinary and human medicine believe it to be very significant and worth considering.

Other advantages include good sedation and calming in animals given combinations. When sedatives are contraindicated or not worth the risk, an analgesic may produce sedation. MAC reduction is expected with most opioids (possibly less consistent with butorphanol).

17. Why are α_2-agonists used so commonly in large animals? Why are they considered a risk in small animals by some anesthesiologists?

Species variations exist. More alternatives exist for small animals.

α_2-Agonists work well as premedication in horses. The cardiovascular depressant effects are recognized and lower doses are used in compromised patients by adding guaifenesin. Good alternatives are not available.

α_2-Agonists show significant respiratory risk that is not dose-dependent in sheep and goats (due to pulmonary macrophage reaction), whereas cattle appear to be more resistant. Thus, other drugs like diazepam or pentobarbital may be chosen in sheep and goats over α_2-agonists. Doses must be watched in bovine, but xylazine works well in healthy cattle. Alternatives are usually used in sick animals.

Morbidity and mortality studies have singled out xylazine as a risk when used for premedication in dogs (less evidence against xylazine/ketamine combinations in cats). New α_2-agonists may appear to be slightly better but retain many of the negative effects. Recognizing complications can be difficult, and noninvasive monitoring may not work as well, due to venous desaturation and vasoconstriction.

Alternative agents exist for small animals to provide sedation, analgesia, and restraint. Because of the multiple negative effects with α_2-agonists (bradycardia, vasoconstriction, reduced cardiac output, perfusion concerns), and lack of consensus on how to deal with such, it may be simpler to select the alternatives. If we ignore such negative effects (sometimes recommended when using α_2-agonists), we would not be treating patients ideally when using other drugs (e.g., bradycardia is best treated when opioids are used during general anesthesia to maintain good cardiac output).

Use of α_2-agonists compared with other premedicants is as different in small animals as the use of methoxyflurane is compared with isoflurane. The question is: "Do we need it?" If we choose to use these agents, we need to understand the significant differences that exist and appreciate the potential risks in certain patients. For some anesthesiologists, it is not worth it.

18. If an animal is difficult to restrain, when is it safe to just administer the premedication intrapatient (without withdrawing on the syringe, thus risking possible intravenous injection)?

Meperidine and morphine are associated with histamine release after rapid intravenous injection. Most other drugs are safe intravenously, although a difference in time to effect or overall effect may be noted. In large animals, often the recommended dose is for intravenous administration.

19. Pain may be associated with administration of premedication. Is there anything that can be done to reduce this concern?

Subcutaneous administration in small animals may be the only practical answer. Local anesthetic creams can be helpful in advance but require time for effect. Fast injections may be preferred in large animals.

Time to effect may be longer and overall effect may be less with subcutaneous injections in vicious animals (area of poorer perfusion). Duration may be longer. Ketamine combinations are not recommended by this route.

Fast injections in large animals are more likely to reduce the discomfort of the handler than that of the animal.

20. When will an animal be sufficiently sedated following premedication administration to allow induction to proceed smoothly?

This depends on the drug, route of administration, and patient disposition. Following intramuscular premedication, 15 minutes is recommended as a minimum, although 30 minutes is often required for full effect (e.g., with vicious animals). Ketamine works in 5 minutes.

Following intravenous premedication, the effects are often observed in 5 minutes, although at least 15 minutes should be allowed if the animal is difficult to handle or maximum pain relief or effect is important to allow handling. Propofol or diazepam/ketamine may be given intravenously in low doses to achieve or add to premedication effect in small animals, and their effect occurs in 15–30 seconds (but is also very short in duration).

Subcutaneous injections require at least 30 minutes for effect.

α_2-Agonists rarely produce as good an effect if animals are disturbed in the initial 15–20 minutes after administration. Caution must still be used, since some profoundly sedated dogs are able to show aggression when stimulated.

21. Is there a safe way to deal with preoxygenation, or the restraint required for induction, in the patient that is insufficiently sedated with the premedication chosen?

Usually. If a catheter is in place, intravenous administration of propofol or diazepam/ketamine in low doses (up to 25% of induction dose) provides more restraint without detrimental effects on respiration allowing preoxygenation or movement of the aggressive or in-pain small animal.

More opioid can be given to achieve a better effect if a μ-agonist was selected. Morphine or hydromorphone work best. Unpublished data indicate the cardiovascular safety of hydromorphone.

Guaifenesin can be administered intravenously while walking the agitated horse until movement behind the swing gate or stopping proves safe. Caution must be used to judge the amount given, avoiding excessive ataxia from the guaifenesin.

22. Are opioids recommended or contraindicated as premedication before endoscopy?

Butorphanol has been tested and shown to cause no increased difficulty to the passage of an endoscope into the duodenum. Sphincter tone may be increased with other opioids (e.g., morphine).

23. If respiratory depression is expected with the use of opioids, is this a concern in animals admitted for neurologic problems?

Not usually. If a neurologic problem involves increased intracranial pressure, then positive pressure ventilation is required if anesthesia is used, regardless of premedication selected.

If an opioid is chosen for premedication, it should be selected and dosed based on the analgesia requirements. Increased cerebrospinal fluid pressure can also occur if pain exists. A trauma case that involves head injury and possible increased intracranial pressure will also need analgesia.

24. Would you select acepromazine as a premedication based on its antiarrhythmic effects?

No. It may be beneficial when anesthetic complications arise in healthy animals (as in equipment problems with associated hypoxia), by resulting in a lessened chance of fibrillation.

The vasodilation and hypotension from acepromazine are usually considered more detrimental than the antiarrhythmic benefit in most animals that have pre-existing arrhythmias.

25. Is there any benefit to the addition of acepromazine to an analgesic given as premedication in a patient in pain?

Yes, if the detrimental effects from acepromazine are acceptable. Sedation and central nervous system depression can intensify the effect from an analgesic. Neurolept-analgesic combinations appear to produce synergistic effects. Acepromazine administration is a common method to improve analgesia in animals showing mild pain postoperatively in spite of reasonable opioid use.

Quieter animals are less likely to resist restraint and therefore are less likely to create pain from such resistance.

Inhalant MAC is reduced by many sedatives as well as analgesics and this can have a beneficial effect through reduction of dose-dependent inhalant depressant effects.

REFERENCES

1. Celly CS, McDonell WN, Young SS, et al: The comparative hypoxaemic effect of four alpha-2 agonists (xylazine, romifidine, detomidine, medetomidine) in sheep. J Vet Pharmacol Therap 20:464–471, 1997.
2. Graham LF, Merkel LK, Hendrix PK: Comparison of three premedication techniques on passage of an endoscope through the pyloric sphincter in dogs. Proceedings of the Annual Meeting of the American College of Veterinary Anesthesiology, Dallas, 1999, p. 13.
3. Hall LW, Clarke KW, Trim CM: Veterinary Anaesthesia, 10th ed. London, W.B. Saunders, 2001.
4. Jones DJ, Stehling LC, Zauder H: Cardiovascular responses to diazepam and midazolam maleate in the dog. Anesthesiology 51:430–434, 1979.
5. Mathews KA (ed): Management of Pain. Vet Clin North Am 30:4, 2000.
6. Mitchell RW, Smith G: The control of acute postoperative pain. Br J Anaesth 63:147–158, 1989.
7. Pettifer G, Dyson D: Hydromorphone: A cost-effective alternative to the use of oxymorphone. Can Vet J 41:135–137, 2000.
8. Torske KE, Dyson DH, Conlon PD: Cardiovascular effects of epidurally administered oxymorphone and an oxymorphone bupivacaine combination in halothane-anesthetized dogs. Am J Vet Res 60:194–200, 1999.

9. ANESTHETIC MACHINES

Tom Doherty M.V.B., M.Sc., D.A.C.V.A.

1. What size of oxygen cylinder is most commonly used on small animal anesthetic machines?
E cylinders are in general use.

2. Before attaching a cylinder to an anesthetic machine, it is recommended that the valve be opened, *briefly*, to vent gas. Why?
Dust, grease or metal filings on the port could cause a flash fire, or explosion, if the cylinder is opened while it is attached to the machine. Venting gas will remove foreign material from the port. Also, venting will prevent these contaminants from being blown into the machine.

3. Once the cylinder is attached to the hanger yoke, it is recommended that the cylinder valve be opened *slowly*. Why?
A build up of heat, between the valve and yoke, may occur if the valve is opened rapidly. The heat results from the rapid recompression of the gas in the confined space (adiabatic compression). This may cause ignition of dust particles or grease, causing a fire or explosion. For this reason, the valve should be opened slowly, allowing time for the heat to dissipate.

4. You have just attached an oxygen cylinder to the hanger yoke and upon opening the cylinder valve, there is a loud hissing noise. What is the most probable source of this noise?
Most probably, the gasket (washer), which fits between the cylinder port and the yoke, is missing or damaged.

5. A pressure gauge may give the pressure reading as psi or psig. What do these letters stand for?
Psi is pounds per square inch. Psig refers to pounds per square inch gauge. This represents the difference between the measured pressure and the atmospheric pressure. Most gauges are calibrated at zero atmospheric pressure.

6. Is it possible to estimate the volume of gas in an oxygen cylinder?
Yes. For E cylinders, cylinder pressure (psig) $\times$ 0.3 gives a close estimate of the liters of oxygen in the cylinder; e.g., 1000 psig $\times$ 0.3 = 300 L of O_2 in cylinder. For the larger H cylinders, multiplying the psig $\times$ 3 estimates the volume in liters.

7. Is it possible to estimate the volume of nitrous oxide remaining in the cylinder by reading the cylinder pressure gauge?
No. Unlike oxygen, which is stored in cylinders entirely in the gaseous form, nitrous oxide is stored partially in liquid form. So for N_2O, the pressure gauge will show a constant pressure until all the liquid has evaporated (assuming a constant temperature); then the pressure will decrease directly as the gas is removed. It is best to replace a N_2O cylinder if the gauge reads < 600 psig.

8. The high-pressure system of the anesthetic machine includes which components?
The hanger yoke, cylinder pressure indicator, and cylinder pressure-reducing device.

9. Since the pressure in the oxygen cylinder decreases as the gas is removed, how is a constant oxygen flow maintained in the anesthetic machine?
The role of the pressure-reducing valve is to reduce pressure in the system to approximately 45 psig; in this way, a constant flow is maintained. To further refine the process, some machines

have a second-stage pressure-reducing valve that reduces the oxygen pressure from the cylinder pressure-reducing valve, or the pipeline, to 14 psig.

10. According to manufacturing standards, an oxygen flush valve must be able to deliver a flow within what range?
   35–75 L/min.

11. What is the danger associated with activating the oxygen flush valve when the patient is connected to the machine?
   The high oxygen flow could cause a dangerous increase in pressure in the breathing circuit, causing barotrauma to the patient's lungs. This is more likely to happen if the patient is small and the pop-off valve is closed. For this reason, the oxygen flush valve must be designed in a manner that protects it from accidental activation and must *not* be capable of being locked in the ON position.

12. What factors determine the rate of flow through a variable-orifice flowmeter?
- The physical properties of the gas (viscosity and density).
- The pressure drop across the constriction, which is constant for all positions in the tube and is equal to the mass of the float divided by the cross-sectional area.
- The area of the annular opening around the float.

13. Why do some types of floats rotate in the flow tube?
   A rotating float has flutes (grooves) in its upper rim. The passage of gas between the wall of the tube and the float impacts on the flutes and causes the float to rotate. As long as the tube is vertical, the rotating float remains in the center of the tube. Rotation of the float reduces the friction between the wall and float, resulting in a decrease in wear and measurement errors.

14. Where is an out-of-circuit vaporizer usually located on the anesthetic machine?
   The most common location is to the right of the flowmeter(s), between the flowmeter(s) and the common gas outlet. One reason to position the vaporizer at this location is to have a secure mounting. Unlike an in-circuit vaporizer, the out-of-circuit vaporizer is not part of the breathing system. It is *not* advisable to position the vaporizer between the common gas outlet and the breathing system. At this location, activation of the oxygen flush would deliver a high concentration of anesthetic to the breathing system.

15. Where is an in-circuit vaporizer located on the anesthetic machine?
   In-circuit means that the vaporizer is part of the breathing system, situated in the inspiratory limb. Because of their location in the breathing system, in-circuit vaporizers must be of low resistance. They are of simple construction, basically consisting of a glass jar and a wick. Rarely used nowadays, most were designed for use with methoxyflurane, an agent with a low vapor pressure. However, some machines (e.g., Stephens) were designed specifically for use with halothane in-circuit, and halothane has a much greater vapor pressure than methoxyflurane. In this case, to prevent inhalation of dangerous concentrations of halothane, the maximum output of halothane from the vaporizer is approximately 3%.

16. What is the function of a pressure-relief valve?
   A pressure-relief valve is present on some anesthetic machines. It is located near the common gas outlet. The valve is designed to prevent high pressure from being delivered to the patient from the machine, and to prevent high pressures from reaching the machine. At a preset pressure, the valve opens and vents to the atmosphere.

17. What is the function of a check valve?
   A check or unidirectional valve is present on some anesthetic machines. It is designed to limit the effects of increases in pressure in the breathing system on vaporizer output. Changes in

pressure can develop when ventilation is controlled or the oxygen flush is activated. The check valve is located between the vaporizer(s) and the common gas outlet.

BIBLIOGRAPHY

1. Bito H, Ikeuchi Y, Ikeda K: Effects of water content of soda lime on compound A concentration in the anesthesia circuit in sevoflurane anesthesia. Anesthesiology 8 (1):66-71, 1998.
2. Dorsch JA, Dorsch SE: The anesthesia machine. In Understanding Anesthetic Equipment, 4th ed. Baltimore, Williams & Wilkins, 1999, pp 75-120.
3. Dorsch JA, Dorsch SE: Medical gas cylinders and containers. In Understanding Anesthetic Equipment, 4th ed. Baltimore, Williams & Wilkins, 1999, pp 3-29.
4. Suter CM, Pascoe PJ, McDonell WN, Wilson B: Resistance and work of breathing in the anesthetized cat: Comparison of a circle breathing system and a coaxial breathing system. In Proceedings of the American College of Veterinary Anesthesiology Annual Meeting, New Orleans, October 1989.

10. ANESTHETIC CIRCUITS

Tom Doherty, M.V.B., M.Sc., D.A.C.V.A., and
Stephen A. Greene, D.V.M., M.S., D.A.C.V.A.

1. How are anesthetic circuits classified?

Anesthetic circuits have been classified in a number of ways. A simple approach first breaks down circuit types based on whether or not rebreathing of exhaled gases occurs; thus, a circuit either allows "rebreathing" or it is "non-rebreathing." Circle circuits are designed to be rebreathing circuits, but not all rebreathing circuits are circle circuits (e.g., coaxial Universal F circuit). Modern anesthesia circuits can also be referred to using nomenclature such as open, semi-open, closed, or semi-closed. Circle circuits are operated as either closed or semi-closed circuits, depending on the oxygen flow rate delivered. When using a circle circuit, an oxygen flow rate equal to the patient's metabolic oxygen consumption rate constitutes a closed circuit. Likewise, an oxygen flow rate greater than the patient's metabolic oxygen consumption rate constitutes a semi-closed circuit. Generally, for operation of a semi-closed circuit, the targeted oxygen flow rate is two to three times the patient's metabolic oxygen consumption rate. Most non-rebreathing circuits are operated as a semi-open circuit.

2. What is the metabolic oxygen consumption rate for dogs and cats?

10 ml/kg/min

3. What components of the circle breathing system contribute most to the resistance to flow?

Since the tubing used in the adult breathing systems has an internal diameter of 22 mm, the major portion of the resistance is not in the tubing but in components such as the one-way valves (inspiratory and expiratory), soda lime canister, and pop-off valves. It is important to remember that the endotracheal tube is a much more important factor than the breathing circuit in contributing to resistance.

4. Is the mechanical dead space in a circle breathing system excessive?

No. The dead space in circle systems extends from the patient port to the partition at the end of the breathing tubes (about 1.5 cm), not, as is sometimes thought, from the unidirectional valves to the patient port. So the length of the tubing does not contribute to dead space, if the valves are competent. In reality, the mechanical dead space in a circle system is the same as in a non-rebreathing system.

5. What are the disadvantages of using high fresh-gas flows (50–100 ml/kg/min) with a circle system?

In addition to the extra cost incurred with oxygen and anesthetic use, there is a loss of heat and moisture from the circuit. Some of the extra cost will be offset by a savings on absorbent. However, a major concern is pollution. Unless adequate scavenging is used, pollution of the surgical area is inevitable. Atmospheric pollution is especially important with N_2O, which has an extremely long half-life.

6. What are the disadvantages of using relatively low (10–20 ml/kg/min) fresh-gas flows with a circle system?

For users unfamiliar with low flows, the main problem is delivering enough anesthetic to the patient, especially in the period immediately following induction. This can be easily overcome by increasing the vaporizer setting. Many people get alarmed upon seeing a high vaporizer setting; but what may not always be understood is that at a low oxygen flow, the animal is inhaling a much lower concentration of anesthetic, especially in the first few minutes of the procedure. This discrepancy between vaporizer settings and inspired anesthetic concentrations becomes clear if you can monitor end-tidal anesthetic concentrations.

7. Is there a circle system available for smaller patients?
     A special pediatric circle system with a small CO_2 absorber was available at one time. Now, more commonly, short, small-diameter tubing is used with a small rebreathing bag. Recently, an anesthetic machine with a built-in respirator has been marketed for use with animals as small as 150 g. The internal diameter of the breathing tubes is 10 mm. The maximum tidal volume of the system is 100 ml.

8. Is it acceptable to use an adult-size circle system for a 5 kg (11 lb) cat?
     Yes. Research on the work of breathing of cats attached to a circle system indicates that it is acceptable to use a circle system with cats as small as 2.5 kg (5.5 lb).

9. How does one determine the size of rebreathing bag to use?
     A bag volume of five times the patient's tidal volume (10–15 ml/kg) is generally suitable.

10. What is the function of the "pop-off valve"?
     The "pop-off valve" is a pressure relief valve with a connection to the waste gas scavenging apparatus. A closed pop-off valve will cause build-up of pressure within the anesthetic circuit and the patient's respiratory tract due to the constant delivery of fresh oxygen. This hazard may result in rupture of the lung or trachea. Cats that spontaneously develop subcutaneous emphysema in the region of the neck or thorax during or after inhalation anesthesia delivered by an endotracheal tube are sometimes the unfortunate victims of this situation. (Trauma to the trachea at the time of intubation may also cause subcutaneous emphysema.) The pop-off valve is left in the open position unless positive pressure ventilation is being administered.

11. Where are the most likely sources of leaks in the circle breathing system?
     Equipment leaks are generally present in the low-pressure components of the machine due to the presence of seals and joints.

- Around the soda lime canister, either because the housing needs to be tightened or because a piece of soda lime has become trapped between the gasket and the canister, causing a leak to occur.
- Around the valve caps.
- The rebreathing bag may have a hole or, more commonly, has become frayed around the neck.
- Most large animal machines have a draining port that must be closed when the machine is in use.

If a leak is occurring while an animal is attached to the machine, first check that the endotracheal tube is properly located and the cuff is adequately inflated.

12. How does one test a circle breathing system for leaks?
     1. Turn off the gas flow.
     2. Close the pop-off valve.
     3. Occlude the patient port.
     4. Fill the rebreathing bag, using the oxygen flush valve, pressurizing the system to 30 cm H_2O. The pressure should not decrease by more than 20 cm H_2O in 10 seconds.

According to the American Society for Testing and Materials, the leak should not exceed 300 ml/min, at a pressure of 30 cm H_2O.

13. What factors influence the inspired anesthetic concentration when using a circle system?

The inspired anesthetic concentration is influenced by many factors including:
- The volume of the system
- The fresh-gas flow
- The concentration of anesthetic in the fresh gas
- The uptake of anesthetic by the patient
- The uptake of anesthetic by elements of the system
- Elimination (e.g., N_2), and uptake (e.g., N_2O) of other gases by the patient

14. Name some toxic substances that may build up in the breathing circuit?

Methane, ethanol, acetone, carbon monoxide, metabolites of volatile anesthetics, compound A, argon, and nitrogen are some of the substances that may accumulate in the breathing circuit. This build-up is more likely to occur with low gas flows and prolonged anesthesia.

15. What are the major differences between rebreathing and non-rebreathing circuits?

Rebreathing circuits allow rebreathing of exhaled gases and non-rebreathing circuits do not. There is slightly more resistance to breathing through the rebreathing circuit because of the presence of valves and the soda-lime canister. This may cause increased work of breathing during anesthesia, especially in very small patients. Many anesthetists use the rule of thumb that patients weighing less than 7 kg are maintained on a non-rebreathing circuit to minimize the work of breathing. In practice, animals that weigh less than 7 kg may breathe quite normally on a rebreathing circuit, especially if the duration of anesthesia is brief.

16. What is the Mapleson system of classification for non-rebreathing anesthetic circuits?

The Mapleson classification system for non-rebreathing circuits was devised by Mapleson to describe systems that have no device for absorbing carbon dioxide. The circuits function as a "flow-controlled breathing system" or a "carbon dioxide washout circuit." The system originally described types A through E, and type F was added later. FGF = fresh gas flow.

Mapleson Systems

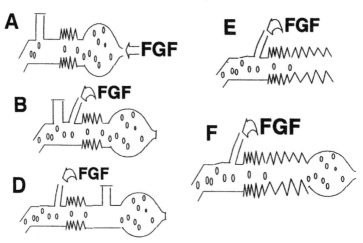

17. What is the composition of soda lime?

Soda lime is a mixture of sodium hydroxide (4%), potassium hydroxide (1%), and water (14–19%), and the remainder is calcium hydroxide. Sodium hydroxide is the more active substance.

18. What is added to soda lime to increase its hardness?
Silica and kieselguhr (diatomaceous earth) are added to increase hardness. Increasing hardness is important to decrease dust formation. Reducing dust formation is important, because dust may get into the breathing system and be inhaled by the patient. It may also cause caking, channeling, and resistance to flow.

19. What is the composition of Baralyme?
It is a mixture of barium hydroxide (20%) and calcium hydroxide (80%).

20. Is it necessary to add a hardening agent to Baralyme?
No. The water of crystallization provides adequate hardness.

21. Describe the reaction of carbon dioxide (CO_2) with soda lime.
Initially, carbon dioxide reacts with water on the surface of the granules to form carbonic acid:
$$CO_2 + H_2O \rightarrow H_2CO_3$$
Sodium and calcium ions combine with carbonate ions to form sodium and calcium carbonate:
$$2NaOH + 2H_2CO_3 + Ca(OH)_2 \rightarrow CaCO_3 + Na_2CO_3 + 4H_2O + Heat$$
Note that heat and water are generated during this process.

22. If soda lime turns purple with use, what indicator is being used?
Ethyl violet (this is the most commonly used indicator).

23. What percentage of the soda lime canister space is occupied by air?
Approximately 50% of the canister space is occupied by air. It is made up of the void space (40–47% of the container volume for soda lime and 45% for Bbaralyme) and the pore space. The latter (about 8%) is the space within the granules, and this decreases as absorption progresses.

24. Do carbon dioxide absorbents react with volatile anesthetics?
Yes. The absorbent degrades all the volatile anesthetics to some extent. The degradation product of sevoflurane, compound A, has received most attention, because of reports of its nephrotoxicity in rats. Its clinical significance is undetermined, however.

25. How can the concentration of compound A in a circuit be reduced?
• Use high gas flows.
• Use lower concentrations of sevoflurane.
• Use soda lime instead of baralyme.
• Decrease the absorbent temperature.
• Increase the moisture content in the absorbent. Spraying 100 ml of distilled water onto each 1 kg of soda lime has been shown to significantly decrease the concentration of compound A in the breathing circle. This effect is not related to a change in temperature of the absorbent.

26. How much carbon dioxide can 100 g of soda lime absorb?
Approximately 26 L of CO_2 are absorbed by 100 g of soda lime.

27. List the advantages of non-rebreathing systems such as a Bain.
• Simple, inexpensive, and most have no moving parts (some have an adjustable pressure-limiting valve).
• The inspired gases are warmed by the exhaled gases, a feature of coaxial tubing.
• Resistance is acceptable, at recommended flows.
• The tubing is lightweight, flexible, and does not distort the position of the head and endotracheal tube.
• It is easy to estimate the inspired anesthetic concentration. If the fresh-gas flow is ade-

quate, rebreathing is minimal, and the inspired anesthetic concentration is a close reflection of the vaporizer setting.

28. What are the disadvantages of the Bain system?
- Increases cost of anesthetic and oxygen.
- Absolute dependence on high fresh-gas flows for CO_2 removal.
- Increases the likelihood of pollution due to high gas flows.
- The system must remain intact to prevent rebreathing. Disconnection of, or holes in, the inner tube will lead to a significant increase in apparatus dead space.

29. How can you determine whether the inner tube of a Bain circuit is intact?
Set the flow meter at 2 L/min. Occlude the inner tube (using a finger or the plunger of a syringe). If the inner tube is intact, the flowmeter indicator will fall.

30. How is nitrous oxide used in a rebreathing or circle circuit?
When nitrous oxide is used, the gas flow must be added to the oxygen flow. Thus, to use 50% nitrous oxide and an oxygen flow rate of 1 L/min, the nitrous oxide flow rate would also be 1 L/min. Using less than the calculated oxygen flow rate may compromise oxygen delivery to the patient.

31. How is nitrous oxide used in a non-rebreathing circuit?
When nitrous oxide is used with a non-rebreathing circuit, the situation is different from that described in question 30. This is because the non-rebreathing circuit requires a high fresh-gas (oxygen) flow rate to ensure that exhaled carbon dioxide is removed from the circuit. It is reasonable to reduce the oxygen flow rate by an amount made up by the nitrous oxide flow rate in this case, to conserve gas and anesthetic utilization. Thus, to deliver 50% nitrous oxide, the calculated oxygen flow rate may be halved and an equivalent flow rate of nitrous oxide added to the fresh-gas mixture.

BIBLIOGRAPHY

1. Dorsch JA, Dorsch SE: Anesthesia machines and breathing systems. In Understanding Anesthetic Equipment, 4th ed. Baltimore, Williams & Wilkins, 1999, pp 75–269.
2. Hartsfield SM: Anesthetic machines and breathing systems. In Thurmon JC, Tranquilli WJ, Benson GJ, (eds) 3rd ed. Lumb and Jones' Veterinary Anesthesia, Baltimore, Williams & Wilkins, 1996, pp 366–408.

11. VAPORIZERS

Stephen A. Greene, D.V.M., M.S., D.A.C.V.A.

1. How are veterinary anesthetic vaporizers classified?

There are basically two types of anesthetic vaporizers: variable bypass and measured flow. Precision and nonprecision are also terms used to describe vaporizers. These terms really refer to the accuracy with which the anesthetist can control the vaporizer output.

Vaporizers are also classified by the method of vaporization: flow-over, bubble-through, or injection.

Finally, modern vaporizers are either thermocompensated or have a supplied heat source. Nearly all concentration-calibrated vaporizers use a thermal element to automatically provide thermocompensation. Some vaporizers (e.g., desflurane) use an electric heater to maintain constant temperature.

2. What is the difference between a variable bypass and a measured flow vaporizer?

Variable bypass vaporizers employ a control dial that adjusts the proportion of fresh-gas flow to be diverted through the vaporizing chamber. All modern, concentration-calibrated vaporizers are variable bypass designs. A measured flow vaporizer uses a separate flowmeter to accurately deliver the desired flow of concentrated anesthetic vapor directly from the vaporizer into a mixing stream with the fresh-gas flow.

All measured flow vaporizers would, by design, be precision vaporizers, since they accurately calculate the anesthetic concentration output. Variable bypass vaporizers may be either precision or nonprecision. The Ohio 8 vaporizer is an example of a variable bypass, nonprecision anesthetic vaporizer. Dräger 19.1 and "tecs" (e.g., Fluotec, Fortec) are variable bypass, precision vaporizers. The measured flow vaporizers include older machines such as the Verni-Trol and the Copper Kettle.

3. Describe the different methods of vaporization.

In a flow-over vaporizer, the fresh-gas stream flows over the surface of the liquid anesthetic. Wicks are often used to improve the efficiency of the gas-liquid interface for vaporization. In a bubble-through vaporizer, the fresh gas is bubbled into the liquid anesthetic much like an aerator for an aquarium. The smaller the bubbles, the greater the gas-liquid interface area. Some vaporizers control the vaporization by injecting liquid anesthetic into precise volumes of gas.

4. What are the advantages and disadvantages of a nonprecision vaporizer?

Nonprecision vaporizers are inexpensive and simple devices. However, the actual percentage of anesthetic agent output from the vaporizer is not known, so there is more guesswork in adjusting the vaporizer dial to deliver anesthetic.

Nonprecision vaporizers are usually located in the breathing circuit rather than outside of the breathing circuit. With this placement, the patient's breathing pattern will affect the vaporizer output. Increased ventilation rate or tidal volume during anesthesia will increase anesthetic delivery to the patient even though the control dial is not changed. (Positive pressure ventilation can dramatically and rapidly increase circuit anesthetic concentration and delivery, resulting in deepening of the anesthetic plane.) This type of vaporizer is inherently more prone to create anesthetic overdose when used by inexperienced anesthetists.

There is no mechanism to compensate for changes in vaporizer output that are associated with alterations in the fresh-gas flow. Decreases in fresh-gas flow are associated with less dilution of the circuit's anesthetic concentration and tend to increase delivery of anesthetic to the patient. Alternatively, an increase in the fresh-gas flow may result in decreased circuit concentration and thus anesthetic depth of the patient. The nonprecision vaporizer does not adjust its output when the ambient temperature changes. Thus, if left at the same dial setting, the vaporizer output will increase as the room temperature increases. Examples of the nonprecision vaporizer are Boyle-pattern, Ohio 8, Goldman, Stephens, and Komesarov.

5. What are the advantages and disadvantages of a precision vaporizer?

The precision vaporizer delivers an accurate output percentage of anesthetic in the fresh gas (usually oxygen). Modern precision vaporizers deliver a constant output over a wide range of fresh-gas flow rates (for most, within 0.5 to 10 L/min). In addition, vaporizer output will remain relatively constant even when the patient's breathing pattern changes, positive pressure ventilation is initiated, or the ambient temperature changes. For this ease of use and high degree of control, precision vaporizers are expensive devices because of their complexity. Precision vaporizers should be serviced regularly for optimal performance.

6. Which vaporizers can use multiple anesthetic agents?

Several vaporizers can use multiple anesthetic agents (one at a time). Such "universal" vaporizers include most of the measured flow type of vaporizers. These vaporizers come with a slide rule that includes settings for both the vaporizer and fresh-gas flow meters at various temperatures for several different anesthetic agents. The Verni-Trol and Copper Kettle are examples of universal agent vaporizers. The simple nonprecision vaporizers, such as the Ohio 8 or the Stephens vaporizer, can be filled with ether, methoxyflurane, halothane, isoflurane, enflurane, or sevoflurane.

7. Is any anesthetic agent preferable in a nonprecision vaporizer?

Ideally, the nonprecision vaporizer is used with an anesthetic that has poor vaporization and/or high blood:gas solubility (ether, methoxyflurane). Ether, with a relatively high vapor pressure compared with methoxyflurane, is safely used in this vaporizer because of its high blood:gas solubility (nearly equivalent to that of methoxyflurane) and its low potency. Methoxyflurane, although very potent, is relatively soluble and, because of its very low vapor pressure, poorly volatile. More highly volatile agents have been used in nonprecision vaporizers with modification of the delivery technique. For example, the wick from the Ohio 8 vaporizer is removed when halothane or isoflurane is used. Such highly volatile anesthetics with low blood:gas solubility can easily lead to anesthetic overdose in the hands of an anesthetist unfamiliar with use of this vaporizer.

8. Describe the Ohio 8 vaporizer.

The Ohio 8 is a ubiquitous vaporizer that for years was the only gas anesthetic delivery device in many veterinary practices. It is essentially an amber or clear glass jar with a corrugated paper wick and a control dial with markings from 0 to 10. The dial markings indicate a relative amount of the fresh-gas flow that is diverted into the vaporizing chamber above the liquid anesthetic. A dial setting of 5 would indicate that 50% of the fresh gas flow was diverted into the vaporizer. The dial settings do not indicate the percentage of anesthetic output.

9. What is a Copper Kettle?

The Copper Kettle is an older example of a universal, measured flow vaporizer. Copper has high thermal conductivity and is used in the construction of the vaporizer jacket to promote ambient heat transfer to the liquid anesthetic within the vaporizing chamber. Many other vaporizers have copper jackets, but their outer surfaces are coated with less corrosive metals that help retain heat in the jacket.

10. What are the hazards associated with soaking cotton balls with liquid anesthetic agents, such as isoflurane, to anesthetize small animals in a chamber?

The vaporization of the liquid anesthetic is unregulated and highly dependent on ambient temperature. High concentrations of anesthetic can be produced (e.g., 33% isoflurane) and overdosing can easily occur. There may also be tissue sensitivity to the direct contact with liquid anesthetic.

11. What is unique about the desflurane vaporizer?

The desflurane vaporizer is specifically designed for an agent with a high vapor pressure (664 mm Hg). Desflurane will boil at near room temperature. The vaporizer is always sealed off from the atmosphere and requires a special filling port for use with the uniquely designed desflurane bottle that utilizes a valve to maintain its seal. The vaporizer is electrically heated to maintain constant temperature during use and employs a back-up battery for alarm functions in case of power failure. A sensor will cease vaporization of desflurane if the vaporizer is tilted more than 10 degrees. The Ohmeda Tec 6 vaporizer is commercially available for use with desflurane. The Tec 6 output dial is marked from 0 to 18% and has a release that must be pressed to obtain output above 12%.

12. How is constant output maintained during temperature fluctuation (thermocompensation) with a precision vaporizer like the Tec or Vapor 19.1?

Thermocompensation for the concentration-calibrated vaporizers is accomplished by use of a bimetallic strip. The use of two metals with different expansion characterics over a range of clinically relevant temperatures provides a mechanical device that will bend. As the temperature changes, the movement of the bimetallic strip is linked to a needle valve in the vaporizing chamber orifice, effectively increasing or decreasing gas flow.

13. What is the difference between the Dräger Vapor 19 and Vapor 19.1 vaporizers?

The Dräger Vapor 19 has manual thermocompensation and the Vapor 19.1 has automatic thermocompensation. Use of the Vapor 19 requires observation of the temperature of the liquid anesthetic via a built-in thermometer. The temperature value is used with a scale printed on the vaporizer dial to adjust the desired output concentration to the measured temperature.

14. Why do some sevoflurane vaporizers have different maximum concentrations indicated on the output dial?

Sevoflurane has a minimal alveolar concentration that is higher than that of halothane or isoflurane (about 2.1% in the dog). Production of new sevoflurane vaporizers with maximum dial concentrations of 8% allows use of the overpressure technique to achieve rapid inductions. Vaporizers originally designed for use with other agents (e.g., enflurane) that are converted to sevoflurane vaporizers may have different maximum dial concentrations engraved, depending on the limitations of the vaporizer or the common practice of the refurbishing facility.

15. What will happen if sevoflurane is inadvertently used to refill an isoflurane vaporizer?

Because sevoflurane has a lower vapor pressure (about two-thirds of that for isoflurane), it will not volatilize as readily. At a vaporizer setting that would produce 2% isoflurane, less sevoflurane would be delivered, about 1.3%.

16. What is a "keyed refilling system"?

This term refers to the use of specifically designed fill ports and bottle fill tubes that match the fill tube with the fill port of the vaporizer. The "lock and key" concept requires that each volatile anesthetic fill tube have a unique size and shape to fit the fill port of the intended vaporizer.

17. What is the Aladin cassette vaporizer?

The Aladin 2222 cassette vaporizer is a precision, variable bypass, agent-specific vaporizer designed as a modular cassette that is easily inserted or removed from the Datex-Engstrom AS/3 anesthesia machine. The cassette feature allows quick exchange of vaporizers for use of a different anesthetic agent. The cassette vaporizer can be handled and stored in any position. A magnetic sensor identifies the specific anesthetic agent in use when inserted in the anesthetic machine. The vaporizer automatically compensates for changes in temperature, fresh-gas flow (0.2 to 10 L/min), or circuit back pressure using electronic flow control circuitry.

18. Why do some vaporizers become very cold when used with high oxygen flows?

The halogenated anesthetics effectively act as refrigerants when used in a fresh-gas flow stream. Higher flows require more vaporization of the anesthetic, drawing more heat from the vaporizer jacket and environment. The effect can be quite dramatic, and some models of vaporizers have been observed to "ice up" when used with fresh-gas flowrates of 8 L/min. Vaporizer output likely is less than expected when this happens. Adjustment of the fresh-gas flow to the lowest rate suitable for safe use will minimize the problem. Use of better materials in the construction of the vaporizer jacket helps to eliminate this occurrence.

19. What causes the halothane vaporizer dial to "stick"?

Halothane is manufactured with a preservative, thymol, that is less volatile than halothane. Thus, over time, the thymol tends to accumulate in the vaporizer. This is why the liquid in the vaporizer refill window turns brown or amber. Thymol is a sticky substance, and its build-up is responsible for the vaporizer dial sticking. The dial can be removed and cleaned with alcohol to remove some of the thymol. The vaporizer should be drained and refilled with fresh anesthetic.

20. What is the effect on anesthetic output when a vaporizer is used at high elevation?

The effects of barometric pressure on vaporizer output are more pronounced for anesthetic agents with low boiling points than those with high boiling points. The following anesthetics are listed in order of increasing boiling points: desflurane, isoflurane, halothane, enflurane, sevoflurane, methoxyflurane. Although gas anesthetic concentrations are commonly expressed as volume percentage, the depth of anesthesia and patient uptake are directly related to the partial pressure of the anesthetic in brain tissue. Partial pressure of a liquid anesthetic depends only on the temperature and is not affected by changes in barometric pressure.

For a concentration-calibrated vaporizer, the vaporizer output concentration of anesthetic will be higher than that from the same vaporizer at the same dial setting when used at sea level, but the partial pressure will remain unchanged. The change in vaporizer concentration output for a vaporizer calibrated at sea level can be calculated as: C_{alt} is $C_{sea}(760/P_{alt})$, where C_{alt} is anesthetic concentration at altitude, C_{sea} is anesthetic concentration at sea level, and P_{alt} is barometric pressure at altitude. Practically, the dial on concentration-calibrated vaporizers used at high elevation would be placed at similar settings as if the vaporizer were in use at sea level. The partial pressure in mm Hg of the anesthetic output from the vaporizer will be the same in both instances, but the volume percentage concentration measured by a gas analyzer will read a higher concentration at altitude as compared to the same dial setting at sea level.

In contrast, the Tec 6 desflurane vaporizer maintains a constant output in volumes percent but variable partial pressure when operated at barometric pressures other than that for which it was calibrated (usually sea level). At high altitude, the Tec 6 will output less partial pressure of desflurane at a given dial setting as compared with operation at sea level.

21. How can I estimate the amount of liquid sevoflurane anesthetic a vaporizer will use over time?

This calculation is useful to help estimate costs associated with changing to a new inhalation agent. Practically, all common inhaled anesthetics will produce about 200 ml of anesthetic vapor from each ml of liquid anesthetic. For example, to calculate the volume of sevoflurane vapor used at 3% for 1 hour at a fresh gas flow rate of 1 L/min: 3/100 × 60 min × 1 L/min = 1.8 L or 1800 ml. Divide by 200 to yield the milliliters of liquid anesthetic used: 1800 ml vapor ÷ 200 ml vapor/ml liquid = 6 ml. Thus, 6 ml of liquid sevoflurane would be required for 1 hour of anesthesia at these settings.

22. What maintenance is recommended for modern vaporizers?

Maintenance for modern vaporizers varies depending on recommendations from the manufacturer and the actual use of the equipment. Anesthetic machines should be tested for leaks at least every 3 months. Servicing should be instituted whenever there is an abrupt change in dial settings required to maintain the desired level of anesthetic depth. If an anesthetic agent analyzer is available, the output of the vaporizer used at different fresh-gas flow rates can be measured to determine the accuracy of the dial. A good rule of thumb is to clean, replace filters or worn parts, and recalibrate the vaporizer annually. The liquid anesthetic must be drained from the vaporizer prior to shipping.

23. How can I convert my halothane vaporizer to use isoflurane?

The concentration-calibrated vaporizers can be converted to use other agents in most instances, depending on the make, model, and specified anesthetic agent of the vaporizer. Halothane vaporizers can nearly always be readily converted to isoflurane by recalibrating and relabeling. Enflurane vaporizers can be converted to isoflurane use but, owing to the required replacement of internal parts, may cost more than converting a halothane vaporizer to isoflurane. Nearly all vaporizers (halothane, isoflurane, or enflurane) can similarly be converted for use with sevoflurane. A qualified service provider should perform the conversion.

BIBLIOGRAPHY

1. Dorsch JA, Dorsch SE: Vaporizers (anesthetic agent delivery devices). In Understanding Anesthesia Equipment, 4th ed. Baltimore, Williams & Wilkins, 1999, pp 121–182.
2. Hartsfield SM: Anesthetic machines and breathing systems. In Lumb and Jones' Veterinary Anesthesia, 3rd ed. Thurmon JC, Tranquilli, WJ, Benson GJ (eds): Baltimore, Williams & Wilkins, 1996, pp 366–408.

III. Pharmacology

12. OPIOIDS

G. John Benson, D.V.M., M.S., D.A.C.V.A.

1. Define the term *narcotic*.

The term *narcotic* often refers to opioids. However, it is actually nonspecific, being derived from the Greek for "stupor" and thus describes any drug that produces sleep. In common usage, the term *narcotic* is used to describe any number of illegally used drugs, whether or not they possess true opioid properties (e.g., cocaine).

2. What are opioids?

Opioids are morphine-like compounds that bind to opioid receptors. Thus they may be opioid receptor agonists, antagonists or agonist-antagonists. Opioids act as agonists of stereospecific presynaptic and postsynaptic receptors in the central nervous system (CNS) (primarily the brain stem and spinal cord) and in other tissues. Opioid receptors are normally activated by endogenous endorphins. By binding to endorphin receptors, opioids activate the endogenous pain-modulating system. Strong binding of the drug to the receptor requires a high degree of ionization, and only the levorotary form is active. The affinity of most opioids for the receptor correlates well with their analgesic potency. Furthermore, increasing opioid receptor occupancy parallels opioid effects. Binding of the opioid to the receptor inhibits adenylate cyclase activity, and hyperpolarization of the neuron results in suppression of spontaneous discharge and evoked responses. Opioids may also interfere with transmembrane transport of calcium ion and act presynaptically to interfere with release of neurotransmitters including acetylcholine, dopamine, norepinephrine, and substance P. Depression of cholinergic transmission in the CNS as a result of opioid-induced inhibition of acetylcholine release may be an important mechanism for the analgesic effects and side effects of opioids. Opioids do not effect responsiveness of afferent nerve endings to noxious stimuli nor impair transmission of impulses along peripheral nerves.

Opioids are the analgesic drug of choice for treatment of severe, acute pain.

3. Are there species differences in the effects of opioids?

Morphine is the prototype opioid to which all others are compared. Although actions and effects of most drugs differ little among mammalian species, there are marked differences in response to selected analgesics (e.g., opioids) that are independent of pharmacokinetics among species. The concentration of opioid receptors in the amygdala and frontal cortex of species that are depressed by opioids (e.g., dogs, primates) is nearly twice as great as in those species that become excited in response to opioids (e.g., horses, cats). By decreasing the dose, excitement can be avoided in those species prone to bizarre reactions. Excitement may result indirectly from increased release of norepinephrine and dopamine. This may explain the mechanism whereby dopaminergic and noradrenergic blocking drugs such as phenothiazine and butyrophenone tranquilizers suppress clinical evidence of opioid-induced excitement. Xylazine and detomidine, α-2 adrenergic agonists, are effective in preventing opioid-induced excitement. Because analgesia and excitement are mediated by different receptors, i.e., μ—analgesia and σ—excitement, they can occur concurrently and are not mutually exclusive.

4. What are the specific effects of opioids?

Opioid analgesics induce CNS depression characterized by miosis, hypothermia, bradycardia, and respiratory depression in primates, dogs, rats, and rabbits. Stimulation occurs in horses, cats, ruminants, and swine, characterized by mydriasis, panting, tachycardia, hyperkinesis, and sweating in horses. Systemic effects of opioids include release of antidiuretic hormone, prolactin, and somatotropin; inhibition of the release of luteinizing hormone; increased vagal tone; release of histamine and attendant hypotension; decreased motility and increased tone of the gastrointestinal tract; spasm of the biliary and pancreatic ducts; spasm of ureteral-smooth muscle and increased bladder tone; and decreased uterine tone.

5. How do opioids work?

Opioids raise the pain threshold or decrease the perception of pain by acting at receptors in the dorsal horn of the spinal cord and mesolimbic system, i.e., brain stem-nucleus raphe magnus and locus coeruleus, midbrain periaquaductal gray matter, and several thalamic and hypothalamic nuclei. In the dorsal horn, opioids induce postsynaptic inhibition of nociceptive projection neurons (T cells). In addition, there is some evidence that opioids may act presynaptically to inhibit release of substance P from primary afferent nerves. Centrally, at the level of the mesencephalon and medulla, opioids activate the descending endogenous antinociceptive system that modulates nociception in the dorsal horn via release of serotonin and perhaps norepinephrine. Opioids act at the limbic system to alter the emotional component of the pain response thus making it more bearable. Opioids decrease cerebral blood flow and intracranial pressure if normocapnea is maintained. The effect of morphine on the electroencephalogram resembles changes associated with normal sleep.

Morphine is well absorbed following parenteral administration, but not following oral administration. Its pharmacologic effects do not correlate well with peak plasma concentrations. Presumably this is due to morphine's low lipid solubility resulting in a slow penetration of the blood-brain barrier. Morphine is conjugated and most of the drug is excreted as the conjugate in the urine.

6. What are the possible side effects of opioids?

Successful use of opioids requires appropriate selection of the drug and dose for the given species to avoid undesirable side effects. They must be used with caution in animals with impaired pulmonary function because they depress the respiratory and cough centers, decrease secretions, and may induce bronchospasm secondary to histamine release. In species that can freely vomit, nausea and vomiting may occur. Repeated doses can result in constipation and ileus and urinary retention. Mice and rats rapidly develop tolerance and physical dependence to opioid agonists. Morphine decreases the number and phagocytic function of macrophages and polymorphonuclear leukocytes in mice and may alter their immune function.

7. Are there any endogenous opioids?

There are several endogenous opioid peptides: beta-endorphin produced in the pituitary; methionine-enkephalin and leucine-enkephalin widely spread in the CNS from the cerebral cortex to the spinal cord, adrenal medulla, and gastrointestinal tract; and dynorphin found primarily in the gut, pituitary, and brain. The location of opioid receptors and endogenous ligands is related to their functions. Those mediating analgesia are located in greater density in areas of the brain and spinal cord involved in pain sensation. The significance of the number of peptides, their locations, and the sites of opioid receptors is not clearly understood.

8. Describe the receptors where opioids express their effects.

There are several types of opioid receptors, each mediating a spectrum of pharmacologic effects in response to activation by an opioid agonist. It appears that there are subpopulations of receptors within each major classification. μ-Receptors are morphine-preferring and principally responsible for superspinal analgesia. Analgesia is associated with the μ_1-receptor subpopulation, whereas μ_2-receptors appear to mediate hypoventilation, bradycardia, physical dependence, euphoria, and ileus. Beta endorphin is the endogenous μ receptor agonist; other μ-agonists include morphine, meperidine, fentanyl, sufentanil, and alfentanil. Naloxone is a μ receptor antagonist, binding to the receptor without activating it. δ-receptors appear to modulate the activity of μ-receptors and bind leuenkephalin. κ-Opioid receptors mediate analgesia (primarily spinal) with little depression of ventilation, sedation, and miosis. Opioid agonist-antagonist drugs, such as butorphanol, nalbuphine buprenorphine, and pentazocine, act at κ-receptors. Lastly, activation of σ-receptors results in excitation, dysphoria, hypertonia, tachycardia, tachypnea and mydriasis. It is postulated that some of ketamine's effects are σ-receptor mediated.

Opioid receptors are located in areas of the brain and spinal cord involved with pain perception, integration of nociceptive activity, and responses to noxious (painful) stimuli, particularly the periaqueductal gray matter of the brain stem, amygdala, corpus striatum, hypothalamus and substantia gelatinosa. Opioids or endorphins inhibit the release of excitatory neurotransmitters from terminals of neurons carrying nociceptive stimuli.

9. What is the difference between efficacy and potency?

Potency is the dose of a drug required to produce an effect of given intensity and is often expressed as ED_{50}, that is, the dose required to produce a given effect in 50% of subjects. Potency varies inversely with dose, in that the lower the dose required to produce the desired effect, the more potent the drug is. Potency of a drug does not necessarily correlate with efficacy or safety. Efficacy refers to the maximal effect the drug can produce.

10. What is meant by equianalgesic dose?

Opioids differ in potency. Thus, for purposes of comparison, the dose required to induce a particular degree of analgesia is expressed as the equianalgesic dose.

11. Name the opioids commonly used in the perioperative setting, their trade names, half-life, equivalent morphine dose, and class.

Opioid	Trade Name	Half-Life	Equivalent Morphine Dose	Class
Morphine	Morphine sulphate	2	10	Agonist
Oxymorphone	Numorphan	—	1	Agonist
Hydromorphone	Dilaudid	2–3	1.2	Agonist
Meperidine	Demerol	3–4	75–100	Agonist
Methadone	Dolophine	15–40	—	Agonist
Fentanyl	Sublimaze	3–4	0.1	Agonist
Sufentanil	Sufenta	2–3	0.01–0.02	Agonist
Alfentanil	Alfenta	1–1.5	0.5–1.0	Agonist
Remifentanil	Ultiva	<1	—	Agonist
Tramodol	Ultram	3–4	100	Partial agonist
Butorphanol	Torbugesic	2.5–3.5	2–3	Agonist-antagonist
Buprenorphine	Buprenex	—	0.3	Partial agonist

12. What are appropriate dosing intervals for opioid analgesics?

Analgesics should be administered as needed and to effect to provide adequate analgesia. That said, the commonly used opioid analgesics—morphine, hydromorphone, oxymorphone and butorphanol—when administered intramuscularly may be supplemented on a 3- to 5-hour schedule. However, more frequent dosing may be needed initially.

13. What are the side effects of opioids?

Morphine's side effects are characteristic of all opioids, although incidence and severity may vary. Morphine is not a direct myocardial depressant and does not induce hypotension in supine normovolemic patients. Morphine reduces sympathetic nervous tone, which can lead to decreased venous tone, pooling of blood in capacitance vessels, and decreased cardiac output and arterial pressure secondary to decreased return. Morphine may indirectly reduce blood pressure via histamine release. Heart rate is decreased as a result of increased vagal tone due to stimulation of the medullary vagal nucleus.

Opioids induce respiratory depression via direct depression of the medullary respiratory center, resulting in a shift of the CO_2 response curve to the right (decreased sensitivity to CO_2). Periodic or altered patterns of breathing are the result of μ-opioid activity at the pontine and medullary centers that regulate rhythm of breathing. Pain counteracts the respiratory effects of opioids.

14. What is meant by tolerance and what are its clinical manifestations?

Tolerance refers to decreased response to the analgesic or side effects of an opioid. Tolerance can begin with the first dose but generally is not clinically manifested until 1 week of exposure to therapeutic doses. Tolerance develops most rapidly in mice and rats. In patients with chronic stable pain, tolerance may require little if any adjustment in dose. Animal studies suggest that tolerance does not develop when opioids are administered during painful stimuli. Should tolerance develop, increasing the dose or switching to a different opioid will effectively provide pain relief. The administration of α_2-adrenergic agonists can be used to "rescue" or reduce tolerance acutely.

15. What is meant by *physical dependence*?

Physical dependence is characterized by an abstinence syndrome upon discontinuation of administration of opioids. The syndrome consists of lacrimation, agitation, tremors, insomnia, fever, tachycardia, hypertension and sympathetic hyperactivity, and diarrhea. When opioids are administered for a painful medical condition, the risk of dependence is very low. *Addiction* refers to psychological dependence in people with abnormal behavior patterns of drug use for effects other than analgesia.

16. Can opioids act peripherally?

There is evidence that opioid receptors develop in inflamed tissue, allowing opioids to have a peripheral effect.

17. Do opioids have a place in regional anesthesia?

Opioid receptors are located in the spinal cord. Therefore, opioids can be used epidurally or intrathecally to induce perioperative analgesia. When used alone, they do not provide appropriate conditions for surgery, unlike the local anesthetics. They do reduce the requirement for inhalant anesthetics. Neuraxial opioids are useful in postoperative pain management. Unlike the local anesthetics, they do not affect the sympathetic nervous system, skeletal muscle function, or proprioception. Epidural morphine induces analgesia similar to that induced by 0.5% bupivicaine but of longer duration and with decreased incidence of hypotension. Neuraxial opioids have greater potency, lower daily requirements, less CNS depression, and fewer gastrointestinal side effects than systemic opioids.

18. Explain the mechanism of neuraxial opioids.

Epidural or intrathecal opioids bind to opioid receptors in the dorsal horn of the spinal cord, principally in the substantia gelatinosa. This area processes afferent pain information and contains μ-, δ-, and κ-receptors. The μ and δ receptors inhibit afferent pain signals from somatic tissues, whereas μ- and κ-receptors inhibit visceral pain. Kappa receptor activation is thought to inhibit release of substance P through blockade of calcium entrance into neurons.

19. What are the side effects of neuraxial opioids?

Pruritis, nausea and vomiting, urinary retention, and ventilatory depression may occur, but at low incidence.

20. Discuss the effect of lipid solubility on neuraxial opioid action.

Increasing lipid solubility decreases spinal cord bioavailability of spinally administered drugs. Highly lipid-soluble opioids such as fentanyl, sufentanil, and alfentanil, when administered epidurally or intrathecally, are rapidly absorbed and exert their effects by systemic uptake and redistribution to the brain. Plasma concentrations are the same whether these drugs are infused intravenously or intrathecally. In addition, as lipid solubility increases, the ability of the opioid to penetrate the spinal cord decreases and increases the amount of drug in the white matter rather than the gray matter. Thus opioids of intermediate lipid solubility such as morphine will effectively reach the dorsal horn and produce spinally mediated analgesia, whereas fentanyl produces analgesia through systemic absorption even when administered spinally.

21. Is it true that opioids should not be used in procedures involving the biliary tract?

No. Opioids have been reported to cause biliary smooth muscle spasm, but the incidence is low. Because of the need for analgesia, opioids should not be withheld because of this theoretical concern.

22. Name the opioid antagonist most commonly used in clinical anesthesia. Discuss its effects.

Naloxone is a pure μ-receptor antagonist. It is used to treat opioid overdose and reverse opioid-induced respiratory depression. Because reversal of respiratory depression also reverses analgesia, it should be used cautiously and only if needed postoperatively. Sudden reversal of analgesia can cause a catecholamine surge, resulting in tachycardia, hypertension, dysrhythmias, and pulmonary edema.

23. What are opioid agonist-antagonists?

Opioid agonist-antagonists are opioids that are either partial agonists or antagonists at μ-receptors while being κ-receptor agonists.

24. How do agonist-antagonist drugs differ from pure opioid agonists?

Agonist-antagonists, because of their low efficacy at μ-receptors, do not induce as profound a degree of analgesia as full agonists. They are used primarily to treat pain of mild to moderate intensity. Because of the lack of μ receptor activity, they induce less respiratory depression as well as analgesia and exhibit a "ceiling effect."

25. What is the advantage of using a partial agonist as an antagonist if naloxone is readily available?

Naloxone reverses analgesia and respiratory depression equally. Because of their partial agonist activity at μ-receprtors and because of their κ-agonist activity, some analgesia is retained when agonist-antagonists are administered to reverse opioid-induced respiratory depression.

BIBLIOGRAPHY

1. Kohn DF, Wixson SK, White WJ, Benson GJ (eds): Anesthesia and Analgesia in Laboratory Animals. New York, American College of Laboratory Animal Medicine Series, Academic Press, 1997.
2. Thurmon JC, Tranquilli WJ, Benson GJ (eds): Lumb and Jones' Veterinary Anesthesia, 3rd ed. Baltimore, Williams & Wilkins, 1996.
3. Stoelting RK: Pharmacology and Physiology in Anesthetic Practice, 2nd ed. Philadelphia, JB Lippincott, 1991.

13. α_2-AGONISTS

William J. Tranquilli, D.V.M., M.S., D.A.C.V.A.

1. Name the α_2-agonists commonly used in companion animals.

The two most widely used α_2-agonists in dogs and cats are xylazine and medetomidine. Xylazine, detomidine, and romifidine are used primarily in horses.

2. How do α_2-agonists produce their effects and how should they be used?

This class of agents produces its sedative-analgesic effects by activating α_2-receptors located within the central nervous system. They are labeled as sedative-analgesics by federal regulatory agencies and produce good muscle relaxation in most patients. This spectrum of effects has made this class of agents popular for use as chemical restraint drugs for short, minor diagnostic procedures. They can also be used as preanesthetics in appropriate patient populations by knowledgeable veterinarians.

3. What effects do α_2-agonists have on blood pressure?

Whether given intravenously or intramuscularly, α_2-agonists typically cause an acute increase in vascular resistance and blood pressure. This increase is associated with activation of α_2-receptors located in several large vascular beds (e.g., skin, mucous membranes, gastrointestinal tract). The typical response to this acute increase in pressure is the development of reflex vagal bradycardia that often reduces pressure to near baseline levels. Within 15 to 30 minutes, the central action of α_2-agonists begins to take effect, causing a decrease in sympathetic neuronal terminal release of norepinephrine. This effect tends to reduce baseline vascular tone and can result in a reduction in blood pressure. In summary, α_2-agonists cause an initial transient increase in blood pressure followed by a longer but also transient decrease in blood pressure.

4. What effects do α_2-agonists have on heart rate?

Generally speaking, all α_2-agonists reflexively decrease heart rate in response to the rapid increase in vascular resistance and pressure. This response is physiologically normal and is mediated by a vagal reflex action that can be antagonized by prior or concomitant anticholinergic administration.

5. When should an anticholinergic agent be used with an α_2-agonist?

The coadministration of an α_2-agonist and an anticholinergic should be restricted to patients with good cardiac function that are exercise tolerant and may be receiving additional agents that enhance vagal activity (such as the opioids). It is common to administer atropine with medetomidine and butorphanol or morphine in healthy, exercise-tolerant dogs.

6. What patients should not be given an α_2-agonist?

Dogs or cats with suspected or potential cardiopulmonary dysfunction should not be given an α_2-agonist. Patients should be exercise tolerant at a minimum and should have no signs of cardiopulmonary disease. Because α_2-agonists will rapidly increase afterload, dogs with dilatative cardiomyopathy and weakened systolic function should never be given an α_2-agonist. Similarly, dogs with mitral valve disease should not be administered agents that increase afterload.

7. Are cats less susceptible than dogs to the cardiopulmonary side effects of α_2-agonists?

Generally speaking, many more practitioners use α_2-agonists in combination with ketamine in cats than in dogs. Veterinarians' collective experience over the years appears to support the safer use of this combination in cats than in dogs. Differences in the rate of untoward events between cats and dogs may be attributable to a variety of reasons, including whether an anticholinergic is coadministered with the α_2-agonist, inherent differences in baseline cardiac function and cardiopulmonary disease-modifying factors in dogs versus cats, and pharmacodynamic differences in α_2-agonist activity between species.

8. Compare the preanesthetic uses of α_2-agonists and acepromazine.

Acepromazine is a commonly used preanesthetic that works by antagonizing dopamine activity within the central nervous system (CNS). The calming effect of acepromazine is accompanied by a degree of vasodilation, minimal analgesia, if any, and little muscle relaxation. In contrast, α_2-agonists typically produce a visible sedative action that is usually accompanied by some hypoalgesia and good muscle relaxation. With either class of agent, it should be remembered that these drugs produce effects through interference or activation of discrete populations of receptors within the CNS, and acute arousal is possible when stimuli exceed a given threshold. A false sense of security concerning the level of CNS depression achieved with these agents has resulted in harm to some veterinary practitioners and hospital personnel following acute arousal.

9. Can α_2-agonists be combined with other sedatives or tranquilizers?

Yes. Although not approved for combination use, α_2-agonists are commonly coadministered with opioids to enhance sedation and analgesia. α_2-Agents have also been combined with ketamine to enhance muscle relaxation and improve analgesia beyond what is achievable with ketamine alone. α_2-Agonists may also be used as preanesthetics prior to gas anesthesia. The preanesthetic use of α_2-agonists reportedly can reduce inhalant anesthetic requirements by as much as 80 to 90%.

10. What influence do α_2-agonists have on cardiac output?

The initial increase in vascular resistance and afterload may reduce cardiac output by 50% or more, often similar to the percentage reduction in heart rate. This decrease in blood flow is tolerated quite well in healthy patients, as the largest reductions occur in vascular beds perfusing peripheral tissues, such as the skin and mucous membranes. These tissues have evolved and are designed to undergo periods of significant reductions in perfusion (which is why α-receptors are located in these vascular beds). Blood flow to vital organs does not appear to mimic the overall decrease in cardiac output. Nevertheless, it would seem prudent to restrict use of this class of agents to procedures of relatively short duration. Repeated redosing of α_2-agonist to produce longer periods of sedation and muscle relaxation is not generally recommended.

11. Where can α_2 receptors be found?

In addition to the CNS, α_2-receptors have been identified in vascular beds (somewhat variable depending on species), sympathetic neuronal terminals, platelets, the gastrointestinal tract, pancreatic beta cells, reproductive tissues, and renal tissues.

12. Why do mucous membranes appear pale following α_2-agonist administration?

This is the result of intense vasoconstriction within the vasculature of the mucous membranes.

13. How do α_2-agonists affect capillary refill time?

Capillary refill time (CRT) is usually prolonged following α_2-agonist administration and is in direct contrast to the decreased CRT following acepromazine administration. α_2-Agonists increase vascular resistance, whereas acepromazine decreases vascular resistance, with which capillary refill time is directly correlated.

14. How do α_2-agonists affect heart rhythm?

The most common arrhythmogenic effects of α_2-agonists include sinoatrial block, atrioventricular (AV) block, bradycardia, first- and second-degree heart block, AV dissociation, and sinus arrhythmia. These arrhythmias are thought to be the result of altered sympathetic and parasympathetic activity on the AV conducting cells and spontaneously depolarizing tissues of the atrium. There does not appear to be an inherent arrhythmogenic action of α_2-agonists upon cardiac myocardial cells.

15. What is the mechanism of action for the analgesic effects produced by α_2-agonists?

α_2-Agonists produce their analgesic effect by effector mechanisms similar to those of opioids. α_2-Receptors are linked to membrane-associated G proteins that induce a chain of events that open potassium channels in the neuronal membrane. Loss of intracellular potassium hyperpolarizes ascending neurons, making them less responsive to excitatory input and inhibiting the passage of painful stimuli through the CNS.

16. How does α_2-receptor activation influence gastrointestinal function?

Decreased gastroesophageal tone has been reported following xylazine administration in dogs. Vomiting is commonly induced after α_2-agonist injection by the subcutaneous route. The incidence appears to be reduced following intravenous injection of most α_2-agonists. Xylazine also prolongs the gastrointestinal transit time in dogs and a number of other species. Similar effects have been seen in horses following detomidine injection. Reduced myoelectric activity may relax the large intestine in horses following xylazine administration. Gastrointestinal function may also be influenced, to some extent, by reduced blood flow.

17. What influences do α_2-receptor agonists have on urine production?

Increased urine output has been observed following xylazine and medetomidine administration in a number of species including dogs and cats. Micturition reflexes appear to remain normal. Increased urine production may be mediated via a decrease in antidiuretic hormone (ADH) release but more likely is the result of inhibition of ADH activity within the kidney or some other local renal mechanism mediated by α_2-receptors.

18. How does the administration of an α_2-agonist influence the insulin-glucose axis?

Transient hypoinsulinemia and hyperglycemia are commonly induced following α_2-agonist administration. The magnitude and duration of these effects appear to be dose-dependent. Inhibition of insulin release is mediated by α_2-receptor activation in pancreatic β cells. α_2-Agonists should be avoided in patients undergoing a glucose tolerance test. α_2-Agonists should not be used in patients suspected of diabetes that are not yet on insulin therapy.

19. Are there differences in dose requirements and potency of various α_2-agonists among domestic species?

Yes. Xylazine most noticeably is efficacious at relatively low doses in domestic cattle, whereas pigs require nearly 10 times this dose to achieve equivalent sedation. Dogs, cats, and horses require relatively similar dosages (higher than cattle but lower than pigs) to achieve sedative-analgesic actions. Medetomidine dose requirement appears to be higher for cats than dogs and similar to the dose reported for pigs.

Dose Range of α_2-Agonists ($\mu g/kg$)

	XYLAZINE	MEDETOMIDINE	DETOMIDINE	ROMIFIDINE
Cattle	20–2,000	20–50	10–40	NA
Dog	200–2,000	5–30	5–20	NA
Cat	200-2,000	10–80	NA	NA
Horse	200–2,000	10–30	5–20	30–80
Pig	2,000–4,000	30–80	NA	NA

20. List the α_2-agonists in clinical use in human medicine.

Clonidine (Duraclon) is used in human medicine as an antihypertensive and analgesic agent.

Dexmedetomidine (Precedex) is approved for use as an antistress and analgesic agent for patients in the critical care setting.

BIBLIOGRAPHY

1. Eisenach JC: Analgesic drug classes in the management of clinical pain: alpha-2 agonists. In Yaksh TL, Lynch C III, Zapol WM, et al (eds): Anesthesia: Biological Foundations. Philadelphia, Lippincott-Raven, 1998, pp 935–942.
2. Thurmon JC, Tranquilli WJ, Benson GJ: Preanesthetics and anesthetic adjuncts. In JC Thurmon, WJ Tranquilli, GJ Benson (eds): Lumb and Jones' Veterinary Anesthesia, 3rd ed. Baltimore, Williams & Wilkins, 1996, pp 183–209.

14. TRANQUILIZERS

David C. Rankin, D.V.M., M.S., D.A.C.V.A.

1. What are tranquilizers?
Tranquilizers are agents that alter perception of the environment and external stimuli, resulting in calmness and decreased anxiety. Some tranquilizers (α_2-agonists) have analgesic effects, but they are the exception when considering classes of tranquilizers. Analgesia is *not* a hallmark of tranquilizers. However, there is evidence that anxiety and stress can heighten pain perception and/or lower the pain threshold for certain stimuli. It would therefore seem that the alleviation of stress and anxiety would benefit patients in pain or patients in the perioperative period. Certainly, tranquilizers work synergistically with opioids in neuroleptoanalgesic combinations.

2. What are the classes of tranquilizers?
Two broad categories are considered in veterinary medicine: major and minor tranquilizers. Chemical structure or site of action further breaks them down into several other classes.

Major	*Minor*
Phenothiazines	Benzodiazepines
(acepromazine, chlorpromazine)	(diazepam, midazolam, zolazepam)
Butyrophenones	
(droperidol)	
α_2-Agonists (detomidine, medetomidine, xylazine; best classified as sedative/analgesic agents; see Chapter 13)	

3. Are the effects of tranquilizers reversible?
There is no reversal agent for acepromazine. Overdoses and side effects are dealt with symptomatically. Flumazenil is a benzodiazepine antagonist that will override the agonists and typically result in reversal without excitement. It is fairly short-acting, and animals may become sedated again depending on the time-frame of agonist administration, half-life, and time of reversal. α_2-Agonists have several reversal agents used in veterinary practice: yohimbine, tolazoline, and atipamezole (see Chapter 13).

4. Is droperidol commonly used in veterinary patients?
Butyrophenones are not commonly used in veterinary medicine. Droperidol was used frequently in a combination with fentanyl (Innovar-Vet) but that proprietary combination is no longer manufactured. Droperidol is a dopamine antagonist like acepromazine but more commonly causes extrapyramidal side effects. Droperidol is available as a stand-alone drug but is not as popular as acepromazine because of its side effects.

5. What are phenothiazines?
Phenothiazines are a class of drug used in veterinary medicine primarily for their sedative/tranquilizer qualities. They have no analgesic properties but may alter reactions to pain by reducing anxiety. They have antihistamine, anticholinergic, and α-adrenergic blocking effects.

6. How do phenothiazines work?
Phenothiazines work primarily by antagonizing dopamine receptors in the central nervous system. This antagonism in the limbic areas of the brain results in tranquilization. Some side effects are mediated by this blockade mechanism as well.

7. What are the common side effects of phenothiazines?

The major side effect is dose-dependent hypotension, mediated by central depression of the vasomotor center as well as peripheral blockade of α_1-adrenoreceptors in the vasculature. This depression is dose-dependent and is occasionally seen with clinically useful doses, particularly in patients with true or relative hypovolemia. The phenothiazine tranquilizers do not typically cause changes in ventilation but may potentiate the respiratory depression of other drugs. The blockade of dopamine and α_1-receptors can result in mild antiemetic and antiarrhythmic properties. In high doses, extrapyramidal signs (rigidity, tremor, spasticity) may be seen. This is not seen typically with clinically relevant doses. Stallions may exhibit transient or permanent penile paralysis.

8. What is the connection between phenothiazines and seizures?

Chlorpromazine has been demonstrated to enhance epileptiform activity in the canine electroencephalogram. Therefore, most clinicians refrain from giving phenothiazine tranquilizers to animals with seizure history, or to animals undergoing myelography.

9. Are phenothiazines useful for skin testing?

Because of their antihistamine effect, acepromazine and similar drugs are often avoided when intradermal skin testing is performed.

10. How are phenothiazines used?

Acepromazine is the most commonly used phenothiazine in veterinary medicine. It can be administered intravenously, intramuscularly, or subcutaneously to achieve sedation. It will reduce the amount of induction and maintenance drugs needed for general anesthesia when used as a premedication. Acepromazine can be used alone but acts synergistically with opioids to produce superior sedation with analgesia (neuroleptoanalgesia). Again, acepromazine alone provides no analgesia.

Oral acepromazine is available and is often used to sedate dogs and cats for a variety of reasons. Oral administration is not a commonly used in the perianesthetic period. Chlorpromazine is used primarily as an antiemetic but has sedative properties as well.

11. What are benzodiazepines?

Another tranquilizer, the benzodiazepines act on the $GABA_A$ receptor, resulting in increased chloride conductance and hyperpolarization of nerve membranes. This results in anxiolysis, muscle relaxation, and anticonvulsant activity. They have no analgesic properties. Diazepam, midazolam, and zolazepam are the most commonly used benzodiazepines in veterinary medicine.

12. Why are benzodiazepines called "minor" tranquilizers?

They tend not to be strong sedatives in veterinary medicine, unless the patient is very old, very young, or very debilitated. Healthy patients can actually become less inhibited with benzodiazepine administration, demonstrating excitement.

13. How are benzodiazepines used?

Diazepam and midazolam are used as anticonvulsants, as muscle relaxants, and as premedication prior to general anesthesia. They may be given with ketamine to abolish the muscle rigidity seen with dissociatives. Both are suitable for intravenous use. They can be given rectally in seizuring patients as an anticonvulsant.

Zolazepam is part of the product Telazol. It is combined in a 50:50 ratio with tiletamine, a dissociative, and used as an intravenous or intramuscular anesthetic induction agent (see chapter 15).

14. What are the differences between midazolam and diazepam?

Midazolam is water-soluble, making it more useful as an intramuscular injection. Diazepam can be given intramuscularly, but its bioavailability is variable when given via this route. Midazolam is considered to be more potent, but shorter acting. It has a half-life ranging from 1–4 hours, unlike diazepam with a half-life of 21–37 hours. Frequent repeated dosing of diazepam can lead to very high plasma concentrations.

15. Is diazepam an appetite stimulant?

Intravenous diazepam has been described as a very short-acting appetite stimulant, particularly in cats. Low doses may stimulate appetite if food is present, but the effect is very short-acting. Because of drug accumulation with frequent redosing and low efficacy, this is not recommended for ongoing appetite stimulation.

16. What are the side effects of benzodiazepines?

The benzodiazepines have very few adverse side effects with clinically relevant doses. Some animals may become excited after intravenous or intramuscular administration of this class. This is likely due to disinhibition as the GABA system is activated. This is less likely in very sick, very young, or very old patients.

Benzodiazepines are very stable in terms of effects in the cardiovascular system, occasionally causing a small and transient drop in blood pressure. Cardiac output may drop slightly, with a rise in heart rate.

The effect on ventilation is negligible, but they may augment the respiratory depressant effects of other drugs. High plasma concentrations may cause drowsiness, ataxia, hypoventilation, or other neuralgic signs. Injectable diazepam is provided in a vehicle of propylene glycol. Propylene glycol has its own potential side effects, including hemolysis and pain on injection.

17. Is oral diazepam often used in veterinary medicine?

It is not used commonly in the perianesthetic period because of its mild effects. Diazepam has been linked to hepatic failure in cats following repeated oral dosing. It is recommended that discontinuation of oral diazepam administration take place if serum aspartate or alanine transaminase levels increase within 5 days of starting the regimen.

Oral diazepam is not typically used as a sole agent for treating idiopathic epilepsy in dogs and cats, as it is difficult to maintain a high enough steady-state plasma concentration. Its use in cats in this fashion has been described, but it is often used along with phenobarbital to control seizures.

18. How are tranquilizers metabolized?

Phenothiazines are oxidized and conjugated in the liver. The metabolites are excreted primarily in urine and can be detected for up to 96 hours. Benzodiazepines are also metabolized in the liver; midazolam is hydrolyzed and diazepam is oxidized. Both produce active metabolites. The active metabolites of midazolam are very weak. In contrast, the metabolites of diazepam are quite potent, adding to the duration of effect of the drug. These metabolites are eventually excreted in the urine.

19. Are there contraindications for the use of tranquilizers?

There are no absolute contraindications for the use of phenothiazines or benzodiazepines, aside from the general avoidance of phenothiazines in seizure-risk patients. Patients with hepatic disease may have decreased clearance; acepromazine and droperidol are often avoided for this reason. Low-dose benzodiazepines (< 0.2 mg/kg) are often considered reasonable for patients with liver disease.

Potential side effects may preclude the use of certain tranquilizers in certain situations. For example, the antihistamine effects of acepromazine will interfere with allergy skin testing. Hypovolemic patients are at higher risk of hypotension produced by acepromazine. Benzodiazepines and acepromazine are sometimes avoided in portosystemic shunt cases because of the potential presence of an endogenous GABA agonist and prolonged clearance times for both drugs. The benefits should be evaluated in comparison to the risk of use or interference with a procedure such as allergy testing.

20. How do I dose tranquilizers?

Dosing of these medications is variable depending on patient attitude, procedure, other drugs administered, disease state, and the desired level of sedation. Typically, animals that are very sick or very old require less drug to achieve the same effect.

21. Will analgesics reduce the necessary dose of tranquilizer?

When administered with an opioid, less tranquilizer is typically required to reach a level of sedation as opposed to the tranquilizer alone (again, this synergistic effect with opioids is known as neuroleptoanalgesia). Recalling that most side effects of tranquilizers are dose dependent, it is often desirable to administer opioids concurrently to reduce the dose, particularly in surgical or in-pain patients. The dose ranges are wide, reflecting the variability of desired level of sedation and patient presentation.

	Dogs	*Cats*	*Horses*	*Ruminants*
Acepromazine	0.02–0.1 mg/kg IV, IM, SQ	0.05–0.2 mg/kg IV, IM, SQ	0.01–0.06 mg/kg IV, IM	0.01–0.06 mg/kg IV, IM
Diazepam	0.2–0.4 mg/kg IV, IM	0.2–0.4 mg/kg IV, IM	0.04–0.1 mg/kg IV	Not commonly used; dose for horses may be appropriate
Midazolam	0.2–0.4 mg/kg IV, IM	0.2–0.4 mg/kg IV, IM	N/A	N/A

BIBLIOGRAPHY

1. Center SA, Elston TH et al: Fulminant hepatic failure associated with oral administration of diazepam in 11 cats. J Am Vet Med Assoc 209: 618–625, 1996.
2. Ettinger SJ, Feldman EC (eds): Textbook of Veterinary Internal Medicine: Diseases of the Dog and Cat, 5th ed. Philadelphia, W. B. Saunders, 2000.
3. Klein LV, Klide AM: Central α_2 adrenergic and benzodiazepine agonists and their antagonists. J Zoo Wildl Med 20(2) 138–153, 1989.
4. Miller RD (ed): Anesthesia, 5th ed. Philadelphia, Churchill Livingstone, 2000.
5. Muir WW, Hubbell JAE, Skarda RT, Bednarski RM (eds): Handbook of Veterinary Anesthesia, 3rd ed. St. Louis, Mosby, 2000.
6. Oliver JE, Lorenz MD, Korengay JN: Handbook of Veterinary Neurology, 3rd ed. Athens, GA, W. B. Saunders, 1997.
7. Redman HC, Wilson GL, Hogan JE: Effect of chlorpromazine combined with intermittent light stimulation on the electroencephalogram and clinical response of the Beagle dog. Am J Vet Res 34(7): 929–936, 1973.
8. Stoelting RK (ed): Pharmacology and Physiology in Anesthetic Practice, 3rd ed. Philadelphia, Lippincott-Raven, 1999.
9. Thurmon JC, Tranquilli WJ, Benson GJ (eds): Essentials of Small Animal Anesthesia and Analgesia, 1st ed. Baltimore, Lippincott Williams & Wilkins, 1999.
10. Thurmon JC, Tranquilli WJ, Benson GJ (eds): Lumb and Jones Veterinary Anesthesia, 3rd ed. Baltimore, Williams & Wilkins, 1996

15. INTRAVENOUS ANESTHETICS

G. John Benson, D.V.M., M.S., D.A.C.V.A.

1. How do intravenous anesthetic agents work?

Barbiturates modulate gamma-aminobutyric acid (GABA) transmission. GABA is the most common inhibitory transmitter in the mammalian nervous system. Activation of postsynaptic GABA receptors increases chloride conductance through the Cl ion channel, resulting in hyperpolarization, thereby inhibiting the postsynaptic neuron. The GABA receptor is an oligomeric complex consisting of the GABA receptor, its associated chloride ion channel, the barbiturate receptor, the benzodiazepine receptor, and the picrotoxin binding site. Binding of barbiturates to their receptor decreases the rate of dissociation of GABA from its receptor, thus prolonging the duration of GABA-induced opening of the chloride channel. Barbiturates appear to be especially capable of depressing activity in the reticular formation whose activity is necessary for maintenance of wakefulness. In addition, barbiturates selectively depress transmission at sympathetic ganglia, which may contribute to decreased blood pressure following their administration. High doses of barbiturates reduce sensitivity of postsynaptic membranes of the neuromuscular junction to acetylcholine thereby interfering with transmission

2. How does propofol work?

Propofol exerts its central nervous system (CNS) effects via modulation of the GABA-activated chloride channel. Its specific site of action appears to be distinct from those of the barbiturates, steroids, benzodiazepines, and GABA.

3. How does etomidate work?

Etomidate is an imidazole compound that appears to depress CNS function via GABA. In contrast to the increased affinity of the GABA receptor induced by barbiturates, etomidate appears to increase the number of GABA receptors, possibly by displacing endogenous inhibitors of GABA binding.

4. How do benzodiazepines work?

Benzodiazepine receptors are located on the α-subunit of the GABA receptor on postsynaptic nerve endings in the CNS. Benzodiazepines bind with their receptors and induce an allosteric modification of the GABA receptors, increasing the efficiency of the GABA receptor/chloride ion channel coupling. As a result, benzodiazepines increase the frequency of ion channel openings produced by GABA. The resulting effect is to enhance the chloride-channel gating effect of GABA. Increased chloride channel conductance leads to hyperpolarization of the cell and decreased (inhibition of) transmission. Benzodiazepine receptors occur nearly exclusively on postsynaptic membranes in the CNS resulting in minimal non-CNS (cardiopulmonary) effects. The highest density of benzodiazepine receptors occurs in the cerebral cortex followed in decreasing order by the hypothalamus, cerebellum, midbrain, hippocampus, medulla, and spinal cord.

5. How does ketamine work?

The mechanism of action of ketamine has not been established. It appears that the cyclohexamines exert their effects via antagonism of CNS muscarinic acetylcholine receptors and by agonism of opioid receptors. Ketamine is thought to be a specific antagonist of N-methyl-D-aspartate glutamate receptors (NMDA). NMDA is the principal excitatory receptor system in the mammalian brain. Blockade of adrenergic and serotonergic receptors attenuate ketamine-induced analgesia. Ketamine is available as a racemic mixture of the two isomers of the drug. The positive isomer has been shown to produce more intense analgesia, more rapid recovery, and a lower incidence of emergence reactions than the negative isomer. Both isomers appear to have a "cocaine-like" effect in that they inhibit uptake of catecholamines into postganglionic sympathetic nerves.

6. Describe the properties of the ideal intravenous anesthetic.

The ideal intravenous anesthetic should be water soluble, have a long shelf-life (>1 year), be stable on exposure to light, and require a small volume for anesthetic induction. It should have a safe (wide) therapeutic index, have a rapid onset of action (one circulation time) and a short duration of action, and be inactivated by rapid metabolism to nontoxic metabolites. It should not induce anaphylaxis or histamine release. Lastly, the ideal intravenous anesthetic would be nontoxic and nonirritating and have no side effects, producing only its primary CNS effects.

7. What are the properties of barbiturates?

Barbiturates induce a dose-dependent state of sedation or hypnosis. Their classification as long-, intermediate-, short-, and ultrashort-acting is misleading in that drug levels persist for several hours even with ultrashort-acting drugs administered to induce anesthesia. Furthermore, species differences in barbiturate pharmacokinetics are responsible for the significant variation in duration of action among species. Currently, barbiturates used in anesthesia are pentobarbital, thiopental, methohexital and thiobutabarbital (Inactin).

8. How does recovery from barbiturates occur?

Recovery from single doses of thiopental and methohexital is due to redistribution of the drug from brain to non-nervous tissues, primarily viscera and skeletal muscle. In the case of methohexital, rapid hepatic metabolism contributes to recovery as well. Redistribution of pentobarbital occurs, but recovery is primarily due to metabolism. Ultimate elimination of barbiturates from the body is by metabolism; less than 1% is recovered unchanged in the urine.

Repeated exposure to barbiturates results in tolerance due to induction of hepatic enzymes. Conversely, drugs such as chloramphenicol that inhibit hepatic microsomal enzyme activity cause sleep time to increase. In rats and mice, sleep time is affected by age, sex, strain, nutritional status, bedding material, and temperature. Administration of drugs that are highly protein bound, such as phenylbutazone and sulfonamides, displace barbiturates from serum protein, resulting in increased sleep time. Administration of certain other agents during recovery can result in renarcotization. This effect is of little clinical significance, but has been reported to occur following administration of glucose, fructose, lactate, pyruvate, glutamate, adrenergic agents, and chloramphenicol.

9. Describe the hemodynamic effects of barbiturates.

The hemodynamic effects of equivalent doses of thiopental and methohexital as administered for intravenous induction are similar. In normal subjects, there is a transient small decrease in arterial blood pressure that is compensated for by an increase in heart rate. Myocardial depression is minimal and far less than would occur with volatile inhalants. The compensatory tachycardia and unchanged myocardial contractility appear to be due to increased peripheral sympathetic activity mediated by the carotid sinus baroreceptor.

10. Describe the negative inotropic effects of barbiturates.

Direct negative inotropic effects occur in the absence of compensatory increases in sympathetic activity. The initial decrease in arterial pressure is due to peripheral vasodilation induced by depression of the medullary vasomotor center and decreased sympathetic outflow. In the absence of carotid sinus baroreceptor activity, or in hypovolemic patients with less ability to compensate for vasodilation, vasodilation results in pooling of blood in large capacitance vessels, decreased venous return, and decreased arterial blood pressure and cardiac output. Arrhythmias occur on induction but are transient and well tolerated. Pentobarbital induces decreased contractility, arterial blood pressure, stroke volume, pulse pressure, and central venous pressure. Heart rate is increased.

11. What effects do barbiturates have on oxygenation?

Barbiturates induce a dose-dependent depression of the medullary and pontine respiratory centers, resulting in decreased hypercapnic and hypoxic drive of ventilation. Apnea may occur, especially in the presence of other depressant drugs, and when breathing resumes it is at a reduced minute volume of ventilation.

Barbiturates decrease cerebral metabolic oxygen requirements by about 50% when the electroencephalogram is isoelectric. This would indicate a reduction in neuronal but not metabolic oxygen needs. Barbiturate-induced decreases in cerebral metabolic oxygen requirements exceed the decrease in cerebral blood flow. This may account for the protective effects against focal cerebral ischemia.

12. Do barbiturates have adverse effects on other organ systems?

Barbiturates have no direct effects on either liver or kidney function. They are neither hepatotoxic nor nephrotoxic. Alterations in liver or kidney function associated with their use is secondary to hemodynamic effects of the drugs and altered perfusion. Placental transfer of barbiturates occurs rapidly. However, when used in proper induction doses, excessive depression of the fetus does not occur.

13. What are the properties and side effects of propofol?

Propofol is an isopropylphenyl compound that is available for intravenous use as a 1% solution in soybean oil, glycerol, and egg phosphatide. It rapidly induces unconsciousness. Recovery is more rapid and complete with minimal residual CNS effects than following induction with thiopental or methohexital. Plasma clearance exceeds hepatic blood flow, indicating that tissue uptake is also important. Less than 0.3% of the drug is excreted unchanged in the urine. There is, however, no evidence of impaired elimination of propofol in either patients with cirrhosis or those with renal impairment. Because of its rapid clearance, propofol can be administered as a continuous infusion to maintain a level of basal narcosis as part of a balanced anesthetic protocol.

Propofol is primarily used as an induction agent and to maintain short periods of unconsciousness for short procedures such as bronchoscopy. It does not induce analgesia; analgesics should accompany propofol when painful manipulations or procedures are performed.

Cerebral blood flow, perfusion pressure, and intracranial pressure decrease following propofol administration. The cardiovascular effects of propofol resemble those of thiopental but are of greater magnitude at comparable doses. Heart rate is less likely to increase with propofol as compared with thiopental. Propofol is a potent respiratory depressant. Apnea is common on induction unless the drug is given slowly. When used as the sole anesthetic agent, apnea occurs at doses required to prevent movement in response to painful manipulation.

14. What are the properties of ketamine?

Ketamine is the most commonly used dissociative agent. Dissociative anesthesia is a state in which the patient is "dissociated" from the environment, resembling a catatonic state; the eyes remain open and the patient is not unconscious. Muscle relaxation is not a feature, and varying degrees of hypertonus and purposeful movement occur independent of surgical stimulation. There is electroencephalographic evidence of dissociation between the neothalamocortical and limbic systems, and differential depression and activation of various areas of the brain. Amnesia is present, and while somatic analgesia may be intense, visceral analgesia is less reliable. Emergence excitement and delirium may occur. The dissociative anesthetics are cyclohexamines. Tiletamine is available in combination with zolazepam (a benzodiazepine) as Telazol. Phencyclidine is no longer available.

Ketamine's pharmacokinetics resemble those of thiopental, being rapid in onset and of short duration. Ketamine is five to 10 times more lipid soluble than thiopental, ensuring rapid transfer to the CNS and recovery through rapid redistribution. Ultimate clearance from the body is dependent on hepatic metabolism. Norketamine, an intermediate metabolite, has one-fifth to one-third the potency of ketamine and may contribute to prolonged effects. There are significant differences among species in the relative amount of free ketamine excreted in the urine. In people, dogs, and horses, metabolism is extensive, whereas in cats, most of the drug appears unchanged in the urine. Ketamine, like the barbiturates, can induce hepatic enzymes with repeated exposure.

15. What are the side effects of ketamine?

The cardiovascular effects of ketamine resemble sympathetic nervous stimulation. Systemic and pulmonary arterial blood pressure, heart rate, cardiac output, cardiac work, and myocardial oxygen consumption increase. These effects are obtunded by prior administration of tranquilizers or sedatives. In intact patients with a functioning CNS, ketamine increases myocardial contractility. In isolated papillary muscle preparations or in denervated hearts, however, myocardial depression occurs. Ketamine's cardiovascular effects are primarily due to direct stimulation of the CNS, leading to increased sympathetic outflow from the CNS. Plasma concentrations of norepinephrine and epinephrine increase transiently following ketamine administration as a result of inhibition of their uptake at postganglionic sympathetic nerve endings. The effect of ketamine on arrhythmogenicity remains controversial. In hypovolemic patients, arterial blood pressure is better maintained with ketamine because of vasoconstriction; however, tissue perfusion may suffer. In critical patients with depleted catecholamine stores and exhaustion of sympathetic compensating mechanisms, ketamine can induce unexpected decreases in arterial blood pressure and cardiac output.

Ketamine does not induce significant respiratory depression. An apneustic pattern of breathing is commonly seen. Bronchial dilation secondary to increased sympathetic tone occurs and protective upper airway reflexes are maintained. Airway and salivary secretions are increased. Ketamine does not significantly affect hepatic or renal function.

Ketamine is a potent cerebral vasodilator. Cerebral blood flow, intracranial pressure, and cerebrospinal pressure increase significantly. The mechanism, while controversial, appears to be secondary to increases in arterial carbon dioxide tension. Controlled ventilation to maintain normocapnea effectively prevents ketamine-induced increases in cerebral blood flow and intracranial pressure. Ketamine induces epileptiform bursts in the thalamus and limbic system, but without spread to cortical areas. Ketamine does not induce seizures in human epileptics and has been shown to increase the seizure threshold in rats and mice. There have been reports of seizures occurring in dogs and cats. Hallucinations and emergence delirium can occur. In cats, emergence reactions are characterized by ataxia, increased motor activity, hyperreflexia, hypersensitivity to touch and inappropriate avoidance behavior, and violent recovery. Although these responses usually cease within several hours, they can be minimized by concurrent treatment or pretreatment with tranquilizers or sedatives. Other reported adverse reactions include hyperthermia and blindness.

16. What is tiletamine?

Tiletamine, a dissociative with potency and duration of action intermediate between ketamine and phencyclidine is available in a 1:1 combination with zolazepam, a benzodiazepine tranquilizer, as Telazol. This combination of drugs represents an effort to provide a longer-acting dissociative agent for dogs and cats without the negative side effects of rough recovery and muscle rigidity. The physiologic side effects are similar to those of ketamine-benzodiazepine combinations. Heart rate and arterial blood pressure increase. Respiration rate decreases transiently, and minute ventilation is well maintained.

17. What are the properties and side effects of etomidate?

Etomidate's duration of action is intermediate between thiopental and methohexital, and recovery from a single dose is rapid, with little residual depression. Like the barbiturates and propofol, etomidate does not induce analgesia. Etomidate induces unconsciousness within one circulation time. Recovery is rapid as a result of extensive redistribution and rapid metabolism. Etomidate is hydrolyzed by hepatic microsomal enzymes and plasma esterases. Less than 3% is recovered unchanged in the urine. Overall clearance rate of etomidate is three to five times that of thiopental.

Etomidate is a potent direct cerebrovascular vasoconstrictor. Cerebral blood flow and oxygen requirements decrease 35 to 45%, decreasing intracranial pressure. Etomidate may activate seizure foci in a manner similar to that of methohexital.

Etomidate is relatively free of cardiovascular depressant effects. Heart rate, stroke volume and cardiac output are minimally affected and blood pressure may decrease slightly secondary to decreased vascular resistance. Unlike other anesthetics, etomidate does not decrease renal blood flow. Hepatic function is not altered. Respiratory depression is less than that induced by thiopental and of shorter duration.

Undesirable side effects of etomidate that may limit its use include pain on injection, myoclonus and adrenocortical suppression lasting 4 to 6 hours following an induction dose.

18. What are the properties and side effects of benzodiazepines?

Benzodiazepines, unlike the phenothiazines and butyrophenones, lack antipsychotic effects in people and as a result are classified as minor tranquilizers. They have potent anxiolytic, anticonvulsant, and muscle relaxant effects. They do not induce the degree of tranquilization-sedation of the other tranquilizers. In veterinary medicine, they are most commonly used as anticonvulsants and as coinduction agents in combination with injectable anesthetics. Benzodiazepines undergo hepatic metabolism and the metabolites are active, contributing to the relatively long duration of action of these drugs. Ultimately, the metabolites are excreted in the urine. Unlike barbiturates, benzodiazepines do not appear to induce hepatic enzyme production. The half-life of these drugs varies among species, being shortest in rodents. The dog appears to clear benzodiazepines more rapidly than the cat. Elimination half-life increases up to fivefold with liver disease. In addition, sensitivity and increased duration of action increases with age, not related to hepatic function.

The electroencephalographic effects are similar to those of the barbiturates: decreased α and increased low β activity. Unlike the barbiturates, tolerance to the electroencephalographic effects of benzodiazepines does occur. Unlike the phenothiazines and butyrophenones, benzodiazepines have a specific antagonist, or reversal drug: flumazenil.

Benzodiazepines have minimal depressant effects on cardiopulmonary, renal, or hepatic function. Although respiratory effects are minimal, they can enhance respiratory depression of other drugs, such as opioids. Benzodiazepines induce minimal decreases in arterial blood pressure, cardiac output, and vascular resistance similar to those observed during natural sleep. Skeletal muscle relaxant effects are caused by decreased transmission at the internuncial neuron in the spinal cord and not at the myoneural junction.

19. Which benzodiazepines are used in veterinary medicine?

The most commonly used benzodiazepines in veterinary medicine are diazepam, midazolam, and zolazepam (available only in combination with tiletamine, i.e., Telazol). Midazolam is more potent than diazepam and is water soluble. It has a shorter half-life than diazepam but is otherwise similar to diazepam in its effects. Zolazepam is a water-soluble benzodiazepine that is available in combination with tiletamine (Telazol). Zolazepam's pharmacokinetics are similar to those of diazepam and midazolam. It produces less tranquilization than diazepam or midazolam and at high doses can induce dysphoria and excitement.

20. Can the adverse effects of benzodiazepines be reversed?

The benzodiazepines can be reversed by flumazenil, a pure benzodiazepine receptor antagonist.

21. Which drugs reduce and which increase intracranial pressure?

Etomidate, thiopental, and propofol reduce intracranial pressure secondary to decreased cerebral metabolic consumption of oxygen and decreased cerebral blood flow. Ketamine and tiletamine increase cerebral blood flow, intracranial pressure, and cerebral metabolism.

BIBLIOGRAPHY

1. Kohn DF, Wixson SK, White WJ, Benson GJ (eds): Anesthesia and Analgesia in Laboratory Animals. New York, American College of Laboratory Animal Medicine Series, Academic Press, 1997.
2. Thurmon JC, Tranquilli WJ, Benson GJ (eds): Lumb and Jones' Veterinary Anesthesia, 3rd ed. Baltimore, Williams & Wilkins, 1996.
3. Stoelting RK: Pharmacology and Physiology in Anesthetic Practice, 2nd ed. Philadelphia, JB Lippincott, 1991.

16. INHALANT ANESTHETICS

Robert D. Keegan, D.V.M., D.A.C.V.A.

1. What inhalant anesthetics are available for veterinary use?

Halothane, isoflurane, and sevoflurane are approved for veterinary use and desflurane is approved for use in humans. Methoxyflurane is also approved for veterinary use but is not currently being manufactured in the U.S.

2. How do sevoflurane and desflurane compare to isoflurane?

Both sevoflurane and desflurane have cardiovascular and respiratory effects similar to those of isoflurane. Like isoflurane, they are less likely than halothane to be associated with the development of anesthetic-induced cardiac arrhythmias. In addition, both sevoflurane and desflurane undergo minimal hepatic metabolism, similar to isoflurane. Despite similarities, both sevoflurane and desflurane are less potent than isoflurane, thus vaporizer settings of 3–4% are typical for sevoflurane while settings of 8–11% are typical for desflurane. Sevoflurane and desflurane are also less soluble in blood compared with isoflurane. The lower blood solubility translates to a more rapid induction, recovery, and changes in the depth of inhalant anesthesia when using sevoflurane or desflurane.

3. What is a MAC value, why is it useful?

The **Minimum Alveolar Concentration** (MAC) is that concentration of inhalant anesthetic within the alveoli that will prevent gross purposeful movement in 50% of a test population. The MAC value of an inhalant anesthetic is thus a measure of anesthetic potency. It is similar to an ED50 value used for injectable drugs. The MAC value is inversely proportional to anesthetic potency: an inhalant anesthetic having a low MAC value is more potent than an inhalant having a high MAC value. Concentrations of anesthetics are frequently reported as multiples of the MAC value since the MAC value inherently provides information about potency; 1.5 MAC of isoflurane provides the same anesthetic potency as 1.5 MAC of sevoflurane. Thus, MAC values permit comparison of different inhalant anesthetics on an equi-potent basis.

4. What is a partition coefficient (PC)? Why is it useful?

The blood/gas partition coefficient (PC) of an inhalant anesthetic is a measure of the anesthetic's solubility in blood. Individual gases have intrinsic solubility in specific liquids. The solubility of a gas in a liquid defines the relationship between the partial pressure of the gas in the liquid and the volume of gas that is dissolved in the liquid as a result of that partial pressure. Highly soluble gases will have a large volume of gas dissolved within the liquid when the partial pressure of the gas within the liquid is small. Poorly soluble gases, on the other hand, will have a relatively small volume of gas dissolved within the liquid when the partial pressure of the gas within the liquid is high. For an inhalant anesthetic to result in general anesthesia, the drug must enter the patient's brain. The quantity that provides the driving force and results in the transfer of anesthetic from the alveoli to the blood and ultimately the brain is the partial pressure of the anesthetic. It is crucial to the understanding of inhalant uptake to realize that inhalant anesthetics within the body move along partial pressure gradients, not along concentration gradients. A highly soluble anesthetic such as methoxyflurane may have a large volume of inhalant dissolved in the blood but, due to the high intrinsic solubility, the partial pressure will be low and therefore the gradient along which the inhalant moves will be small even though the concentrations within the blood may be quite high. If a high blood concentration is not accompanied by a sufficiently high partial pressure, transfer of inhalant anesthetic from the blood to the brain will occur slowly.

As a result, induction of anesthesia will be delayed. A similar line of reasoning allows us to predict that highly soluble inhalant anesthetics will result in longer recoveries from anesthesia and will provide for slower changes in anesthetic depth when the anesthetic vaporizer setting is altered. The PC value of an inhalant anesthetic is a measure of its solubility.

5. I read that isoflurane may be delivered from a halothane vaporizer. Is this true?

Yes. Isoflurane and halothane are commonly delivered using agent-specific, precision, variable bypass vaporizers. These vaporizers are designed to deliver precise concentrations of a specific inhalant anesthetic having a specific vapor pressure. The vapor pressure of an inhalant anesthetic is an inherent property that determines the maximum attainable concentration of that anesthetic. The vapor pressure is some percentage of atmospheric pressure (760 mm Hg at sea level) and thus specifically determines the maximum percentage of 1 atmosphere that may be attained with any given inhalant anesthetic. For example, the vapor pressure of isoflurane at 20° C is 238 mm Hg. The maximum attainable concentration of isoflurane at 20° C is thus 238/760 = 0.32 of 1 atmosphere or 32%. Since the vapor pressure of halothane at 20° C is similar to that of isoflurane at 243 mm Hg, or 33% of 1 atmosphere, a halothane vaporizer will deliver predictable, clinically useful concentrations of isoflurane. The procedure of converting a vaporizer is simple. Empty the vaporizer of the halothane and fill it with ether or medical grade alcohol overnight. The ether or alcohol will remove residual halothane and thymol, a halothane preservative, from the vaporizer. After emptying the ether or alcohol from the vaporizer, run oxygen at a flow rate of 1–2 L/min through the vaporizer while the dial is set to deliver 5% overnight. After the vaporizer has been flushed of any residual ether or alcohol, it may be filled with isoflurane, relabeled, and placed in use.

6. I have heard that mask inductions are frequently "rough." If so, why do clinicians use them?

Inducing a patient into general anesthesia with an inhalant anesthetic has the advantage of not requiring the patient to metabolize the anesthetic agent to permit him or her to regain consciousness. Inhalant anesthetics such as isoflurane and sevoflurane are inert substances that undergo limited hepatic metabolism. When administration of inhalant is discontinued, the patient's cardiac output and minute ventilation remove the inhalant anesthetic from the patient's body, lowering the brain anesthetic partial pressure, thus permitting recovery from anesthesia. Hepatic metabolism is not strictly necessary for recovery from anesthesia. This feature is advantageous in patients having impaired hepatic metabolism where injectable anesthetics may result in prolonged recovery from anesthesia. Uptake of inhalant anesthetics having low blood solubility, while fairly rapid, is still much slower than induction of anesthesia with a rapidly acting injectable anesthetic such as thiopental or ketamine. The relatively slower induction into anesthesia with the inhalant anesthetics allows the patient to have a prolonged excitement phase of anesthesia and this is manifest as struggling during the induction. The incidence of excitement during mask induction of anesthesia may be markedly reduced through the use of preanesthetic sedative/analgesics and proper technique. A technique that works well for mask inductions in small animals is to administer low concentrations of inhalant anesthetic to sedated or debilitated patients at the start of the induction and to gradually increase the concentration as the induction progresses. As most inhalant anesthetics can be quite pungent and unpleasant to breathe in higher concentrations, the lower initial concentration of the inhalant at the start of the induction facilitates acceptance of the anesthetic drug. Administration of nitrous oxide at the appropriate time during the mask induction may be used to advantage and facilitate a smooth induction into anesthesia (see Question 10). Disadvantages of mask inductions include the possibility of struggling, with resultant rough induction and the possibility of exposure of operating room personnel to anesthetic vapor during the mask induction procedure.

7. Most modern vaporizers look quite similar. Why is the desflurane TEC 6 vaporizer radically different?

Variable bypass precision vaporizers are designed for use with an agent having a specific vapor pressure. These vaporizers perform the function of converting a liquid inhalant anesthetic into a vapor. The maximum concentration of anesthetic that can be generated from the liquid inhalant is a function of the vapor pressure of the inhalant and of the ambient temperature. The higher the vapor pressure or the higher the ambient temperature, the greater the concentration will be output from the vaporizer. Desflurane has a vapor pressure much higher (643 mm Hg at 20° C) than any currently used inhalant anesthetic. The high vapor pressure and steep vapor pressure curve of desflurane translates to large changes in vaporizer output concentration resulting from comparatively small changes in ambient temperature. Most variable bypass precision vaporizers are able to compensate for changes in ambient temperature by controlling the quantity of inhalant that is vaporized. The steep vapor pressure curve of desflurane makes conventional means of compensation impractical, thus the TEC-6 desflurane vaporizer heats the liquid desflurane to a constant 41° C. Since the vapor pressure of desflurane is 1400 mm Hg at 41° C, desflurane may be metered from the vaporizer in gaseous form. Constancy of the output desflurane vaporizer concentration is achieved. Heating is accomplished through the use of an electrically heated vaporization chamber.

8. What is low-flow anesthesia? What are its benefits?

Low-flow anesthesia refers to the use of minimal oxygen carrier gas flows during inhalant anesthesia. The oxygen flow required during inhalant anesthesia varies with the breathing circuit that is employed; however, systems that do not permit rebreathing of exhaled gases require a higher fresh gas flow than systems that do permit significant rebreathing. A low-flow technique is one in which fresh gas flows sufficient to meet metabolic oxygen demand are delivered to the breathing circuit. The patient consumes the oxygen delivered into the breathing circuit, exhaled carbon dioxide is removed by a carbon dioxide absorbent, and the remaining circuit gases including the inhalant anesthetics recirculate and are rebreathed. The amount of inhalant anesthetic vaporized is directly proportional to the fresh gas flow rate presented to the vaporizer; at a fresh gas flow rate of 2 L/min the amount of liquid anesthetic vaporized for any given vaporizer setting is twice as great as when the fresh gas flow rate is 1 L/min. A delivered fresh gas flow rate in excess of patient metabolic demand is wasteful because some fresh gas and some vaporized inhalant anesthetic escape the breathing circuit through the APL (pop-off) Valve and are captured by the waste gas scavenging unit. Thus, a big advantage of minimal fresh gas flow techniques is economic: if delivering flows in excess of those required to meet metabolic demand is not beneficial, why waste liquid inhalant anesthetic and fresh gases such as oxygen and nitrous oxide? In addition to the economic advantages of minimal flow techniques, significant rebreathing of exhaled gases permits patients to retain body heat and moisture to a greater degree compared with conventional higher flow techniques. Limitations to the use of minimal flow techniques include an increased risk of administration of a hypoxic gas mixture, a limitation on the ability to deliver nitrous oxide into the breathing mixture and difficulties experienced during induction, recovery, and changes in the depth of anesthesia.

9. I have tried using low-flow techniques, but my patients keep waking up. Why?

A low-flow technique is one in which the oxygen flow supplied to the circuit is just sufficient to meet the metabolic oxygen demand of the patient. Typically, low-flow techniques are delivered through relatively high-volume circle breathing circuits which permit significant rebreathing of exhaled gases. The typical internal volume of these circuits is surprisingly large, comprising approximately 7 liters. A low initial inspired concentration is seen because the patient inspires from the breathing circuit and not directly from the anesthetic vaporizer. The rate at which the circle and therefore the inspired anesthetic concentration may be increased is directly dependent upon the fresh gas flow rate transiting the vaporizer and entering the breathing circuit (see Question 13). The higher the fresh gas flow rate, the more rapidly the circuit and thus the inspired concentrations will approach what is exiting the vaporizer. A technique that uses minimal or low carrier gas flows to deliver the inhalant anesthetic to the breathing circuit results in a relatively slow approach of circuit concentrations to those exiting the vaporizer. Since most IV induction agents may be expected to be associated with a 10–15 minute period of unconsciousness, uptake of the inhalant anesthetic must occur rapidly and effect sufficient CNS depression before the patient awakens prematurely. It is not possible to achieve the high inspired inhalant concentrations within the time afforded by IV induction anesthetics at fresh gas flow rates that match the patient's metabolic oxygen demand. Instead of trying to run a patient on a closed circuit immediately following induction of anesthesia, increase the fresh gas flow rate (to 3–5 L/min) into the breathing circuit for the first 5–15 minutes following induction using typical vaporizer settings. The high fresh gas flow rate will make the circuit concentration approach the concentration of inhalant anesthetic exiting the vaporizer much more rapidly than the lower flow rates used with closed circuits. This rapid achievement of high circuit anesthetic concentrations will permit rapid uptake of inhalant anesthetic and result in a smooth transition from IV to inhalant anesthesia. Once the patient is in a stable plane of anesthesia and patient uptake of inhalant from the breathing circuit is decreased (usually 10–15 minutes for isoflurane), the fresh gas flow rate may be gradually reduced to the low and economical flow rates associated with closed circuit anesthesia.

10. What are the advantages to the use of nitrous oxide in veterinary patients?
    Nitrous oxide may be used in conjunction with oxygen as the fresh gas flow into the breathing circuit. In addition to flowing through the anesthetic vaporizer and delivering the inhaled anesthetic to the breathing circuit, nitrous oxide has the ability to cause CNS depression and to provide analgesia when administered to veterinary patients. Although nitrous oxide is an inhaled analgesic, it is not potent enough to achieve anesthesia under normal circumstances. The so-called potent inhalant anesthetic agents all have MAC values well below 10%, while the MAC value of nitrous oxide in humans is 105% and is considerable higher (180%–200%) in most animal species. The low potency of nitrous oxide necessitates administration of high concentrations if any beneficial effect is to be realized. Administered concentrations of between 50% and 70% are common when using nitrous oxide. The potential beneficial effects of administration of nitrous oxide include improved analgesia, enhanced CNS depression, a more stable plane of anesthesia, and a more rapid induction into anesthesia via the second gas effect. Clinicians who favor the use of nitrous oxide feel that the anesthetic adds additional analgesia and sedation without resultant depression of the patient's cardiovascular system. An additional advantage to the use of nitrous oxide particularly during the induction of anesthesia is the so-called second gas effect.

11. What is the second gas effect?
    The second gas effect refers to the enhanced uptake of potent inhalant agents such as isoflurane when administered concomitantly with high concentrations of nitrous oxide. The high partial pressure gradient generated by the administration of high concentrations of nitrous oxide results in the rapid uptake of nitrous oxide from the alveoli into the blood. The rapid removal of nitrous oxide decreases the total volume of gas present within the alveoli such that the isoflurane becomes a larger proportion of the total volume within the alveoli, hence its concentration has increased at the alveolar level. The higher concentration of isoflurane results in a larger partial pressure gradient promoting the transfer of isoflurane from the alveoli into the blood. The net result is a more rapid uptake of isoflurane and a more rapid induction into inhalant anesthesia. Nitrous oxide's second gas effect is often useful during mask inductions in small animals. As the anesthetic vaporizer is gradually increased during the induction, nitrous oxide may be introduced to invoke the second gas effect as the animal loses consciousness in an effort to carry the patient rapidly through the excitement phase of induction. Although several past and recent studies have validated the existence of the second gas effect and the beneficial effects have been in widespread clinical use, at least one study has disputed the validity of the second gas effect.

12. What are the disadvantages to the use of nitrous oxide in veterinary patients?
    Nitrous oxide is a gaseous anesthetic that must be administered in high concentrations because of low anesthetic potency. The high concentrations of nitrous oxide necessarily limit the concentration of oxygen which may be administered concurrently. Patients presenting with dis-

turbances in oxygen transport may require a high-inspired oxygen concentration to insure adequate oxygenation during anesthesia. The low potency of nitrous oxide necessitates administration of high-inspired concentrations to gain any beneficial effect. The high-inspired concentrations of nitrous oxide necessarily reduce the inspired oxygen concentration and may thus promote hypoxemia in the patient having impaired oxygen exchange. An additional consequence of the necessarily high concentrations of nitrous oxide is the tendency of nitrous oxide to pool into air-filled spaces within the patient's body. The administered nitrous oxide may accumulate in closed, air-containing pockets to such a degree that the volume of those pockets markedly increases. The increased volume of an air-containing pneumothorax or intestinal volvulus may interfere with venous return to the heart, thus impeding cardiac output, and it may inhibit chest expansion, making it difficult or impossible to achieve a normal minute ventilation. In practice, nitrous oxide is the only medical gas in which the phenomenon of closed space pooling occurs. This phenomenon, however, is not linked to some unusual property that is unique to nitrous oxide. Any inspired gas will exhibit this behavior provided both that the gas is inspired in high enough concentrations and that the gas has sufficient solubility in blood. The closed pockets within the body contain large quantities of nitrogen from ambient air. Although nitrogen is present in high quantities in ambient air, it is a poorly soluble gas in blood, meaning that the blood has a limited capacity to serve as a solvent for nitrogen and thus cannot transport large quantities of nitrogen. As mentioned, nitrous oxide is the only inhalant anesthetic that is administered in concentrations ranging from 50% to 70%. This high concentration of inspired nitrous oxide coupled with the 34 times greater blood solubility of nitrous oxide compared to that of nitrogen translates to a much larger quantity of nitrous oxide carried in the blood compared to nitrogen. When administration of nitrous oxide is begun, the high partial pressure of nitrous oxide in the lung creates a large partial pressure gradient that favors the uptake of nitrous oxide into the blood. The comparatively higher blood solubility of nitrous oxide dictates that a large volume of nitrous oxide will dissolve in the blood and be carried throughout the body. When blood carrying large volumes of nitrous oxide perfuses the closed pocket containing large quantities of nitrogen, the partial pressure gradient for nitrous oxide favors movement of nitrous oxide into the pocket while the partial pressure gradient for nitrogen favors the movement of nitrogen out of the pocket and into the blood. Due to the differences in blood solubility of nitrous oxide and nitrogen, the circulating blood flow will carry a much greater volume of nitrous oxide to the pocket than it will carry nitrogen away from the pocket. The net result is an increase in the volume of the pocket (if the walls of the pocket are distensible) due to the differential delivery and removal of nitrous oxide and nitrogen. If the walls of the air-containing space are non-compliant, as is found in facial sinuses, the differential delivery and removal still occurs, with the result being an increase in the pressure within the space rather than an increase in volume.

13. How important is oxygen flow rate in determining the speed of induction when administering inhalation anesthesia?

When administering inhalant anesthesia using a rebreathing circuit, the carrier gas flow rate is a major factor influencing speed of inhalant induction and the rapidity at which the depth of anesthesia may be altered. The patient draws their respiratory gases not directly from the vaporizer but from the breathing circuit. The breathing circuit inserts a relatively large volume to act as a buffer area between the anesthetic vaporizer and the patient. Changes in vaporizer dial settings are not immediately "seen" by the patient because of the presence of the circuit buffer. The higher the carrier gas flow rate transiting the vaporizer, the more rapidly the circuit concentration (and therefore the inspired concentration) will approach the concentration exiting the vaporizer. The rate of rise of the circuit concentration may be calculated from the time constant equation: $1 - 1/e^{KT}$ where e is the base of the natural logarithms, K is a constant equal to flow/volume (for 1 time constant K is thus equal to 1), and T is time. From the equation it may be calculated that a carrier gas flow rate of 7 L/min transiting a container having a 7 L volume will effect a 63% change in circuit anesthetic concentration in 1 minute. That is, after 1 minute the anesthetic concentration within the breathing circuit will be 63% of the concentration that is leaving the vaporizer. Further, it may be shown that after 2 minutes of a 7 L/min flow into a 7 L circuit, the anesthetic concentration within the breathing circuit will be 86% of the concentration leaving the vaporizer, while after 3 minutes the concentration within the breathing circuit has reached 95% of the vaporizer output concentration. When administering anesthesia through a rebreathing circuit, the setting of the vaporizer controls the maximum or minimum concentration that will be inspired by the patient while the fresh gas flow transiting the vaporizer effectively controls the rate at which the inspired circuit concentration will rise to approach that set by the vaporizer.

14. Is there any advantage to the use of epidurally administered analgesics concurrent with inhalant anesthesia?

Definitely! Epidurally administered analgesics have been reported to reduce the MAC value for inhalant anesthetics. The combination of the epidurally administered analgesic and the lower inspired anesthetic concentration usually translates to better cardiovascular conditions particularly in patients presenting with cardiovascular compromise. Patients receiving epidurally administered analgesics prior to the beginning of the surgical procedure tend to be much more stable patients during the surgery. Physiologic responses to pain that occur during anesthesia to facilitate painful surgical procedures are blunted because the patient's perception of pain is markedly reduced. Even during normally painful orthopedic manipulations, patients given epidural analgesics remain adequately anesthetized and nonresponsive to painful procedures at very low vaporizer settings. In addition, administration of analgesics prior to the start of surgery (so called preemptive analgesia) has been shown to decrease or prevent the central and peripheral sensitization that occurs once painful impulses are transmitted to the brain. Sensitization enhances the pain-transmitting pathways in the CNS, widening the range of stimuli which are perceived as painful, resulting in a patient who is more refractory to the analgesic effect of opioids and other analgesics. As a result, patients experiencing sensitization require much higher doses of post-operative analgesics and a much longer course of analgesic therapy. Human studies have shown that pre-emptively administered analgesics, such as epidural opioids, reduce the length of hospital stays following surgical procedures. In dogs, morphine at a dose of 0.1 mg/kg in 0.25 ml/kg of saline injected into the lumbosacral epidural space provides analgesic effects for up to 24 hours.

15. I have read that sevoflurane can be degraded in the presence of soda lime with resultant production of a toxic compound. How serious is this problem and under what conditions is the toxin likely to be produced?

Sevoflurane can react with carbon dioxide absorbent (soda lime or Baralyme) in rebreathing anesthetic circuits to produce a vinyl ether known as "Compound A." High doses of Compound A have been demonstrated to be associated with renal tubular necrosis and subsequent death. Significant production of Compound A in clinical anesthesia is problematic only if low-flow anesthesia is administered for a prolonged period of time. If it is desired to administer sevoflurane using low-flow or closed circuit techniques, it is recommended that fresh gas flow rates be increased periodically to flush out any accumulations of Compound A that may occur within the circuit. The toxic production of Compound A must be recognized but should not dissuade the practitioner from the use of sevoflurane, even in low flow systems. No human volunteer study undertaken to date has produced any evidence that administration of sevoflurane for long periods of time using low-flow circuits is associated with clinical or subclinical organ toxicity.

16. I've noticed that the most recently introduced inhalants for veterinary use, isoflurane and sevoflurane, have low blood solubility and thus have the potential to allow anesthetic depth to be changed very rapidly. Is this a trend and is low blood solubility always advantageous?

It does seem to be a trend that the recently introduced inhalant anesthetics have lower blood solubility when compared to the older inhalants such as halothane and methoxyflurane. Solubility in the patient's blood is the primary factor in determining speed of induction, speed of recovery and the ability to change depth of anesthesia rapidly. The CNS depressant effect achieved by inhalant anesthetics is directly related to the partial pressure that the anesthetic exerts on the CNS, not necessarily to the absolute concentration of inhalant anesthetic in the blood. Inhalant anesthetics that are highly soluble in blood have a large concentration of anesthetic dissolved within the circulating blood volume, but this large dissolved volume of inhalant generates a comparatively small partial pressure, and thus the degree of CNS depression is small. Conversely, an inhalant that is relatively insoluble in blood requires relatively small volumes of anesthetic to be dissolved within the circulating blood volume to generate a comparatively high partial pressure and therefore anesthetic effect. Since high blood solubility delays the development of a comparatively high anesthetic partial pressure, agents having low blood solubility generate high partial pressures much more rapidly compared with agents having high blood solubility. An advantage of using anesthetics that possess low blood solubility is the ability to rapidly adjust the administered partial pressure and thus the degree of CNS depression. Depth of anesthesia of the patient is thus much more responsive to changes in inspired anesthetic concentration when highly insoluble inhalant anesthetics are administered. This is particularly advantageous in critical patients when an anesthetist is monitoring the patient constantly. Low blood solubility and the ability to rapidly change anesthetic depth is not always advantageous, however, particularly when an anesthetist is not available to constantly monitor the patient. In this situation, it may be more advantageous to administer an anesthetic having higher blood solubility such that depth of anesthesia changes more slowly in response to changes in inspired anesthetic concentrations. Without a trained anesthetist immediately available to respond to changes in patient depth, an inhalant which was associated with comparatively slow changes in anesthetic partial pressure may be advantageous. A final consideration of the differences in inhalant anesthetic solubility is the total amount of anesthetic absorbed by the patient during a surgical procedure. Large volumes of highly soluble inhalant anesthetics will be absorbed by the various tissue groups of the patient. The longer the period of anesthesia and the higher the solubility of the inhalant, the larger the volume of administered anesthetic will be absorbed. The large volumes of soluble anesthetics absorbed by the various tissues increase the opportunity for the patient to metabolize the anesthetic, which in turn increases the likelihood that reactive or toxic metabolites may be produced in the course of metabolism.

Properties of Inhalant Anesthetics

PROPERTY	HALOTHANE	ISOFLURANE	SEVOFLURANE	DESFLURANE	NITROUS OXIDE
MAC (Dog)	0.87	1.30	2.36	7.20	188
Partition coefficient					
(blood/gas solubility)	2.54	1.46	0.68	0.42	0.47
Vapor pressure at 20° C	243	240	160	664	—

BIBLIOGRAPHY

1. Sun X-G, Su F, Lee C: The "second gas effect" is not a valid concept. Anesth Analg 88:188-192, 1999.
2. Eger EI 2nd: Anesthetic Uptake and Action. Baltimore, Williams and Wilkins, 1975.
3. Brown B: Sevoflurane: Introduction and overview. Anesth Analg 81:S1-S3, 1995.
4. Woolf CJ, Chong M: Preemptive analgesia: Treating postoperative pain by preventing the establishment of central sensitization. Anesth Analg 77:362-369, 1993.
5. Malan TP: Sevoflurane and renal function. Anesth Analg 81:S39-S45, 1995.
6. Eger EI 2nd: Nitrous Oxide. New York, Elsevier, 1985.
7. Dobromylskyj P, Flecknell PA, Lascelles BD, et al: Management of postoperative and other acute pain. In Flecknell PA, Waterman-Pearson A (eds): Pain Management in Animals. London, W. B. Saunders, 2000, pp 81-145.
8. Kharash ED: Biotransformation of sevoflurane. Anesth Analg 81:S27-S38, 1995.
9. Steffey EP: Inhalation anesthetics. In Thurmon JC, Tranquilli WJ, Benson GJ (eds): Lumb and Jones' Veterinary Anesthesia, 3rd ed. Baltimore, Williams & Wilkins, 1996, pp 297-329.
10. Kenna JG, Jones RM: The organ toxicity of inhaled anesthetics. Anesth Analg 81:S51-S66, 1995.
11. Baden JM, Rice SA: Metabolism and toxicity. In Miller RD (ed): Anesthesia, 3rd ed. New York, Churchill-Livingstone, 1990, pp 135-170.

17. LOCAL ANESTHETICS

Leigh A. Lamont, D.V.M.

1. What was the first local anesthetic to be discovered?

Cocaine is an alkaloid present in the leaves of *Erythroxylon coca,* a shrub that grows in the Andes Mountains, some 1000 to 3000 m above sea level. Inhabitants of the Peruvian highlands chew or suck the leaves primed with plant ash to obtain the sense of well-being it produces. The pure alkaloid was first isolated in 1860; however, the compound was not used clinically until 1884, when Sigmund Freud and Karl Koller published a general study of the physiologic effects of cocaine, noting that instillation of the drug into the conjunctival sac produced anesthesia of the eye. This prompted efforts to develop chemical substitutes for cocaine that were less addictive and toxic but retained local anesthetic activity. This ultimately led to the synthesis of procaine in 1905 by Einhorn, followed some 40 years later by the synthesis of lidocaine in 1943 by Lofgren.

2. What is the general chemical structure of local anesthetics?

The basic local anesthetic molecule has three parts: a hydrophilic end, which confers water solubility, a lipophilic end, which provides lipid solubility, and an intermediate hydrocarbon chain connecting the two ends. The hydrophilic end is usually a tertiary amine (that is, a nitrogen atom with three attached organic groups), but there are a few examples of secondary amines. The lipophilic end is aromatic and is derived from either benzoic acid or aniline.

3. What are the two main categories of local anesthetics based on chemical structure?

Local anesthetics are typically classified as either esters (e.g., procaine) or amides (e.g., lidocaine, bupivacaine) based on the structure of the intermediate chain and its linkage to the aromatic group. Ester-linked compounds are derived from benzoic acid, while amide-linked compounds are derived from aniline.

4. How does the chemical structure of local anesthetics affect their activity?

Increasing the lipophilicity of the compound increases both the potency and the duration of action of local anesthetics. This is a result of more extensive association of the drug at lipophilic (hydrophobic) sites, which decreases the rate of hydrolysis by plasma esterases and enhances the partitioning of the drug to its sites of action. Lipophilicity also tends to increase potential toxicity for these same reasons.

5. What is the effect of protein binding on local anesthetic activity?

Protein binding is believed to be the primary determinant of local anesthetic duration. The greater the binding affinity for axonal membrane protein, the longer local anesthetic activity persists.

6. How does pH affect local anesthetic activity?

The acid dissociation constant (pK_a) of a local anesthetic is important in determining the rate of onset of action. At physiologic pH, local anesthetics exist in solution as both a charged cation and an uncharged base. With pK_a values in the 8 to 9 range, local anesthetics are weak bases, with most of the drug existing in the hydrophilic protonated form. The charged cation does not readily penetrate lipid membranes compared to the uncharged base; thus, drugs with lower pK_a values (that is, closer to physiologic pH) tend to have a more rapid onset of action.

7. Describe the events underlying normal nerve impulse conduction.

Nerve fibers have a lipoprotein membrane that separates the intracellular matrix from the extracellular phase. A concentration gradient between the intracellular fluid (containing mainly potassium) and the extracellular fluid (containing mainly sodium) is maintained by an active metabolic process involving Na$^+$-K$^+$-ATPase. In the resting state, the membrane is polarized, with a potential of -70 to -90mV, with the exterior positive relative to the interior. During an action potential, voltage-gated Na$^+$ channels that are in the activated state open briefly, allowing influx of extracellular Na$^+$ ions to flow into the cell. The membrane potential is transiently elevated to its threshold and depolarization occurs, which is spread electrically to adjacent areas of membrane. Membrane repolarization is mediated by voltage-gated K$^+$ channels, which conduct an outward K$^+$ current that restores electrical neutrality.

8. How do local anesthetics prevent transmission of nerve impulses?

Local anesthetics produce conduction blockade by inhibiting voltage-gated Na$^+$ channels located on nerve cell membranes. A portion of the Na$^+$ channel itself found within the intracellular half of the transmembrane pore, forms a specific receptor for local anesthetics. Binding of both protonated and neutral local anesthetic molecules effectively interferes with the conformational changes, known as "gating," that underlie the process of channel activation. Suspended in the inactivated state, the subsequent failure of Na$^+$ channel permeability to increase slows the rate of depolarization such that threshold potential is not reached and an action potential is not propagated. Despite earlier popular theories, actual occlusion of open Na$^+$ channels by local anesthetic molecules appears to contribute little to overall channel inhibition and reduced ionic current flow.

9. What is meant by the terms *frequency-dependent* and *voltage-dependent* blockade?

The degree of blockade produced by a given concentration of local anesthetic depends on how the nerve has been stimulated and on its resting membrane potential. A higher frequency of stimulation and more positive membrane potential results in more intense blockade. Conversely, resting nerves are much less sensitive to local anesthetics. These frequency- and voltage-dependent effects occur because the local anesthetic molecule in its charged form gains access to its binding site only when the Na$^+$ channel is in its activated ("open") state, and because the local anesthetic binds more avidly to the inactivated state of the channel, thereby stabilizing it. The degree to which a given local anesthetic exhibits these two phenomena depends on its physicochemical properties, including pKa, lipid solubility, and molecular size.

10. Does the type of nerve fiber influence sensitivity to blockade by local anesthetics?

Yes. Nerve size appears to be a critical factor in determining sensitivity to local anesthetic block. In general, small unmyelinated C fibers (mediating pain sensations) are blocked before small myelinated Aδ fibers (mediating pain and temperature sensations), which are in turn blocked before larger myelinated Aγ, Aβ, and Aα fibers (carrying touch, pressure, and motor information). Smaller nonmyelinated fibers are preferentially blocked because the critical length over which an impulse can propagate passively is shorter. In myelinated nerves, it is generally agreed that local anesthetic concentrations great enough to block three consecutive nodes of Ranvier are required to stop electric transmission through an axon, which favors blockade in fibers with shorter internodal distances.

11. What effect does the addition of epinephrine have on neuronal blockade?

The duration of action of a local anesthetic is proportional to the time during which it is in contact with the nerve. Thus, in the past, preparations containing vasoconstrictors (usually epinephrine) were employed to minimize systemic absorption, prolong the duration of local anesthetic action, and localize the effects of the anesthetic to the desired site, which in turn may reduce potential toxicity. In light of the availability of longer-acting agents with higher margins of safety (such as bupivacaine, ropivacaine), the addition of vasoconstrictors to local anesthetic preparations offers fewer advantages in current clinical practice.

12. How are local anesthetics absorbed?

The systemic absorption of local anesthetics is primarily a function of dose and route of administration. Uptake from mucosal, pleural, and peritoneal surfaces is rapid and complete. Similarly, absorption after epidural administration is also relatively quick, whereas uptake following subcutaneous deposition is much slower. The addition of a vasoconstrictor, such as epinephrine, to the local anesthetic preparation may slow the rate of systemic absorption.

13. How are local anesthetics distributed throughout the body?

The liver and the lungs are the primary sites for plasma clearance of local anesthetics. Protein binding may also influence drug distribution by confining local anesthetic to the tissue compartment into which it was administered.

14. How are local anesthetics metabolized and excreted?

Most local anesthetics undergo enzymatic hydrolysis. Aminoesters are hydrolyzed and inactivated primarily by plasma cholinesterase, and the metabolites are excreted in the urine. As plasma cholinesterase is synthesized in the liver, hepatic function can indirectly affect hydrolysis of this group of local anesthetics. Aminoamides, for the most part, are degraded by the hepatic endoplasmic reticulum via an initial N-dealkylation reaction followed by hydrolysis, with metabolites excreted in the urine.

15. In addition to blocking conduction in nerve axons in the peripheral nervous system, what other organ systems do local anesthetics affect?

Local anesthetics may interfere with the function of all organs in which the conduction or transmission of impulses occurs. They have important effects on the central nervous system, the autonomic ganglia, the neuromuscular junction, the myocardium, and smooth muscle function.

16. What are most common types of systemic toxicity associated with local anesthetic administration?

Acute systemic toxicity is most often the result of accidental intravenous injection and manifests as central nervous system stimulation. Restlessness and muscle tremors are usually the first signs of toxicity, which, depending on dose, may progress to generalized seizures and even unconsciousness and respiratory arrest. At higher doses, cardiovascular toxicity arising from direct cardiac and vascular effects, as well as conduction blockade of autonomic fibers, may be seen. Local anesthetics target the myocardium primarily, causing decreases in electrical excitability, conduction rate, and force of contraction. Arterial vasodilation resulting in profound hypotension may also be noted. Evidence suggests that bupivacaine affects the heart somewhat differently than do other local anesthetics, making it the most cardiotoxic of all drugs in its class.

17. What types of localized tissue toxicity can be seen?

Both neural structures and skeletal muscle are susceptible to cytotoxic damage secondary to local anesthetic administration. The more potent, highly concentrated local anesthetics, as well as those preparations containing the preservative sodium bisulfite, can be neurotoxic. Skeletal muscle changes have been observed after intramuscular administration of a variety of commonly used local anesthetics, including lidocaine and bupivacaine. The use of products containing a vasoconstrictor may also contribute to delayed wound healing and promote tissue necrosis, especially if administered to distal extremities that have limited collateral circulation.

18. What are the maximum recommended dosages of the most commonly used local anesthetics in companion animal practice?

Based on experimental evidence and clinical experience, the following dosages constitute safe upper limits for perineural and infiltrative administration. In most situations, doses much lower than these are necessary to achieve the desired effect. It should be noted that bupivacaine should not be administered intravenously at any dose.

	Dogs	*Cats*
Lidocaine	up to 10 mg/kg	up to 6 mg/kg
Bupivacaine	up to 3 mg/kg	up to 2 mg/kg

19. Which local anesthetics have been associated with methemoglobinemia?

Although prilocaine has traditionally been considered unique in its propensity to cause methemoglobinemia, reports have implicated benzocaine, procaine, and even lidocaine as other potential causative agents. Development of methemoglobinemia is dose-dependent and results when ferrous iron (Fe^{2+}) in hemoglobin is oxidized to the ferric form (Fe^{3+}).

20. Are allergic reactions to local anesthetics common?

No, they are very uncommon. The aminoesters (e.g., procaine) are derived from p-amino benzoic acid, a common allergen, and have been documented to induce both local and systemic anaphylactic reactions in rare instances. In addition, solutions containing the preservative methyl-paraben have also been implicated as the cause of allergic reactions.

21. What local anesthetic techniques are most frequently employed in companion animal practice?

Local anesthetics are commonly administered topically, epidurally, interpleurally, intra-artic-ularly, infiltratively, intravenously (regional anesthesia), and perineurally (including brachial plexus blockade, dental nerve blockade, and intercostal nerve blockade).

22. What local anesthetic techniques are most frequently employed in equine practice?

Local anesthetics are commonly administered topically, infiltratively, intra-articularly, and perineurally (most often to produce regional anesthesia of the foot or head). In this species par-ticularly, local anesthetic techniques are essential diagnostic tools, as well as effective and eco-nomic methods for supplementing anesthesia and analgesia.

23. What local anesthetic techniques are most frequently employed in ruminants and swine?

Local anesthetics are commonly administered topically, infiltratively, epidurally, perineu-rally (including paravertebral blocks), and intravenously (to produce regional anesthesia). Owing to the technical difficulties and considerable cost associated with general anesthesia in these species, local or regional techniques are the preferred methods for producing surgical anesthesia/analgesia.

24. Can local anesthetics be administered systemically to provide analgesia?

Yes. Lidocaine can be administered intravenously in low doses as a constant rate infusion to supplement analgesia and improve bowel motility. Because of its cardiovascular toxicity, bupi-vacaine should never be administered intravenously at any dose.

25. Compare the physical, chemical, and pharmacologic properties of the commonly used local anesthetics in companion animal practice.

Agent	Molecular Weight	Lipid Solubility	Relative Potency	pKa	Onset of Action	Plasma Protein Binding (%)	Duration (min)
Procaine	236	1	1	8.9	slow	6	60–90
Lidocaine	234	3.6	2	7.7	fast	65	90–200
Mepivacaine	246	2	2	7.6	fast	75	120–240
Bupivacaine	288	30	8	8.1	intermediate	95	180–300
Etidocaine	276	140	6	7.7	fast	95	180–300
Ropivacaine	274	10	8	8.1	fast	94	180–300

BIBLIOGRAPHY

1. Butterworth JF, Strichartz GR: Molecular mechanisms of local anesthesia: A review. Anesthesiology 72:711–734, 1990.
2. Catterall W, Mackie K: Local anesthetics. In Goodman Gilman A, Rall TW, Nies AS, Taylor P (eds): Goodman and Gilman's The Pharmacological Basis of Therapeutics, 9th ed. New York, Pergamon Press, 1995, pp 331–341.
3. Heavner JE: Local anesthetics. In Thurmon JC, Tranquilli WJ, Benson GJ (eds): Lumb and Jones Veteri-nary Anesthesia, 3rd ed. Baltimore, Williams and Wilkins, 1996, pp 330–336.
4. Lemke KA, Dawson SD: Local and regional anesthesia. Vet Clin North Am 30(4):839–857, 2000.
5. Stoelting RK: Local anesthetics. In Pharmacology and Physiology in Anesthetic Practice, 3rd ed. Philadel-phia, Lippincott-Raven, 1999, pp 158–181.

18. NEUROMUSCULAR BLOCKING AGENTS

Elizabeth A. Martinez, D.V.M., D.A.C.V.A.

1. Why use neuromuscular blocking agents in veterinary anesthesia?

Neuromuscular blocking agents (NMBAs) can be administered prior to intubation when rapid control of the animal's airway is needed without coughing, gagging, or laryngospasm and can be given intraoperatively when mechanical ventilation is used, for relaxation during fracture or luxation reductions, or to ensure a motionless eye during ophthalmologic procedures.

2. Do NMBAs provide sedation or analgesia?

No. Therefore, it is very important that a patient given a NMBA be monitored closely to ensure that an adequate plane of anesthesia is present. NMBAs should never be given alone for immobilization for any reason.

3. How are NMBAs classified?

NMBAs are divided into two groups: depolarizing and nondepolarizing drugs.

4. Describe the mechanism of action of depolarizing NMBAs.

Depolarizing drugs act by binding to postsynaptic acetylcholine (ACh) receptors at the neuromuscular junction, in the same way ACh does, causing transient muscle fasciculations followed by persistent depolarization of the muscle fiber.

5. Describe the mechanism of action of nondepolarizing NMBAs.

Nondepolarizing NMBAs interfere with the postsynaptic action of ACh by binding to ACh receptors, preventing depolarization and muscle contraction of the muscle fiber.

6. What depolarizing NMBAs are used in veterinary anesthesia?

Succinylcholine is the only depolarizing drug used in veterinary anesthesia. Its use is limited due to a rapid onset and short duration of action. Termination of its effects is from hydrolysis by plasma cholinesterase. Anything that decreases plasma cholinesterase levels (organophosphates, malnutrition, liver disease) will prolong succinylcholine's duration of action.

7. What nondepolarizing NMBAs are used in veterinary anesthesia?

Several nondepolarizing drugs are available that are commonly used in veterinary anesthesia. The one selected depends on the desired duration of action, possible side effects, and how the drug is metabolized.

- **Atracurium**
  - Intermediate duration of action (20–35 minutes).
  - Termination of effects primarily from Hoffman elimination.
  - Histamine release can occur following administration of high doses.
  - Laudanosine, a metabolite of atracurium can cause central nervous system stimulation or cardiovascular depression.
- **Vecuronium**
  - Intermediate duration of action (25 minutes).
  - Lack of histamine-releasing or cardiovascular side effects.
  - Hepatic metabolism.
- **Pancuronium**
  - Long duration of effect (30–45 minutes).
  - Possible sympathetic and vagolytic effects: tachycardia, increased arterial blood pressure.
  - Primary route of elimination is via the kidneys.

- **Mivacurium**
  - Duration of action is 15 to 20 minutes.
  - Rapid onset of action.
  - Histamine release can occur.
  - Metabolism via plasma cholinesterase.
- **Cisatracurium**
  - A stereoisomer of atracurium, with approximately 10 times the potency.
  - At equipotent doses, a similar onset and duration of action as atracurium.
  - Lack of histamine release.
  - Undergoes Hoffman elimination.

8. What are the doses for the commonly used nondepolarizing NMBAs in dogs and cats?

Drug	Dose (mg/kg IV)
Atracurium	0.22
Vecuronium	0.1
Pancuronium	0.044–0.11
Mivacurium	ND
Cisatracurium	ND

9. How is the degree of neuromuscular blockade monitored?

The method most commonly used to monitor the degree of neuromuscular blockade is by observation of evoked responses following supramaximal nerve stimulation using a peripheral nerve stimulator. The nerves most commonly stimulated in small animal veterinary patients are the ulnar and peroneal facial nerves.

10. Describe the train-of-four pattern of stimulation.

The train-of-four pattern of stimulation delivers four supramaximal impulses at a frequency of two per second (2 Hz). The degree of muscle relaxation can then be evaluated by comparing the fourth to the first twitch response in the train-of-four. The prerelaxant ratio is approximately 1.0 (the first and fourth twitch being equal in strength). As the degree of relaxation deepens, the ratio decreases, followed by the loss of one or more twitches in the train-of-four. The fourth, third, second, and first twitches disappear, in this order, as the block becomes more profound. During recovery from neuromuscular blockade, the first twitch returns first, followed by the second, third, and forth twitches. The twitches will gradually return to prerelaxant strength during the recovery period. A fourth to first twitch ratio of greater than 0.7 correlates with clinical signs of adequate recovery.

11. Can the effects of NMBAs be antagonized?

Yes. Residual blockade following administration of a nondepolarizing drug can be reversed with the use of anticholinesterase drugs (neostigmine, pyridostigmine, edrophonium). These drugs act by inhibiting acetylcholinesterase, which allows for the build-up of ACh at the neuromuscular junction and the restoration of neuromuscular transmission.

12. Why should an anticholinergic drug be given immediately prior to or concurrently with the reversal agent?

Anticholinesterase drugs have both nicotinic and cholinergic effects which can cause significant bradycardia. This may be prevented or attenuated with the administration of an anticholinergic drug (atropine, glycopyrrolate).

13. What are possible complications during the anesthesia recovery period in patients given NMBAs?

Respiratory depression and muscle weakness due to residual paralysis can occur, even in patients given an anticholinesterase drug. It is very important to observe these patients closely to ensure adequate ventilation and muscle strength.

BIBLIOGRAPHY

1. Benson GJ, Thurmon JC: Clinical pharmacology of succinylcholine. J Am Vet Med Assoc 176(7): 646–647, 1980.
2. Brand JB, Cullen DJ, Wilson NF, et al: Spontaneous recovery from nondepolarizing neuromuscular blockade: Correlation between clinical and evoked response. Anesth Analg 56:55–58, 1977.
3. Fisher DM, Canfell PC, Fahey MR, et al: Elimination of atracurium in humans: contribution of Hofmann elimination and ester hydrolysis versus organ-based elimination. Anesthesiology 65:6–12, 1986.
4. Martinez EA, Mealey KA: Muscle relaxants. In Boothe DM (ed): Small Animal Pharmacology and Therapeutics. Philadelphia, W.B. Saunders, 2001, pp 473–481.
5. Miller RD, Rupp SM, Fisher DM, et al: Clinical pharmacology of vecuronium and atracurium. Anesthesiology 61:444–453, 1984.
6. Mirakhur RK: Newer neuromuscular blocking drugs: An overview of their clinical pharmacology and therapeutic use. Drugs 44(2):182–199, 1992.
7. Nimbex (cisatracurium besylate) injection prescribing information. Research Triangle Park, NC, Glaxo Wellcome Inc., 1996.
8. Plumb DC: Drug monographs. In Veterinary Drug Handbook. White Bear Lake, Pharma Vet Publishing, 1995.
9. Scott RPF, Savarese JJ, Basta SJ, et al: Atracurium: Clinical strategies for preventing histamine release and attenuating the hemodynamic response. Br J Anaesth 57:550–553, 1985.
10. Silverman DG, Mirakhur RK: Nondepolarizing relaxants of long duration. In Silverman DG (ed): Neuromuscular Block in Perioperative and Intensive Care. Philadelphia, JB Lippincott, 1994, p 174.
11. Stoelting RK: The hemodynamic effects of pancuronium with d-tubocurarine in anesthetized patients. Anesthesiology 36:612–615, 1972.

IV. Patient Monitoring

19. RESPIRATORY MONITORING

Deborah V. Wilson, B.V.Sc., M.S., D.A.C.V.A.

1. What is the definition of respiration? Why do we care?

Respiration is the sum total of the chemical and physical processes in an organism by which oxygen is conveyed to the tissues and the oxidation products—carbon dioxide and water—are given off. Most of the ways that we can monitor respiration relate to the measurement of gas tensions, or to the physical act of moving respiratory gases out of the lungs. We care because patients with inadequate respiration or gas exchange could die without appropriate intervention.

2. What options do you have for monitoring respiration in the anesthetized patient?

There are many ways to monitor respiration. Each technique has limitations that must be considered in the context of the patient's disease and likely information required to maintain the patient's well-being. These techniques range from the very simple, such as auscultation of the chest and examination of the mucous membranes, to the use of complex technology, such as pulse oximetry, capnography, and mass spectroscopy. The choice of technology applied will be determined in part by cost and by the patient population in which the monitors will be applied.

3. Which patients would benefit most from respiratory monitoring?

Those patients with pre-existing respiratory disease and those undergoing procedures that may change respiratory function, including the following:

- Thoracotomy, thoracoscopy
- Diaphragmatic hernia
- Possible pneumothorax
- Pneumonia
- Asthma/heaves
- Critically ill—sepsis, shock
- Trauma

4. What is the most expensive respiratory monitor available?

You, the well-trained and observant veterinarian. No one will argue that the cost of your education far exceeds the cost of all the commercially available respiratory monitors. By observing your patients closely, you can frequently detect problems more rapidly than any monitor.

5. What are the cost benefits of monitoring respiration in the anesthetized patient?

Monitoring of this type will pay off for patients who are at higher risk of an adverse outcome from anesthesia. Usually these patients are encountered in a high volume facility that handles more complex cases. If your caseload is made up of healthy patients for elective neutering or dental procedures, there are other variables to monitor which will have a greater impact on patient survival.

6. Why would you monitor respiration?

How about to prevent the lawyers from taking your hard-earned cash? The American College of Veterinary Anesthesiologists has published a position paper on monitoring in the veterinary patient. This paper does not define standard of care but offers suggestions for monitoring to help ensure optimal outcomes. If you have an anesthetized patient that stops breathing and then dies because you did not detect and treat in time, you are liable for the outcome.

How about for greater peace of mind? Many veterinarians are not comfortable with anesthetic agents. In such circumstances, the more information you have telling you that your patient is doing well, the better.

7. Are there any disadvantages to respiratory monitoring?

If you are going to monitor a variable, you must be able to do something with the information that is generated. It is important that the data generated be analyzed by a well-trained caregiver, especially before any radical intervention is considered.

A physical limitation to the use of in-line respiratory monitors in small patients is the increased equipment dead space that occurs with insertion of the sampling connector.

Other consequences of the use of respiratory monitors include the increased potential for leaks in the breathing system, dealing with any sampled gas removed from the breathing system, and possible spread of contamination with reusable sampling connectors.

Adverse effects of monitoring occur very rarely, but no intervention is risk-free. Some of the types of adverse events associated with monitoring follow: patient burns have been reported from the sensor of a capnograph. A near-fatal case of pneumothorax, pneumomediastinum, and subcutaneous emphysema in a cat has been reported with the use of a Bain system and a respiration monitor. This situation arose because the connector of the respiratory monitor fit too tightly and occluded the exhalation port of the Bain breathing system. Incautious application of erroneous data from a malfunctioning monitor may also lead to patient harm.

8. What information can you get from examining the mucous membranes?

Mucous membranes can come in variations of pink, pale, red, congested, mottled, or blue. The color of the membranes is affected both by respiratory and circulatory factors so makes a poor indicator of the function of either system alone. Estimating the capillary refill time can give some guide to the status of peripheral vascular tone.

9. Your patient is not cyanotic. Can it be hypoxic?

For cyanosis to be present, at least 5 g/dl of deoxygenated hemoglobin must be present (see Chapter 2). If a patient is anemic, severe hypoxemia may be present without any easily discernable change in the color of the mucous membranes.

Most hypoxic patients go undetected and untreated. This is particularly so in the recovery period following anesthesia and surgery. The fact that hypoxia is often clinically silent is one of the primary reasons that pulse oximetry and other methods of measuring the effectiveness of gas exchange are so important.

10. What information can the respiratory rate give you?

Within a large range of normal values, the only information provided is that your patient is breathing, which is good to know. A rate that is abnormally low (< 4 bpm) in an anesthetized patient usually indicates anesthetic-induced respiratory depression—lighten up the patient! A respiratory rate that is abnormally high should initiate some troubleshooting in an attempt to determine cause. Tachypnea can indicate physiologic stress of many causes, most treatable.

11. What information can the character of a patient's respiration give you?

- Two phase exhalation in the horse—indicates light plane of anesthesia.
- Irregular rate—light plane of anesthesia, or patient with compromise of the respiratory centers in the medulla.
- Cheyne-Stokes respiration—Breaths get cyclically larger, then smaller, followed by a period of apnea. Can be seen following administration of anesthetic agents such as ketamine and halothane. Usually an indication of abnormal responses of the respiratory center in the cerebral medulla.
- Biot's respiration—Cyclic hyperventilation and apnea. A sign of serious disturbance in control of respiration. Often an incidental observation in anesthetized foals.
- Agonal gasping—when large inspiratory efforts are seen that utilize mainly accessory muscles of respiration, something is very badly wrong. May be airway obstruction, may be cardiac arrest. Check your patient!
- Apneustic respiration—cyclic variation between tachypnea and breath-holding in inspiration. Often associated with administration of ketamine, especially in cats and horses.

12. What information can you get from auscultation of the chest?

Auscultation of the chest is an important part of any physical examination. It identifies the presence of air flow in the lungs and any abnormalities. Auscultation also provides information on the nonpulmonary structures within the chest. Large areas of pulmonary consolidation, the presence of pleural fluid, air, or intestinal tract can all be identified. Also, the presence of fluid in the large or small airways will be apparent, as will the presence of any bronchoconstriction.

13. What information can you get from the esophageal stethoscope?

The esophageal stethoscope can be used to obtain information about breathing and heart function. For a fee, this device has also been adapted to provide information about body temperature and the electrical activity of the heart. Analysis of sound from the esophageal stethoscope at various depths reveals that placement within the chest greatly affects the respiratory and cardiac sounds obtained.

This monitor indicates whether the patient is breathing and gives an indication of the character of the respiration. Amplified esophageal stethoscopy has been used to aid the solo veterinary practitioner in monitoring the anesthetized patient. Instead of listening to tunes while you do surgery, you can listen to heart and breath sounds.

14. What information can you get from the capnograph?

The capnograph provides digital and analog information about the respiratory rate in both intubated and nonintubated patients. The amount of carbon dioxide exhaled and inhaled allows evaluation of respiratory depression and any rebreathing. Evaluation of the curves produced by this monitor allows detection of leaks in the breathing system, bronchospasm, apnea and numerous other more subtle problems with respiration.

Evaluating the arterial–end-tidal gradient in a given patient allows tracking of any changes in dead space ventilation. This gradient will tend to remain constant in any given patient over time, unless something physically changes, such as opening the chest.

Remember that delivery of CO_2 to the lungs requires blood flow. One of the earliest and most sensitive signs of cardiovascular collapse or cardiac arrest is an abrupt decrease in end-tidal CO_2. Remember also that progressive hypoventilation that occurs as a pneumothorax progresses will be indicated by rising end-tidal CO_2 and increasing arterial–end-tidal CO_2 gradient.

15. What are the advantages and disadvantages of the mainstream and sidestream gas monitors?

With a mainstream (nondiverting) gas monitor, the patient's respiratory gas passes through a wide-bore chamber with two windows and is analyzed right there by the attached heated sensor. Advantages of the mainstream gas monitor include fast response, no scavenging of sampled gases, less problem with water and secretions, and use of fewer disposable items. Disadvantages of this system include weight of the sensor, increased potential for leaks or disconnects in system, interference of secretions with the sensor, increased vulnerability of the sensor to damage, longer warm-up time.

A sidestream (diverting) gas monitor uses a pump to pull gas from the breathing system to the sensor that is located in the body of the monitor. Advantages of this system include faster warm-up, lightweight patient interface, and ability to measure several respiratory gases at once. Also, the monitor can be remote from patient (e.g., MRI), and sampling from nonintubated patients is possible. Disadvantages include obstruction of sample tubing with water, blood or secretions; delay in response; dealing with sampled gas; use of more disposable items; need for calibration of the gas source.

Both systems require a connector in the breathing system that will add dead space to the breathing system.

16. How will you know if the capnograph is accurate?

The following specifications are standard requirements for accuracy of capnometers.

- The CO_2 reading shall be within 12% of actual, or ± 4 mm Hg, whichever is greater, over its full range.
- Any interference by O_2, nitrous oxide, halothane, ethanol, acetone, or chlorodifluoromethane must be disclosed.

Most of the commercially available units use infrared absorption. The main cause of inaccuracy in a capnometer is lack of calibration. Sensor malfunction can also occur.

17. When could the capnograph mislead you?

Systems using sidestream sampling of gas are vulnerable to blockage of the sample line, which usually causes false apnea alarms. Monitors using mainstream gas measurement are vulnerable to accumulation of secretions in the measuring chamber, which usually produces a zero reading.

Some respiratory gas monitors combine measuring carbon dioxide with other gaseous anesthetic agents such as halothane, enflurane, and isoflurane. They also use infrared absorption to measure these gases. The presence of nitrous oxide, ethanol, acetone or chlorodifluromethane in the breathing system can all produce erroneous data, usually seen as abnormally high levels of inhaled anesthetic agent.

18. What is the cause of this tracing from a capnograph?

This one is normal! The trace shows normal end tidal carbon dioxide levels during quiet tidal breathing. Scale is mm Hg.

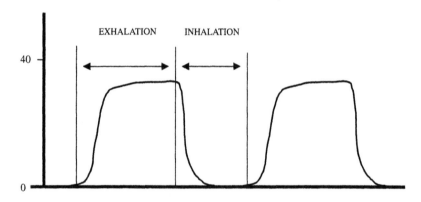

19. What is the cause of this abnormal tracing from a capnograph?

This tracing shows rebreathing of CO_2, such as when the soda lime is exhausted. Note that the inspiratory concentration of carbon dioxide is elevated above normal, as is the end-tidal level. Scale is in mm Hg.

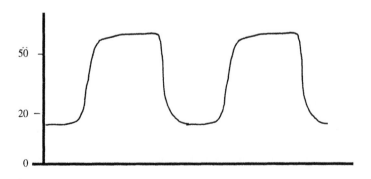

20. What is the cause of this abnormal tracing from a capnograph?

This trace shows cardiogenic mixing of exhaled gases. This phenomenon is more pronounced when the heart rate is high and the respiratory rate is slow. Scale is mm Hg.

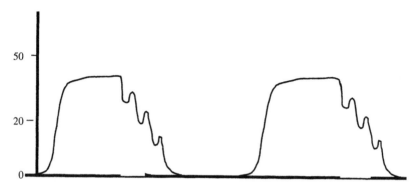

21. What are the most common causes of hypoventilation in the anesthetized patient?

Hypoventilation is diagnosed by an increased level of CO_2 in arterial blood ($PaCO_2$). The most common causes are:

- Barbiturates
- Opiates
- Inhaled agents
- Too deep anesthetic plane

22. What are the most common causes of apnea in the anesthetized patient?

- Pressure relief valve (pop-off valve) left closed
- Overzealous ventilation
- Iatrogenic hyperventilation of patient
- Cardiac arrest

23. What would you do if a patient were hypercarbic?

Detecting elevated levels of CO_2 in end-tidal gas or arterial blood always indicates an imbalance between the carbon dioxide produced and its respiratory excretion. An increased metabolic rate due to pyrexia or malignant hyperthermia would be the least likely cause of this condition. Depression of ventilation and decreased respiratory minute volume would be the more common cause.

In an anesthetized patient, the normal first response is to decrease the anesthetic depth. In a patient that will not tolerate any elevation of $PaCO_2$, or in a patient with severe elevations of $PaCO_2$ (usually > 60 mm Hg), the appropriate treatment is mechanical or manual (controlled) ventilation.

You would also be wise to check your equipment. Some equipment problems that can cause increased $PaCO_2$ include channeling or exhaustion of soda lime, as well as missing or stuck one-way valves in the breathing system. These conditions will cause rebreathing of exhaled gas and contribute to an elevation of $PaCO_2$.

24. What are the most common causes of hyperventilation in the anesthetized patient?

Hyperventilation is diagnosed by a decreased $PaCO_2$. The most common causes are

- Pain
- Surgical stimulation
- Hypoxia
- Hypotension

25. What is rebreathing and why is it important?

Rebreathing implies that some or all of the gas that was exhaled with the last breath is present in the gas that is inhaled. This occurs with every anesthesia circle system and is safe because the soda lime removes carbon dioxide from the exhaled gas. Carbon dioxide is the marker for rebreathing of exhaled gas in situations other than the anesthesia breathing circle.

Rebreathing can occur when there is excessive equipment dead space, such as with an over-long endotracheal tube or an excessively large airway connector for a gas monitor. The gas in these areas moves back and forth and does not get exhaled from the system.

26. What is dead space? Why is it important?

Dead space in the breathing system contains gas that does not participate in gas exchange. It is composed of gas from the equipment dead space and gas in the connecting airways in the lungs. Also included is gas that reaches alveoli in areas of the lung that are ventilated but not perfused.

As the volume of dead space increases in proportion to the tidal volume of the patient the effectiveness of gas exchange will decrease. A normal tidal volume would be 10 to 20 ml/kg. Normal dead space in an anesthetized healthy dog would be 2 ml/kg. This gives a ratio of 0.2 (20%). Patients with dead space ratios of 0.30 to 0.5 will have difficulty maintaining normal levels of carbon dioxide. Their respiratory efficiency is significantly lower than normal.

27. What is a normal tidal volume for an anesthetized patient? How can it be measured?

Irrespective of species, the normal tidal volume for a mammal is 10 to 20 ml/kg. This can be measured by watching the bellows travel if the patient is on a mechanical ventilator. Tidal volume can be estimated by watching the movement of the reservoir bag in a patient under anesthesia. Accurate measurement of tidal volume involves the use of a spirometer or the collection of the actual gas and measurement of its volume by some other means. Most modern spirometers measure flow and integrate the tidal volume from this information.

28. When would you want to use a mass spectrometer?

The mass spectrometer can be used to measure inspired and end-tidal concentrations of oxygen, CO_2, nitrous oxide, nitrogen, and the volatile anesthetic agents. Argon and helium can be measured on some units. This device measures gases as volume percentage, which can present a problem if a gas is present that the mass spectrometer cannot measure. Cost is the usual prohibiting factor to the use of these monitors.

Advantages of this monitoring system include multi-gas and multi-agent capabilities and the ability to measure nitrogen. Other advantages include fast response time, convenience, and reliability.

29. What information can you get from arterial blood gas analysis?

This measuring technique will provide data on the patient's gas exchange (oxygenation and removal of carbon dioxide) and metabolic status. Analysis of venous blood will only provide reliable data concerning the metabolic status of the patient.

30. What information can you get from the pulse oximeter?

This monitoring device uses infrared absorption at several wavelengths. It provides a measure of the hemoglobin saturation in blood. It also provides evidence of pulsatile blood flow where the probe is placed. Indicated hemoglobin saturation of 100% is normal. Assuming normal functioning of the equipment, decreased hemoglobin saturation (< 85%) indicates a patient in need of intervention.

31. When could the pulse oximeter mislead you?

These monitors are vulnerable to a number of causes of artifactual error. Movement, bright ambient lighting, and compression of the probe site will all cause abnormal readings. Endogenous sources of error include the presence of significant levels of carboxyhemoglobin and methemoglobin. Both of these abnormal hemoglobins cause errors in the hemoglobin saturation that is reported.

32. What will it cost to monitor respiration?

As in the rest of life, you get what you pay for. The price also depends on whether you buy new or secondhand. There is a burgeoning market in refurbished monitors for the veterinarian. A simple monitor that makes a noise each time the patient inhales and exhales can be purchased for about $300. An amplifier that attaches to an esophageal stethoscope will set you back about $500. Stand-alone capnographs are getting smaller and cheaper every year. They can be obtained currently for about $1000. Larger systems, especially if combined with other modules measuring electrocardiographic activity, blood pressure, and pulse oximetry can range from $4000 to $10,000.

33. If you could only afford to buy one monitor for use in your anesthetized patients, what would it be?

If you are planning to anesthetize primarily healthy patients, then a pulse oximeter is likely the most useful monitor for you. As you tackle patients with more complex problems, you will add more monitors to your inventory, including blood pressure and a capnograph.

BIBLIOGRAPHY

1. American College of Veterinary Anesthesiologists: Suggestions for monitoring anesthetized Veterinary patients. J Am Vet Med Assoc 206:936–937, 1995.
2. Dorsch JA, Dorsch SE: Understanding anesthesia equipment, 4th ed. Baltimore, Lippincott, Williams & Wilkins, 2000.
3. Evans AT: Anesthesia case of the month: Pneumothorax, pneumomediastinum and subcutaneous emphysema in a cat due to barotrauma after equipment failure during anesthesia. J Am Vet Med Assoc 212:30–32, 1998.
4. Manecke GR Jr, Poppers PJ: Esophageal stethoscope placement depth: Its effect on heart and lung sound monitoring during general anesthesia. Anesth Analg 86:1276–1279, 1998.

20. PULSE OXIMETRY

Tamara Grubb, D.V.M., M.S., D.A.C.V.A.

1. What is pulse oximetry?

Pulse oximetry is the noninvasive measurement of the percentage of hemoglobin (Hb) saturated with oxygen in arterial blood.

2. What abbreviations are used to present the data obtained by a pulse oximeter?

The saturation value obtained *in vivo* by the pulse oximeter is often abbreviated SpO_2 to differentiate it from the saturation value obtained *in vitro* from hemolyzed arterial blood by an oximeter (SaO_2).

3. How does pulse oximetry work?

Pulse oximetry works on the principle that hemoglobin absorbs red and infrared light at different wavelengths, depending on whether the light is bound to oxygen (infrared light, 920–940 nm) or deoxygenated (red light, 660 nm).

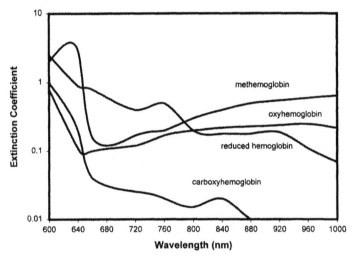

Hemoglobin extinction curves.

The pulse oximeter uses two light-emitting diodes (LEDs) that pulse red and infrared light through perfused tissue several hundred times per second. The amount of light absorbed at each wavelength is measured by sensitive photodetectors, and the absorption data are expressed as a percentage of oxygenated to total hemoglobin.

4. What principle of physics is pulse oximetry based on?

Pulse oximetry is based on the Beer-Lambert law, which states that the absorption of light by a homogeneous solution is a function of the concentration of the solution.

5. How does the pulse oximeter differentiate arterial from venous blood?

Pulse oximeters are designed with the assumption that arterial blood is pulsatile while venous blood and tissue beds are not. With each pulse, the influx of arterial blood into the capillary bed increases the total absorption of light, allowing the pulse oximeter to distinguish systole (arterial blood + venous blood + tissue) from diastole (venous blood + tissue). Data are collected during both systole and diastole, and the diastolic absorption values are subtracted from the systolic absorption values, allowing the pulse oximeter to eliminate all data except that produced by arterial blood. The ability to distinguish pulsatile flow has given this technology its name, "pulse" oximetry.

6. What information will the pulse oximeter provide?

The pulse oximeter will display the percentage of oxygenated hemoglobin in arterial blood. Most pulse oximeters also display heart rate. Many pulse oximeters also provide information about the strength of the signal that the oximeter is receiving through the display of bar graphs or pulse waveforms.

7. What does the saturation value tell me about the physiologic status of the patient?

Percentage of saturation gives an indication of the adequacy both of ventilation and of circulation. Ventilation must be adequate to provide alveolar oxygen for hemoglobin saturation. Circulation must be adequate (1) to perfuse the lungs so that hemoglobin can be exposed to oxygen and (2) to perfuse the tissues so that the pulse oximeter can detect a signal.

8. What saturation value is normal?

Saturation should be maintained ≥ 90%, as this keeps the saturation on the flat part of the oxygen-hemoglobin dissociation curve, where the patient is unlikely to desaturate. If the patient is breathing 100% oxygen, saturation values ≥ 95% may be more appropriate.

9. What is the oxygen-hemoglobin dissociation curve?

The oxygen-hemoglobin dissociation curve is a graphic representation of the relationship between percentage of oxygen saturation of hemoglobin (SaO_2 or SpO_2) and the partial pressure of oxygen in arterial blood (PaO_2).

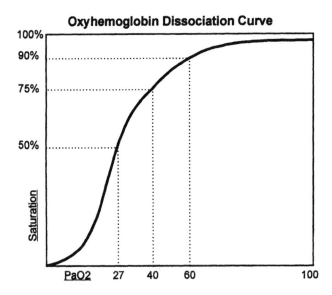

The oxyhemoglobin dissociation curve describes the nonlinear relationship between PaO_2 and percentage saturation of hemoglobin with oxygen (SaO_2). Note that in the steep part of the curve (50% region), small changes in PaO_2 result in large changes in SaO_2. The converse is true when PaO_2 rises above 60 mm Hg. Three regions of the curve have been marked. From Goldman JM: Pulse Oximetry. In Duke J (ed): Anesthesia Secrets, 2nd ed. Philadelphia, Hanley & Belfus, 2000, with permission.

The flat part of the curve on the upper right represents the area where PaO_2 is so high that even large changes in PaO_2 result in minimal to no changes in SpO_2 / SaO_2. Below 90% saturation, the curve becomes steep, and this portion represents the area where even a minimal change in SpO_2 / SaO_2 is equivalent to large drops in PaO_2, an area where the patient is in danger of rapid desaturation.

10. How should I respond to a low saturation?
The response should be rapid. First, you should ensure adequate ventilation by evaluating patency of the airway, respiratory rate, and tidal volume. If the airway is patent and respiratory rate and tidal volume are appropriate, ensure that there are no interruptions of oxygen flow or accumulations of carbon dioxide in the anesthetic machine. If oxygen is supplied at less than 100%, increase the FIO_2. If nitrous oxide is in use, discontinue use. Institute mechanical ventilation if necessary.

If ventilation and oxygen delivery are satisfactory, ensure that cardiac output is adequate. Cardiac output is rarely measured in veterinary patients, but arterial blood pressure, pulse quality, mucous membrane color, and capillary refill time can be used as crude indicators of output. If neither ventilation nor circulation appears to be impaired, address issues such as positioning of the animal (e.g., dorsal recumbency, especially in large animals), surgical procedure (e.g., thoracotomy with open thorax), and medical conditions of the patient (e.g., anemia, methemoglobinemia, pulmonary disease). If possible, saturation values should be confirmed with values obtained by a co-oximeter.

11. How accurate are the saturation data provided by the pulse oximeter?
Pulse oximeters are reported to be accurate within 2 to 6% in the 80 to 100% saturation range. At an oxygen saturation of greater than 90%, SpO_2 tends to be slightly lower than SaO_2, and at an oxygen saturation of less than 70%, SpO_2 tends to be slightly higher than SaO_2. The accuracy of SpO_2 may deteriorate substantially as SaO_2 continues to decrease. This may be explained in part by the fact that the lower SpO_2 values are often extrapolated from the saturation data from healthy volunteers with SaO_2 values of >70% (see question 12).

12. Is it necessary to calibrate the pulse oximeter?
No. Pulse oximeters are empirically calibrated by the manufacturer using absorption data obtained from a large group of healthy human volunteers (generally with arterial SaO_2 values > 70%). Because the optical properties of blood are similar among mammalian individuals and between mammalian species, no individual instrument calibration is required in the field. However, because each brand of pulse oximeter is calibrated using a different data set, different brands of pulse oximeters may display slightly different saturation values for the same patient.

13. Does the pulse oximeter always provide reliable saturation data?
No. Numerous factors cause SpO_2 to deviate from SaO_2. The main factors can be divided into two groups: intrinsic (dysfunctional hemoglobins, intravascular dyes) and extrinsic (patient motion, electrocautery, and ambient light).

14. What is meant by "dysfunctional hemoglobins"?
There are many types of hemoglobin, but not all types transport oxygen; these are termed "dysfunctional hemoglobins." There are five main types of hemoglobin: fetal hemoglobin (HbF) and four types of adult hemoglobin (oxyhemoglobin [O_2Hb], deoxyhemoglobin, carboxyhemoglobin [COHb], and methemoglobin [MetHb]). Only COHb and MetHb fail to transport oxygen. Since the pulse oximeter uses only two light wavelengths, only oxyhemoglobin and deoxyhemoglobin are measured. However, all moieties of hemoglobin can be measured using a co-oximeter that uses multiple light wavelengths.

15. How does the presence of different types of hemoglobin affect the accuracy of the pulse oximeter?
Fetal hemoglobin does not affect the accuracy of the pulse oximeter. Although HbF has a greater affinity for oxygen than adult hemoglobin, the absorption coefficients for HbF and adult

Hb are similar and the presence of HbF does not affect saturation values. However, both COHb and MetHb may cause SpO_2 errors. Carboxyhemoglobin has an absorbance spectrum similar to that of HbO_2, so most pulse oximeters will overestimate the percentage saturation by the amount of COHb that is present. The absorbance coefficient of MetHb, on the other hand, is similar in both the red and infrared bands. Thus, the presence of a large amount of MetHb causes the ratio of the red to infrared absorbance to approach 1, which corresponds to a saturation value of approximately 85%. Therefore, large amounts of MetHb will drive the SpO_2 to 85%, regardless of the true saturation value. Fortunately, large concentrations of COHb and MetHb are rarely encountered in veterinary medicine.

16. How does the presence of intravascular dyes affect the accuracy of the pulse oximeter?
Methylene blue, which is commonly used to treat methemoglobinemia, causes a large absorbance peak at 670 nm. Because this value is close to the 660 nm wavelength of red light, low SpO_2 values will be recorded. However, dyes rapidly equilibrate in the blood and tissue bed and become part of the nonpulsatile background, thus eliminating their effects.

17. How do the extrinsic factors cause pulse oximetry inaccuracies?
Generally, movement of the patient reduces or eliminates the ability of the pulse oximeter to detect a pulse. Thus, the pulse oximeter does not register a pulse at all or indicates motion artifacts by displaying an erratic heart rate. If the transient motion mimics a heart beat, the instrument may be unable to differentiate between the pulsations that are due to motion artifacts and the normal arterial pulsations. Patient movement has been described as the main limitation of pulse oximetry in both human beings and animals. Ambient light can interfere with the photosensor and can cause failure of the pulse oximeter to produce data or can cause erroneous SpO_2 readings, most commonly approaching 85%. Some xenon arc surgery lights may cause 100% SpO_2 readings and a pulse rate of 180–255 bpm without the pulse oximeter probe even being attached to a patient.

18. What can be done to alleviate the interference from extrinsic factors?
Averaging pulse oximetry readings over longer periods of time (5–10 seconds) helps to decrease motion artifact due to patient movement. Decreasing the size of probes and designing the probes to fit better have also decreased motion artifacts in human beings. Finally, some pulse oximeters are gated on the R wave of the electrocardiogram and interpret data relayed only at the time of the inscription of the R wave, thereby decreasing motion artifact. Under low-perfusion conditions, pulse oximeters are more susceptible to motion artifacts; thus, improving cardiac output may decrease interference from movement. Ambient light interference can most easily be eliminated by simply shielding the probe from room light. In some pulse oximetry units, the effect of stray light is mathematically eliminated by the subtraction of background measurements taken when both of the LEDs in the sensor are turned off from measurements taken when either one of the LEDs is turned on.

19. How can I be sure that the pulse oximeter is providing accurate saturation data?
You can't always be sure. You can be sure that the pulse oximeter is indeed detecting a pulse by observing that the heart rate displayed by the pulse oximeter matches the actual heart rate of the patient (or double the heart rate in the case of some horses; see question 24). Also, if an indicator of pulse strength is displayed, the strength of the signal should be strong.

20. Are there conditions that would cause the pulse oximeter to completely fail to detect a pulse?
Yes. Arterial pulses must be of adequate strength to be detected by the pulse oximeter. Thus, any significant decrease in peripheral vascular pulsation can produce a signal too weak to be detected. The most common examples of this include hypotension, hypovolemia, vasoconstriction, and hypothermia. However, remember that overall perfusion may not be poor but the probe site may have poor intrinsic perfusion and the probe may need to be moved to a site with better

perfusion (see question 22).

21. Are there different types of pulse oximeter probes?

Yes, there are two types: (1) the transmittance type, in which the LEDs and the photodetector are placed on opposite sides of a tissue bed; and (2) the reflectance type, in which the LEDs and the photodetector are positioned side-by-side on the skin or mucosa. Most pulse oximeters use transmittance type probes. The transmittance probe can be provided as a clip type (such as those designed for the human ear) or a C-clamp type (such as those designed for the nasal septum of large animals). "Finger" probes are also available; however, these have a concave surface and generally do not make adequate tissue contact, and thus pulse detection is often difficult for this type of probe.

22. Where is the best site to place the pulse oximeter probe?

Any pulsating arteriolar bed may be used for attachment of probes; however, probe placement is often tricky because it is imperative that the tissue be without hair, nonpigmented, and fairly thin, but not too thin. For most veterinary species, placing a transmittance probe on the tongue of anesthetized patients tends to produce the most reliable and repeatable data. Other sites that can be used if they are clipped free of hair and are relatively nonpigmented include the lip, vulva, prepuce, toe web, fold of the flank, pinna of the ear, metacarpus, digits, and tail. The nostril and nasal septum can also be used in large animals. The reflectance type probe has been used with some success on the rectal mucosa. Animal skin is often thicker than the skin of human beings, making probe placement more difficult in veterinary species.

23. Is pulse oximetry useful in all species?

To our knowledge, pulse oximetry should be useful in most mammals because of the similarity of the spectral properties of mammalian hemoglobin between species. Pulse oximetry has been validated in a number of veterinary species, including dogs, horses, pigs, and sheep.

24. Are their any species-specific considerations when using pulse oximetry?

Yes. The pulse rate displayed by pulse oximeters in horses is often double the actual patient pulse rate. This is because the dichrotic notch in the pulse wave is large and is often counted as a second cardiac contraction. Many pulse oximetry units may be unable to detect a pulse in species with a heart rate greater than 250 bpm. Some pulse oximeters programmed for use in human beings are programmed to provide data only when the heart rate counted by the pulse oximeter is in a physiologically normal range for human beings. These oximeters may not display data for species with heart rates that are lower (e.g., horses) or higher (e.g., some cats, birds, pocket pets) than the normal heart rate range in human beings. Also, because of the small size of vessels, the ability of the pulse oximeter to detect a pulse may be limited in very small patients.

25. Is the pulse oximeter useful in situations other than monitoring saturation during anesthesia?

Yes, pulse oximetry is useful in measuring oxygen saturation in a variety of settings, including in critical care patients with questionable respiratory function (e.g., patients recovering from anesthesia, patients with pneumothorax) and patients requiring or being weaned from supplemental oxygen and/or ventilatory support. However, movement will interfere with data acquisition, making pulse oximetry in conscious animals somewhat difficult. Nonetheless, reliable saturation data have been obtained in conscious patients during times of minimal movement. Probes in conscious animals reportedly work best when placed on the lip (clip-type probe), tail, or toe (circumferential probe for the latter two sites). Pulse oximetry has also been used to measure fetal oxygen saturation during dystocia and to assess intestinal viability during surgery.

26. What are the advantages of pulse oximetry?

First, pulse oximetry is easy to use, requires minimal site preparation, and does not require special training. Second, pulse oximetry is noninvasive. Because pulse oximetry does not require collection of blood, there is no discomfort to the patient and no delay in data collection. Thus, pulse oximetry provides virtually continuous measurement of saturation. Third, pulse oximetry provides information about both the respiratory and cardiovascular systems. Finally, pulse oximetry units are generally affordable, fairly mobile, and convenient to use.

27. The limitations and disadvantages of pulse oximetry have been discussed. Are there any dangers or times when pulse oximetry would be an inadequate form of monitoring?

With high oxygen partial pressures, SpO_2 may not adequately warn the anesthesiologist of impending hypoxic events. Normal oxygen saturation can be achieved in a hypoventilating patient breathing a high inspired oxygen concentration. Thus, the adequacy of ventilation should be assessed separately from the adequacy of saturation.

28. Is pulse oximetry commonly used to monitor anesthetized human beings?

Yes. On Jan 1, 1990, the American Society of Anesthesiologists (ASA) included intraoperative monitoring with pulse oximetry as part of its standards of care. Two years later, the ASA added monitoring with pulse oximetry to its postanesthesia recovery standards of care.

BIBLIOGRAPHY

1. Dorsch JA, Dorsch SE. Understanding anesthesia equipment,4th ed. Baltimore, Williams & Wilkins, 1999, pp 811–849.
2. Ehrhardt W, Hipp LC, von Hegel G, et al: The use of pulse oximetry in clinical veterinary anesthesia. J Assoc Vet Anaesthesiol 68:30–31, 1990.
3. Fairman N: Evaluation of pulse oximetry as a continuous monitoring technique in critically ill dogs in the small animal intensive care unit. J Vet Emerg Crit Care 2(2):50–56, 1992.
4. Huss BT, Anderson MA, Branson KR, et al: Evaluation of pulse oximeter probes and probe placement in healthy dogs. JAMA 31:9–14, 1995.
5. Jacobson JD, Miller MW, Hartsfield SM, et al: Evaluation of accuracy of pulse oximetry in dogs. Am J Vet Res 53(4):537–539, 1992.
6. Mendelson Y: Pulse oximetry: Theory and applications for noninvasive monitoring. Clin Chem 38(9): 1601–1607, 1992.
7. Reich DL, Timcenko A, Bodian CA, et al: Predictors of pulse oximetry data failure. Anesthesiology 84: 859–864, 1996.
8. Whitehair KJ, Watney GCG, Leith DE, et al: Pulse oximetry in horses. Vet Surg 19(3):243-248, 1990.
9. Wright B, Hellyer P: Respiratory monitoring during anesthesia: Pulse oximetry and capnography. Compendium 18:1083–1097, 1996.

21. NEUROMUSCULAR MONITORING

Stephen A. Greene, D.V.M., M.S., D.A.C.V.A.

1. Why monitor neuromuscular blockade?

Neuromuscular blockade should be monitored to determine when additional doses of the neuromuscular blocker agent are required and to verify that adequate recovery from the blockade has occurred when desired. Published durations of effect for neuromuscular blocking agents can vary significantly among individuals, across species, and under variable environmental conditions (e.g., extreme temperatures). Observation of the return of respiratory effort when neuromuscular blockade is wearing off can mislead the anesthetist to cease controlled ventilation prematurely, resulting in hypoventilation and/or hypoxemia.

2. What are some examples of commercially available peripheral nerve stimulators?

Stimulator	*Manufacturer*
MiniStim	Professional Instruments Co., Houston, Texas
Innervator Model NS 252	Fisher & Paykel Healthcare, Auckland, New Zealand
TOF-Guard	Biometer, Turnhout, Belgium
Accelograph Model US 1	Biometer International A/S, DK-5210 Odense NV, Denmark

3. How is peripheral nerve stimulation evaluated during neuromuscular blockade?

Use of a peripheral nerve stimulator for monitoring neuromuscular blockade is described in Chapter 20. Observation of muscle twitches or graphic representation of the twitches is used to interpret the degree of neuromuscular blockade. The simplest and most commonly used method for evaluation of neuromuscular block is seeing or feeling the muscle contraction. Despite the fact that many studies have shown that train-of-four fade or tetanic fade is not detected by visual or tactile means when the T_4 / T_1 is as low as 0.3, these simple methods of interpretation remain in common practice because of their clinical ease of use.

4. What are characteristics of a depolarizing neuromuscular block?

The depolarizing neuromuscular block is characterized by decreased single twitch height, lack of fade with train-of-four stimulation or tetany, and lack of post-tetanic facilitation.

Response	*Depolarizing Block*	*Nondepolarizing Block*	*Phase II Block*
Single twitch height	Decreased	Decreased	Decreased
Tetanic height	Decreased	Decreased	Decreased
Tetanic fade	Minimal or none	Yes	Yes
Train-of-four fade	Minimal or none	Yes	Yes
Post-tetanic facilitation	Minimal or none	Yes	Yes
Effect of anticholinesterase administration	Prolongation of block	Antagonism of block	Antagonism of block

5. What are characteristics of a nondepolarizing neuromuscular block?

The nondepolarizing neuromuscular block is characterized by decreased single twitch height, fade with train-of-four stimulation, and post-tetanic facilitation.

6. What percentage of functional acetylcholine receptors must be blocked to decrease the height of a single twitch?

Between 75 and 80% of the receptors must be blocked to decrease the single twitch height. Between 90 and 95% of the receptors will be blocked when the twitch height is 0.

7. What is "fade"?
"Fade" indicates that the response is diminishing over time.

8. What is "tetany"?
"Tetany" is defined as intermittent tonic muscular contraction. Responses to tetanic stimulation generally yield more accurate assessment of neuromuscular function than train-of-four patterns. However, the high frequency of stimulation used for tetanic stimulation may cause arousal in lightly anesthetized patients.

9. What is "post-tetanic facilitation"?
"Post-tetanic facilitation" is the phenomenon of increased single twitch height observed about 5 seconds after tetanic stimulation during incomplete, nondepolarizing neuromuscular blockade, as compared to a pretetanic single twitch height. This is the earliest clinical indication that recovery from complete neuromuscular blockade has begun. With a complete neuromuscular blockade, post-tetanic facilitation likely will not be observed.

10. What is "TOF"?
"TOF" stands for "train-of-four" stimulations administered at a frequency of 2 Hz. See Chapter 20 for more about train-of-four stimulation.

11. What are "phase I" and "phase II" blocks?
These terms are used in describing characteristics of depolarizing neuromuscular blockade. The early (single dose) blockade following succinylcholine is a phase I block. The characteristics of the phase I block are the same as those listed for the depolarizing block (see table at question 2). Attempts to antagonize succinylcholine with anticholinesterases during phase I block will result in extended duration of the block. A phase II block occurs during prolonged administration of succinylcholine by continuous infusion or repeated bolusing. The characteristics of the phase II block are similar to those of the nondepolarizing block. Although the mechanism of the phase II block is not precisely known, it may be related to desensitization, physical obstruction of the ionophore by the succinylcholine molecule, or disturbed production/release of acetylcholine.

12. What are shortcomings of neuromuscular blockade monitoring?
Use of peripheral nerve stimulation for monitoring the whole-body effect of neuromuscular blocking agents is not perfect. Some groups of muscles are more resistant to neuromuscular blockade than others. The operative site may require a different level of neuromuscular blockade compared with the site used for peripheral nerve stimulation monitoring. Species variability exists in muscle responses to neuromuscular block and peripheral nerve stimulation. The preanesthetic physical status of the patient may affect the required degree of neuromuscular blockade; a severely debilitated patient may not need complete neuromuscular blockade to achieve the same degree of relaxation as a healthy patient.

13. Which muscle groups are least sensitive to neuromuscular blockade?
The diaphragm and laryngeal muscles are more resistant to neuromuscular blockade than peripheral muscle groups on the extremities.

14. Which drugs potentiate the activity of nondepolarizing neuromuscular blockers?
Concurrent medications may affect the duration of action of neuromuscular blocking agents. Drugs that potentiate activity of nondepolarizing neuromuscular blockers include lidocaine, aminoglycoside antibiotics, clindamycin, tetracycline, procainamide, quinidine, magnesium, calcium channel blockers, beta-adrenoceptor antagonists, dantrolene, furosemide, and cyclosporine.

15. What ancillary medications antagonize the activity of nondepolarizing neuromuscular blockers?
In addition to the anticholinesterases mentioned in Chapter 18, concurrent medication with the following agents may antagonize neuromuscular blockers: carbamazepine, phenytoin, raniti-

dine, theophylline. Tachyphylaxis has been observed with chronic exposure to nondepolarizing neuromuscular blockers.

BIBLIOGRAPHY

1. Cullen LK: Muscle relaxants and neuromuscular block. In Thurmon JC, Tranquilli WJ, Benson GJ (eds): Lumb and Jones' Veterinary Anesthesia, 3rd ed. Baltimore: Williams & Wilkins, 1996, pp 337–364.
2. Wall MH, Prielipp RC: Monitoring the neuromuscular junction. In Lake CL, Hines RL, Blitt CD (eds): Clinical Monitoring Practical Applications for Anesthesia and Critical Care. Philadelphia: W.B. Saunders, 2001, pp 119–131.

line, theophylline. Tachyphylaxis has been observed with chronic exposure to nondepolarizing neuromuscular blockers.

BIBLIOGRAPHY

1. [illegible] Muscle relaxants and neuromuscular blockers. In: [illegible] [illegible]
2. [illegible] Monitoring the neuromuscular junction. In: [illegible] [illegible]

22. MONITORING THE ELECTROENCEPHALOGRAM

Stephen A. Greene, D.V.M., M.S., D.A.C.V.A.

1. What creates the electrical signal measured by the electroencephalograph?

The electrical fields generated from synaptic activity in the brain are measured at the level of the skin as the electroencephalogram (EEG). Energy from brain activity in the cerebral cortex is primarily responsible for the EEG. The bioelectric potential observed on the skin or from subdermally placed electrodes is caused by flow of ionic electrical currents. The relatively slowly changing currents from postsynaptic potentials constitute the basis of the raw EEG waveform. The magnitude of the postsynaptic potential is directly proportional to the number of receptors that have bound agonist neurotransmitters. The time for decay of these postsynaptic potentials is on the order of milliseconds to seconds.

Cortical neurons, primarily pyramidal cells, are aligned with uniformly aligned dendrites. Because of the unique architecture of the pyramidal cortical neurons, electrical current loops generated by these cells combine additively in the extracellular fluid. This phenomenon creates large current flows within regions of the brain that can be detected by its voltage on the skin of the head.

2. How is the EEG monitored in animals?

In animals, EEG is monitored in ways that are basically similar to those used in people. Electrodes are attached to the skin or placed in the subdermal tissues over the brain. Electrodes are typically made of a conductive metal such as platinum or an ionically conducting gel. The electrodes are connected to an amplifier for generation of a waveform that corresponds to the brain's electrical activity. The wave can be viewed as a graph on paper or on the screen of a monitor. The waveform can also be digitized to allow further processing of the EEG.

3. What is an epoch of EEG?

An epoch of EEG is an arbitrary period of time for which the characteristics of the EEG are described.

4. What causes interference with acquisition of EEG?

Besides the current generated by brain electrical activity, internal signals from the electrocardiogram or electromyogram (EMG) and external signals radiating from nearby power lines may distort the EEG. EEG is measured in microvolts (μV), and EMG is measured in millivolts (mV). Spontaneous movement of the patient (e.g., blinking) will introduce artifact into the EEG. A differential EEG amplifier can attenuate most unwanted signals. Artifacts from the electromyogram can be filtered by selecting a bandwidth of EEG that is different from the EMG. This is not always possible, however, and EMG must be eliminated by other means.

5. How can EMG be eliminated from EEG?

If band-pass filtering is not effective in elimination of EMG, other techniques that may help to generate an artifact-free EEG signal include topical or intramuscular injection of local anesthetic solution around the offending electrode, use of a systemic neuromuscular blocking agent, or use of a semipermanent neuromuscular blocker such as botulinum toxin.

6. What is meant by "processed" EEG?

"Processed EEG" is a general term indicating that the raw or analog EEG wave data have been digitized so that a specific feature associated with the EEG that is correlated with the physiologic or pharmacologic factor of immediate interest can be better recognized. Signal processors by necessity must trade off some degree of accuracy compared to the raw or analog signal to allow a workable size of digital data to be generated. Processing of the EEG into a digital form has allowed new applications for EEG data. Quantitative EEG is an end-product of processed EEG that can be specifically tailored to yield information about myriad features associated with the nature and relationship of the EEG wave. These features may include data about power, frequency, synchronicity, or coherence of the EEG.

7. What is the "fast Fourier transformation"?

A Fourier transformation generates a histogram of amplitudes of EEG as a function of the frequency (i.e., δ, θ, α, or β). It is based on the theorem that any repetitive waveform can be constructed from, or deconstructed to, a series of simple sinusoidal wave harmonics. Harmonics are sine waves that possess frequencies that are integer multiples of the slowest component. An algorithm written to efficiently determine the Fourier transformationss using computers and digitized EEG has become known as the fast Fourier transformation.

8. What is "spectral edge frequency 95," or SEF$_{95}$?

"Spectral edge frequency" (SEF) refers to the highest frequency of EEG. SEF can be defined to encompass a specified fraction of the entire EEG. Thus, the SEF$_{95}$ represents the highest frequency that includes 95% of all frequencies in an epoch of EEG.

9. How does absolute power of EEG relate to anesthetic depth?

Absolute power or amplitude of the EEG can be related to anesthetic depth by describing the frequency shift that occurs with increasing depth. In general, the awake patient will have more fast-wave (e.g., α and β) activity and the deeply anesthetized patient with have more slow wave (δ) activity. There are differences in EEG patterns that are associated with the specific anesthetic used and the degree of external stimulation. Limitations exist in the utility of absolute power as a reliable indicator of anesthetic depth for all anesthetic agents.

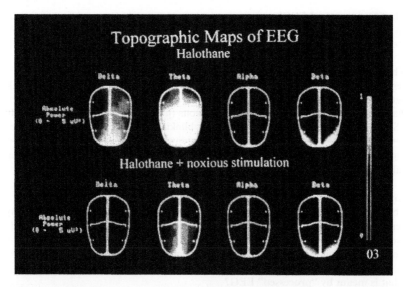

Topographic maps of the absolute power of EEG in a dog anesthetized with 1.5 minimal alveolar concentration halothane without (above) and with (below) noxious stimulation applied to a paw. White areas represent high and dark areas represent low absolute power values. The maps are created using a 21-lead linked ear montage.

10. How does spectral edge frequency relate to anesthetic depth?

Just as the absolute power of EEG can be related in general terms to the anesthetic depth, the spectral edge frequency can describe the same pattern. That is, as an animal becomes more deeply anesthetized, there likely will be less fast-wave and more slow-wave activity. Thus, the SEF for a given percentage of the EEG waves will shift toward 0 as the anesthetic depth is increased.

11. How does β-to-δ ratio relate to anesthetic depth?

A lightly anesthetized patient would be expected to exhibit more β activity and less δ activity compared with a deeply anesthetized patient. Therefore, in general, the β:δ ratio would be expected to decrease as anesthetic depth is increased.

12. Which anesthetics are typically associated with seizure activity?

Inhaled anesthetics have the potential to elicit seizure-like activity on the EEG at deep levels of anesthesia. Of the inhaled anesthetics, enflurane is most likely to cause epileptiform activity on the EEG. Myoclonic movement may accompany the EEG seizure activity.

13. What is "burst suppression"?

Burst suppression is a pattern of EEG observed during deep planes of anesthesia. It may occur with a wide variety of anesthetics. The pattern is characterized by epochs of normal or high-voltage activity that alternate with epochs of isoelectic or very low-voltage activity.

14. What is the burst suppression ratio?

The burst suppression ratio (BSR) is the fraction of an epoch of EEG in which the waveform is suppressed or isoelectic. For quantitative purposes, suppression is defined as a period of time longer that 0.5 seconds for which the EEG voltage does not exceed ±5 mV.

15. What is "bispectral index," or BIS?

Bispectral index (BIS) is a proprietary algorithm developed to measure the degree of "awakeness" in people. The BIS is determined from digitized EEG that is fast-Fourier transformed to yield subparameters related to time, frequency, and synchrony of waveforms. These subparameters have been weighted and incorporated into a multivariate statistical model that creates a final composite parameter, the BIS.

BIS values derived from a vast library of artifact-free EEGs collected during various stages of different anesthetic regimens have been correlated with behavior associated with the same human subjects. The quantified EEG features that describe power, frequency, bicoherence, β activation, and burst suppression are combined to give a statistically valid prediction of sedation or hypnosis during anesthesia. The resulting regression equation has been transformed into a scale from 0 to 100, where 0 is isoelectric activity and 100 is awake. Surgical patients have a very low probability of awareness when anesthesia is maintained such that the BIS value is between 40 and 60.

16. What is an auditory evoked potential?

An auditory evoked potential is a response measured by EEG following an auditory stimulus such as a "click" transmitted through earphones. A brain stem auditory evoked potential will provide information about the integrity of the auditory pathway and brain stem structures between the pons and the upper midbrain but not the cerebral cortex.

17. What is meant by middle latency auditory evoked potential?

The middle latency auditory evoked potential is synonymous with intermediate latency auditory evoked potential. The evoked potential can be described in terms related to the time from the stimulus to the peak of the potential wave. Middle latency evoked potentials are generated with latencies between 1 and 4 msec. Typically there are five measured middle latency evoked potentials measured with a brain stem auditory evoked potential.

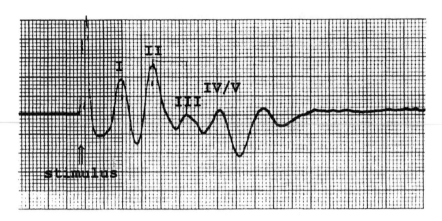

Brain stem auditory evoked potential from a normal dog.

BIBLIOGRAPHY

1. Iselin-Chavez IA, El Moalem HE, Gan TJ, et al: Changes in auditory evoked potentials and the bispectral index following propofol or propofol and alfentanil. Anesthesiology 92:1300–1310, 2000.
2. Lam AM: Do evoked potentials have any value in anesthesia? Anesthesiol Clin North Am 10:657–682, 1992.
3. Rampil IJ: What every neuroanesthesiologist should know about electroencephalograms and computerized monitors. Anesthesiol Clin North Am 10:683–718, 1992.
4. Rampil IJ: A primer for EEG signal processing in anesthesia. Anesthesiology 89:980–1002, 1998.
5. Schwender D, Daunderer M, Klasing S, et al: Power spectral analysis of the electroencephalogram during increasing end-expiratory concentrations of isoflurane, desflurane and sevoflurane. Anaesthesia 53:335–342, 1998.

V. Perianesthetic Complications

23. HYPOTENSION

Lesley J. Smith, D.V.M., D.A.C.V.A.

1. What are acceptable lower limits for blood pressure in anesthetized animals?

Mean arterial pressure is the driving force for blood flow (perfusion) through capillaries that supply oxygen to organs and tissue beds of the body. In small animals, mean arterial pressures lower than 60 mm Hg result in compromised perfusion of visceral organs and peripheral tissues, potentially leading to whole-organ, or regional, ischemia. In large animals, perfusion of skeletal muscle (especially skeletal muscle in recumbent areas of the body) is compromised at mean arterial pressures lower than 70 mm Hg. Thus, an anesthetized horse with mean arterial pressures consistently lower than 70 mm Hg for a significant length of time is at risk for skeletal muscle ischemia, which could result in postanesthetic myopathy. In all species, mean arterial pressures lower than 40 mm Hg are associated with inadequate perfusion of vessel-rich organs such as the heart, lungs, and central nervous system (CNS).

2. Summarize the anesthetic and postanesthetic risks that are posed by hypotension.

Clinically significant hypotension can lead to renal failure, reduced hepatic metabolism of drugs, worsening of ventilation/perfusion mismatch and hypoxemia, delayed recovery from anesthesia, neuromuscular complications during recovery (especially large animals), and CNS abnormalities, including blindness after anesthesia that may or may not resolve with time. Untreated hypotension can lead to cardiac and respiratory arrest.

3. What defines hypotension?

Hypotension, to the anesthetist, is defined as a mean arterial pressure lower than 60 mm Hg for small animals, and lower than 70 mm Hg for large animals.

4. How can I estimate mean arterial pressure from systolic blood pressure?

Mean arterial pressure = diastolic pressure + 1/3(systolic pressure – diastolic pressure). Most indirect blood pressure monitors provide data for systolic pressure (e.g., Doppler method) or systolic, diastolic, and mean arterial pressure (e.g., oscillometric devices). Roughly, the mean arterial pressure is 20 to 30 mm of Hg less than the measured systolic pressure on a Doppler reading in most species. Thus, a Doppler reading of 80 to 90 mm Hg correlates with a mean arterial pressure that would be considered hypotensive. The exception to this rule is in cats smaller than 4 to 5 kg (and likely other small mammals), in which the Doppler reading correlates most closely with mean arterial pressure.

5. What determines mean arterial pressure?

Mean arterial pressure = cardiac output × systemic vascular resistance. In thinking about causes of hypotension, it is useful to break this equation down into its various components and then assess the effects of anesthetic drugs or the animal's physiologic state on each component. Cardiac output = heart rate × stroke volume. Thus, a drug that reduces contractility (e.g., isoflurane) will lower stroke volume and can then contribute to a lower cardiac output, which may result in low mean arterial pressure if systemic vascular resistance has not increased. The following schematic demonstrates the relationship between components that determine mean arterial pressure:

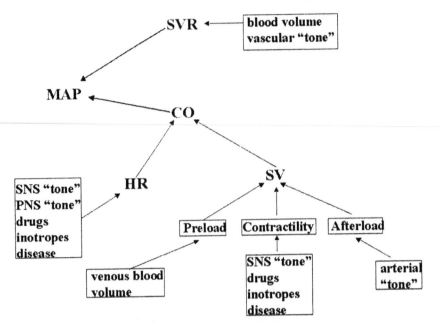

CO, cardiac output; HR, heart rate; MAP, mean arterial pressure; PNS, peripheral nervous system; SNS, sympathetic nervous system; XV, stroke volume; SVR, systemic vascular resistance.

6. Name commonly administered anesthetic drugs that decrease systemic vascular resistance and thus might lead to hypotension.
- Acepromazine
- Thiobarbiturates
- Propofol
- Isoflurane
- Sevoflurane
- Desflurane
- Halothane

All of the above listed drugs decrease systemic vascular resistance (SVR) in a dose-dependent fashion. Thus, higher doses of acepromazine, as might be used for preanesthetic sedation in a fractious dog, could lead to hypotension because of a profound decrease in SVR. The injectable anesthetics decrease SVR transiently because of rapid redistribution.

7. Name other factors that might reduce blood volume and/or vascular tone and lead to a decrease in systemic vascular resistance in an anesthetized patient or one presented for anesthesia.
- Hemorrhage
- Inadequate volume administration or replacement
- Dehydration
- Endotoxemic shock
- Overwhelming sepsis
- Cardiogenic shock
- Neurogenic shock
- Anaphylaxis
- Histamine release
- Severe hypercapnia

8. List physiologic states and common anesthetic drugs that might decrease heart rate.
- Physiologic bradycardia (e.g., athletic equine)
- High cervical disease
- Hypothermia
- Fasting (cattle only)
- Intracranial disease
- Electrolyte imbalances
- Opioids
- α_2 Agonists
- Inhalants
- Acetylcholinesterase inhibitors (e.g. edrophonium)
- Anticholinesterases (transient, paradoxical; increase in heart rate usually follows)

As with drugs that decrease systemic vascular resistance, bradycardia caused by anesthetic drugs is usually dose-dependent and will be most profound in animals that have pre-existing bradycardia.

9. What are factors that reduce preload, and thus indirectly reduce stroke volume?
- Reduction in venous blood volume from blood loss, dehydration, inadequate fluid replacement
- Vasodilation and "relative" hypovolemia from peripheral vascular pooling (e.g., inhalant anesthesia)
- Occlusion of vessels of venous return

A common cause of reduced preload in anesthetized animals is positive pressure ventilation. During the inspiratory phase of positive pressure ventilation, peak airway pressure is reflected as peak intrathoracic pressure, which may be high enough to transiently compress the cranial and caudal venae cavae as they enter the thorax. This results in reduced right atrial filling during inspiration and will lead to lower stroke volume on the subsequent ventricular systole.

10. Afterload and stroke volume are inversely related. What physiologic factors or drugs might increase afterload and thus reduce stroke volume?
- High sympathetic tone
- Pheochromocytoma
- Hyperthyroidism
- Cardiac outflow tract stenosis (e.g., pulmonic stenosis, heartworm disease)
- Exogenous epinephrine administration
- Phenylephrine
- α_2 Agonists (transiently, early after administration, most common after IV administration)
- Ketamine, tiletamine (telazol)

11. List anesthetic drugs or disease states that reduce contractility.
- Inhalants (halothane > isoflurane = sevoflurane > desflurane)
- Thiobarbiturates
- Propofol
- α_2 Agonists
- Intrinsic cardiac disease (e.g., dilated cardiomyopathy)
- Pericardial disease
- Severe sepsis or endotoxemia
- Electrolyte imbalances
- Severe acidemia
- β blocking drugs (e.g., propranolol)
- Profound hypothermia

Reductions in contractility are dose-dependent. Among the commonly administered anesthetic drugs, inhalants probably have the most profound effect on contractility, with reductions of up to 50% at surgical planes of anesthesia. The induction drugs listed also reduce contractility, but their effect is more transient and less profound than that seen with the inhalants.

12. Summarize the major players that reduce mean arterial pressure and may lead to hypotension.

Anything that reduces systemic vascular resistance, heart rate, or stroke volume can contribute to hypotension. Thus, when developing treatment approaches for hypotension, you should consider these three major players and rule in or out factors that affect them in the anesthetized animal.

13. You've decided your anesthetized patient is hypotensive. Devise a generalized treatment algorithm.

When faced with a hypotensive patient, look for drugs or physiologic/pathologic factors as listed above that may reduce (1) systemic vascular resistance, (2) heart rate, or (3) stroke volume (primarily preload and contractility).

14. Can I treat low systemic vascular resistance with crystalloids?

Almost by definition, an animal anesthetized with inhalants (especially isoflurane and sevoflurane) will have some degree of reduction in systemic vascular resistance. Premedication with acepromazine further reduces SVR. One approach is to "fill the space" with aggressive administration of intravenous crystalloids. Before doing this, however, you must assess the animal's anesthetic depth, since reducing the administered dose of inhalant will help to increase SVR.

In inhalant-anesthetized patients with normal cardiac and renal function a standard crystalloid administration rate *before* hypotension develops is 10–20 ml/kg/h. This allows for filling of the increased vascular volume caused by vasodilation by the inhalant. If further increases in vascular volume are deemed necessary, and the patient has normal cardiac and renal function, you can increase the crystalloid rate to 50–70 ml/kg/hr (cats, large animals) and 70–90 ml/kg/hr (dogs) for 15 minutes and then assess the response to treatment.

If mean arterial pressure has not increased at this point, then you should return to the algorithm. When administering aggressive fluid therapy, it is advisable to monitor packed cell volume compared with total plasma (PCV/ TP), electrolyte status, acid-base status, and lung sounds to prevent pulmonary edema.

15. Can I increase systemic vascular resistance with drugs?

It is rarely necessary to increase SVR with drugs. Usually, in hypotensive patients that do not respond to fluid therapy, the cause can be found in stroke volume or, less often, heart rate. However, occasionally ephedrine is used to increase SVR when other parameters in the algorithm have already been addressed. Ephedrine increases vascular tone by indirectly stimulating α_1 receptors in vascular smooth muscle through release of norepinephrine. The recommended dose of ephedrine is 0.03 to 0.07 mg/kg IV as a slow bolus. Since the drug's mechanism of action is indirect, it can take 20 to 30 minutes to induce a response.

16. When does bradycardia cause hypotension?

Bradycardia can be friend or foe when dealing with hypotension. On the one hand, a slow heart rate allows for generous right atrial filling, which in turn provides optimal diastolic ventricular filling and stroke volume on the subsequent systole. Since coronary blood flow (and myocardial oxygenation) occur during diastole, bradycardia and a long diastolic period help to optimize myocardial oxygen supply. However, if bradycardia is coupled with less than optimal contractility (either from anesthetic drugs or disease) it is sometimes necessary to increase the heart rate to treat hypotension.

17. What are treatment approaches for bradycardia?

Bradycardia is common in anesthetized patients, especially when systemic opioids are used concurrently for analgesia. The first approach to treating bradycardia is to reduce administered doses of inhalant, if possible. You can also consider reversal of systemic opioids, if present, with naloxone or nalbuphine. However, since opioids were likely given to provide analgesia, reversal may not be desirable for patient comfort and recovery. One should also ensure that the patient is normothermic, as bradycardia secondary to hypothermia will usually not respond to pharmacologic intervention. Finally, one should address electrolyte or acid-base abnormalities that may be contributing to bradycardia.

18. What drugs will increase heart rate?

Anticholinergics such as atropine or glycopyrrolate will increase heart rate in all species. Atropine is more potent than glycopyrrolate, and as such is more likely to cause undesirable tachycardia. For this reason, atropine is more often used for life-threatening bradycardia. Both drugs can be given intravenously or intramuscularly. The dose for atropine is 0.02–0.04 mg/kg; glycopyrrolate is 0.005–0.01 mg/kg. Paradoxical bradycardia and atrioventricular block are occasionally seen soon after drug administration, especially with glycopyrrolate given intravenously. This effect is usually overridden as the plasma concentration of glycopyrrolate reaches therapeutic levels.

19. Are there risks to treating bradycardia with anticholinergics?

Administration of anticholinergics can result in tachycardia. Severe tachycardia may worsen hypotension, since diastolic filling and stroke volume are compromised. However, if tachycardia develops after anticholinergic administration, it usually resolves within 10–20 minutes. Other side effects of anticholinergic administration include ileus (especially in large animals), decreased salivation (which may or may not be desirable in a given patient), pupillary dilation, bronchodilation, and reduced mucociliary transport in the trachea.

20. What are treatment approaches for reduced preload?

Reduced preload should be addressed first by eliminating factors that might mechanically cause it, such as positive pressure ventilation to high airway pressures, abdominal distension, etc. If this is not possible, then preload can be increased with intravenous crystalloids, as discussed in question 14. Occasionally, crystalloid administration is insufficient to increase preload, owing to low oncotic pressure (e.g., hypoalbuminemia) or blood loss.

21. How can I increase preload with fluids other than crystalloids?

Fluid therapy and blood products are discussed in detail in Chapters 5 and 6, respectively. Briefly, if the animal has reduced preload that is not improved with crystalloids, oncotic agents will help to maintain venous blood volume by reducing leakage of water into the interstitial spaces. Oncotic agents commonly used in anesthetized animals include fresh whole blood, plasma, hetastarch, and dextran 40 and 70. These agents are particularly useful in animals that are hypoproteinemic or have suffered blood loss. They should not, with rare exceptions, be used exclusively for volume replacement, but rather as an adjunct to crystalloids to enhance total venous blood volume.

22. How can I improve stroke volume by enhancing contractility?

If poor contractility is suspected, one should first address, if possible, the physiologic and pathologic causes. For example, if the animal is severely acidemic, that condition should be corrected prior to other manipulations to increase contractility. As mentioned previously, inhalants are the most common causes of poor contractility in normal, anesthetized animals. Thus, a logical approach to improving contractility is to reduce or eliminate the inhalant. However, eliminating the inhalant entirely is rarely feasible.

One option is to reduce the inhalant's MAC by supplementing with systemic opioids. For example, a patient anesthetized with isoflurane can be given intermittent boluses of intravenous opioids such as oxymorphone or hydromorphone to reduce the delivered inhalant concentration while maintaining surgical anesthetic depth. Recommended doses for oxymorphone are 0.025–0.05 mg/kg; and 0.05–0.1 mg/kg for hydromorphone; either drug can be given in this dosage range as needed to reduce the inhalant and thereby improve contractility.

A "fine tuned" alternative is to deliver fentanyl as a constant rate infusion in dose ranges of 2.5–20 µg/kg/hour (note units). This can be accomplished using a syringe pump or buretrol. Fentanyl constant rate infusions allow you to titrate the opioid up or down to maintain adequate depth. With fentanyl doses of 20 μg/kg/hour or higher, especially in sick patients, anesthetic inhalant requirement may be reduced by 100%. In other words, the MAC of isoflurane in a patient receiving fentanyl can be as low as 0.5%.

23. Are there drugs that directly improve contractility and that are safe to use in anesthetized patients?

Inotropes such as dopamine and dobutamine can be given to increase contractility. However, these drugs should not be used without attention to ensuring adequate vascular volume as well. Additionally, before administration of an inotrope, you should seek to minimize inhalant doses as described in question 22. Dopamine and dobutamine stimulate β_1-receptors in the myocardium, thus enhancing myofilament shortening and ventricular contractility. These drugs are given as infusions, at a dose range of 1–10 μg/kg/min. Individual animal sensitivity varies greatly, so you should always start with the lowest recommended dose. The half-life of these drugs is short (3–5 minutes) so their effect is short-lived once the infusion is discontinued.

24. Are there risks associated with giving inotropes?

Dobutamine is a synthetic catecholamine, and dopamine is a precursor to epinephrine and norepinephrine. As such, these drugs exert effects similar to endogenous catecholamines. The most common side effects noticed in anesthetized animals are tachycardia (especially with dopamine) and occasionally atrial and ventricular arrhythmias. Because the half-life of these drugs is short, termination of the infusion or reduction of the dose usually results in resolution of these complications.

25. How can I prevent hypotension when I plan anesthetic management for my patients?

- Ensure adequate volume status prior to anesthesia.
- Correct underlying acid-base and electrolyte abnormalities.
- Correct underlying pathologic states if possible.
- Use the lowest possible dose required of acepromazine or α-2 agonists, or eliminate them altogether.
- Premedicate with agonist opioids for preemptive analgesia and reduction of inhalant requirement.
- Reduce induction drug requirements with intravenous benzodiazapines and opioids immediately prior to induction.
- Consider supplemental opioids during anesthetic maintenance, as needed.
- Look for alternative methods to provide analgesia for surgery, such as epidurals, local blocks etc.
- Give intravenous crystalloids to all patients receiving inhalant anesthetics.
- Monitor blood pressure! The best way to prevent hypotension is to detect reductions in blood pressure as soon as they occur.

BIBLIOGRAPHY

1. Berne RM, Levy MN (eds): Cardiovascular Physiology, 7th ed. St. Louis, Mosby-Year Book, 1997.
2. Caulkett NA, Cantwell SL, Houston DM: A comparison of indirect blood pressure monitoring techniques in the anesthetized cat. Vet Surg 27:370–377, 1999.
3. Grosenbaugh DA, Muir WW: Accuracy of noninvasive oxyhemoglobin saturation, end-tidal carbon dioxide concentration, and blood pressure monitoring during experimentally induced hypoxemia, hypotension, or hypertension in anesthetized dogs. Am J Vet Res 59:205–212, 1998.
4. Hennig GE, Court MH: Equine postanesthetic myopathy: An update. Compend Contin Ed Vet Med 13(11):1709–1716, 1991.
5. Stoelting RK (ed): Pharmacology and Physiology in Anesthetic Practice, 2nd ed. Philadelphia, JB Lippincott, 1991.
6. Thurmon JC, Tranquilli WJ, Benson GJ (eds): Lumb and Jones' Veterinary Anesthesia, 3rd ed. Baltimore, Williams & Wilkins, 1996.

24. CARDIAC DYSRHYTHMIAS

Kris T. Kruse-Elliott, D.V.M., Ph.D., D.A.C.V.A.

1. How does electrocardiography in an anesthetized patient differ from that in a nonanesthetized patient?

The electrocardiogram (ECG) is particularly useful for monitoring electrical activity of the heart. In anesthetized patients, it is generally applied for detection of dysrhythmias, whereas in conscious patients, there are other diagnostic uses for this monitor. In contrast to the traditional diagnostic ECG done on awake patients as part of an overall evaluation of cardiovascular status, during anesthesia and surgery the leads are placed wherever they will not interfere with the surgical procedure. Additionally, the animal may be placed in a variety of positions to accommodate the surgical or medical procedure. In general, lead II is the preferred lead to use given the usual familiarity with normal patterns in this lead. However, when necessary, the other leads (I, III, aVR, aVL, or aVF) may be used to assist in monitoring for arrhythmias.

2. Describe the limitations of using an electrocardiogram to monitor cardiovascular status in an anesthetized patient.

An ECG used as a monitor during anesthesia will not provide accurate and reliable information regarding chamber size in the heart. Additionally, it is important that you be very aware that the ECG does not provide information regarding mechanical (e.g. muscular) activity of the heart and so should not be the sole monitor employed to evaluate cardiovascular status in a patient. Thus, during the perianesthetic period, the ECG should be used strictly for detection of dysrhythmias.

3. Describe a simple, systematic approach to interpretation of the ECG for the diagnosis of arrhythmias.

- Locate a complex and identify the P, QRS, and T waves.
- Is there a P wave for every QRST? If not, then does the QRST look normal or abnormal in configuration and duration?
- Is there a QRST for every P wave? If not, then does the QRST look normal or abnormal in configuration?
- Is the R wave to R wave interval constant or does it vary? If it varies, is there a pattern to the variation?
- Are there complexes that occur earlier than expected? If so, is there an abnormality in either the P wave or the QRST? Is there a pause after these early beats?
- And finally, don't be afraid to call the ECG normal!

4. What are the physiologic consequences of bradycardia or tachycardia?

Keep in mind that cardiac output (CO) is dependent in part on heart rate (HR) and also that blood pressure depends on CO and systemic vascular resistance (SVR). The following formulas are useful to keep in mind when considering the physiologic consequences of bradycardia or tachycardia:

$$CO = SV \times HR \text{ (SV is stroke volume)}$$
$$MAP = CO \times SVR \text{ (MAP is mean arterial pressure)}$$

Thus, you can predict that at a very low HR, CO will decline and result in a lowered MAP; whereas a very high HR will decrease filling time and hence decrease SV, which will result in a lower CO and decline in MAP. Normal HR ranges for dogs and cats are 60–160 and 80–180 bpm, respectively. However, expect a lower range of normal HR in large-breed dogs and a higher range in small-breed dogs. For example, a 2 year-old healthy, relatively fit, athletic Labrador retriever may have a normal resting rate in the low 50s.

5. List the possible causes of this dysrhythmia in an anesthetized patient (exclude causes related to primary disease and focus on those specifically related to anesthesia and surgery).

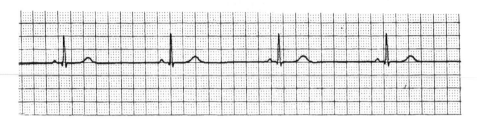

This pattern represents sinus bradycardia (rate of 35 bpm, paper speed 25 mm/sec). Note that there is a linkage between every P wave and every QRST, and the R to R interval is regular, but the HR is slow. In anesthetized patients, there are a variety of causes for bradycardia, including, but not limited to the following:

- Excessive vagal tone induced by intubation, traction or pressure on the orbit, traction on the viscera.
- Drug-induced (opioids, α_2-agonists, high doses of inhaled anesthetics)
- Hypothermia
- Profound hypoxemia

6. Describe the rhythm presented here.

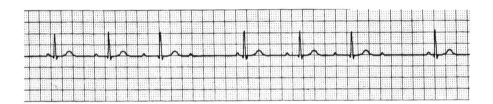

Remember the step-by-step approach to evaluating an ECG:
- Locate a complex and identify the P, QRS, and T waves
- Is there a P wave for every QRST? *Yes*
- Is there a QRST for every P wave? *No*
- Is the R to R wave interval constant or does it vary? If it varies, is there a pattern to the variation? *Yes, it varies. There is evidence of a missed QRST complex that fits within the normal R to R interval.*
- Are there complexes that occur earlier than expected? *No, in fact there are missing complexes where you would expect them to occur.*

This is second-degree atrioventricular block, type I. The most obvious clue to diagnosis is the presence of P waves that do not have an accompanying QRST complex. Also note the progressively longer P-R interval until finally atrioventricular conduction does not occur. This is typical of increased vagal tone in an anesthetized patient or other causes of bradycardia as described in question 5.

7. What treatment should you consider for the rhythms observed in the two readings given in questions 5 and 6?

Anticholinergics are the treatment of choice in both situations. Additionally the suspected cause should be considered and removed if possible. Treatment is considered necessary when the bradycardia or bradyarrhythmia is severe enough to have a negative impact on cardiac output.

8. What are two commonly used drugs in the drug class of choice? What are the important differences between them?

Anticholinergics commonly used in veterinary anesthesia are atropine and glycopyrrolate. These drugs antagonize the effect of acetylcholine at the postganglionic terminations of cholinergic fibers within the autonomic nervous system (e.g., muscarinic receptors). Unlike glycopyrrolate, atropine crosses the blood-brain barrier and thus may have some initial vagal stimulatory effects, which will briefly slow heart rate before it's peripheral parasympatholytic action takes effect. This is particularly true at low doses of atropine (e.g., less than 0.01 mg/kg). The duration of action of atropine is around 1 hour, whereas glycopyrrolate lasts 2 to 3 hours.

9. This reading is from an anesthetized, 20 kg, 2-year-old Greyhound (resting heart rate prior to anesthesia was 52 bpm). What is this rhythm? What are some possible causes for it in this particular patient?

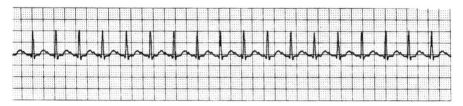

This is sinus tachycardia, HR is 140 bpm(paper speed is 25 mm/sec). There is a linkage of every P with a QRST; however, because of the rate it is difficult to recognize. Look closely at the T waves and you will see a notch that represents the P wave. In a large-breed dog, an HR of 140 bpm is generally considered to be too high, particularly when the normal resting HR is 52. Clinically significant tachycardia is further noted by hypotension due to a reduction in CO. The reduction in CO occurs because SV falls due to a decrease in diastolic filling time. In anesthetized patients, some causes of tachycardia include
- Response to stimulation, e.g., anesthesia level is too light
- Ketamine
- Hypoxemia and/or hypercarbia
- Hyperthermia
- Various preexisting diseases such as pheochromocytoma, hyperthyroidism, cardiac failure, central nervous system disease, etc.

10. Identify this dysrhythmia.

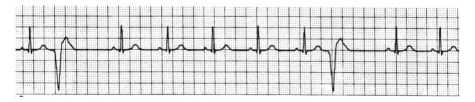

Ventricular premature complex (VPC). Again, remember the systematic process to evaluating this rhythm strip.
- Locate a complex and identify the P, QRS, and T waves.
- Is there a P wave for every QRST? *No*
- Is there a QRST for every P wave? *Yes*
- Is the R to R wave interval constant or does it vary? If it varies, is there a pattern to the variation? *Yes, it varies. There is an abnormal complex that appears earlier than normal. This is followed by a pause until the next normal PQRST complex, e.g., a compensatory pause.*

11. What is this rhythm disturbance? How would you treat it?

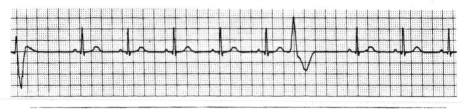

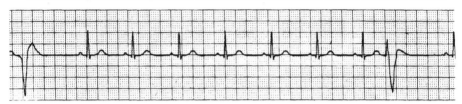

These are multifocal VPCs. Note the variation in shape and direction of the premature complexes. This indicates several origins of abnormal electrical activity in the ventricles.

If the cause is known and can be eliminated, this should be attempted concomitant with antiarrhythmic therapy. Basic support such as supplemental oxygenation, ensuring appropriate anesthetic depth, eliminating arrhythmogenic drugs (such as halothane, thiamylal, inotropes), and fluid therapy should be included. Intravenous lidocaine is the drug of choice for initial therapy of multifocal VPCs. Alternative therapies for ventricular arrhythmias include procainamide, quinidine, propranolol, and various newer antiarrhythmic agents currently under investigation.

12. What are some common causes of multifocal ventricular premature complexes in dogs?

Multifocal VPCs may occur in association with primary cardiac disease, trauma and shock, traumatic myocarditis, hypoxemia, ischemia, electrolyte and acid-base disturbances, digitalis toxicity, and gastric dilation-volvulus or other major abdominal diseases that result in visceral organ failure.

13. List the indications for using lidocaine.
- When the frequency of unifocal VPCs exceeds 20–30 per minute, or there is a significant negative impact on cardiac output
- Runs of VPCs
- Ventricular bigeminy, trigeminy, or similar repetitive situations
- Multifocal VPCs
- Ventricular tachycardia
- R on T phenomenon (the VPC occurs within the QT interval of the previous complex or embedded in the T wave—this is often a prelude to ventricular fibrillation)

14. What is the dose of lidocaine for dogs versus cats?

In dogs, the initial intravenous bolus dose of lidocaine is 1–2 mg/kg, which can be administered every 20 minutes, or an infusion of 50–80 µg/kg/min may be started. In cats, the dose is 0.25 mg/kg and should not exceed 1 mg/kg over a 1-hour period.

15. Name this rhythm disturbance.

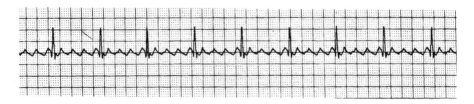

This is an example of atrial flutter, a relatively uncommon dysrhythmia, which is characterized by the sawtooth pattern observed. Cardiac output can decline significantly if the ventricular rate associated with this arrhythmia becomes too high. This is also true for atrial fibrillation.

16. How can you differentiate between atrial fibrillation and baseline noise from muscle fasciculations?

The key hint that a patient is in atrial fibrillation is that the ventricular rate appears "irregularly irregular" (look at the R to R interval); there is no distinct pattern to the irregularity. Generally this is also easily noticed when palpating pulses in these patients. In contrast, respiratory sinus arrhythmia is a good example of a regularly irregular R to R interval.

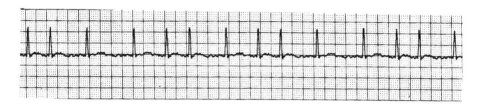

When you evaluate a rhythm strip from a patient with muscle fasciculations, you should observe a regular R to R interval.

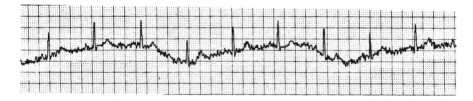

17. What is happening in this ECG?

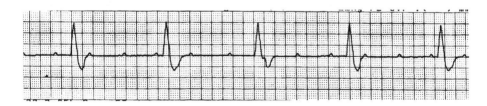

This is an example of third-degree atrioventricular (AV) blockade, or complete heart block. There is no conduction through the AV node and you can observe P waves that do not have a QRST complex associated with them. Additionally, ventricular complexes are evident, which represent ventricular escape beats. Third-degree AV block generally is the result of cardiac disease at the AV node but may also occur with digitalis toxicity or hyperkalemia. This patient represents a poor risk for anesthesia in its current condition.

18. During cardiac arrest, what types of rhythm disturbances might you observe?

- *Electromechanical dissociation*: also known as pulseless electrical activity. Often the rhythm is abnormal, with wide and bizarre QRS complexes, although it may also appear as relatively normal PQRST complexes. The key problem is the lack of mechanical activity and therefore no cardiac output associated with the electrical activity.

- *Ventricular fibrillation* (see ECG): can occur as either course or fine fibrillation and may be difficult to recognize in certain leads (where it may appear as asystole). The electrical activity is random and disorderly, and no functional mechanical activity results.

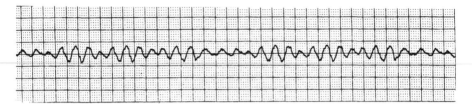

- *Asystole* (see ECG): there is no electrical activity observed in any lead; that is, the ECG is a flat line.

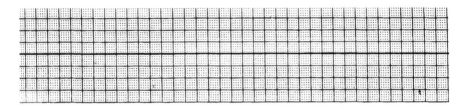

19. Should you be concerned about what you are observing in this ECG?

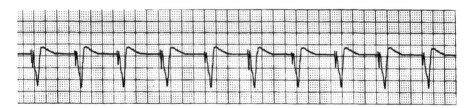

No. This is a dog with sick sinus syndrome and a ventricular pacemaker implanted as treatment. If you look closely, you can see the pacing spike that happens immediately before the ventricular complex.

20. What is the rhythm from this ECG?

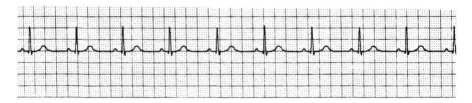

Go through this ECG systematically:
- Can you locate and identify a complex with P, QRS, and T waves?
- Is there a P wave for every QRST and vice versa? Does the QRST look normal or abnormal in configuration and duration?
- Is the R to R interval constant or does it vary, and, if it varies, is there a pattern?

- Do any complexes occur earlier than expected?
- And finally, remember: "don't be afraid to call it normal!"

Diagnosis: normal sinus rhythm. *Gottcha!* Remember, do not be afraid to call it normal. Note there is a PQRST that is regular, a P for every QRST and vice versa, and a regular R to R interval.

21. What is the differential diagnosis for the dysrhythmia shown?

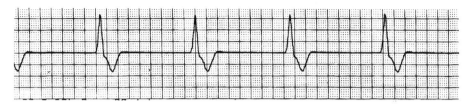

Ventricular escape beats or idioventricular rhythm that may be associated with: AV nodal disease, sick sinus syndrome, persistent atrial standstill, atrial standstill due to hyperkalemia, or atrial fibrillation with complete heart block.

22. Should lidocaine or other antiarrhythmic drugs be used to treat the dysrhythmia at question 21?

No. This ventricular rhythm should not be suppressed by antiarrhythmic agents because it represents an adaptation of the heart's electrical activity to a situation of disturbed impulse formation or conduction. Cardiac output and perfusion in this patient are dependent on continuation of this abnormal rhythm, until the underlying cause is determined and treated appropriately.

23. What is demonstrated in this rhythm strip?

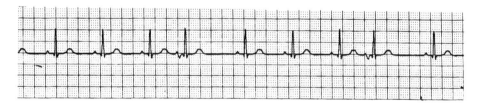

Atrial premature complexes. Remember to evaluate the R to R interval. Note that there are two beats in this strip that occur early, that is, prematurely. Also note that the QRST of these early complexes is of normal configuration and duration; however, there is a P wave associated with these complexes that is abnormal. It has a biphasic appearance.

24. What is the rhythm shown? What commonly used anesthetic induction drug may be associated with increased incidence of this dysrhythmia?

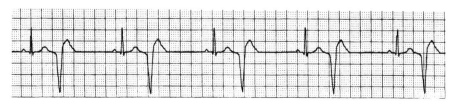

Ventricular bigeminy. There are a variety of situations in which ventricular bigeminy may be observed, but it is not uncommon in association with high doses of thiobarbiturates for intravenous induction (thiamylal or thiopental). Generally this dysrhythmia will resolve given adequate time for redistribution of the induction drug and lowering of blood drug levels. However, if there is a significant negative impact on cardiac output and blood pressure, then a single bolus of lidocaine intravenously should resolve this into normal sinus rhythm. One dose of lidocaine should outlast the duration of high blood levels of the offending anesthetic agent. This rhythm is infrequently observed when premedication is used to aid in reducing the dose of thiobarbiturate required for anesthetic induction.

BIBLIOGRAPHY

1. Carr AP, Tilley LP, Miller MS: Treatment of cardiac arrhythmias and conduction disturbances. In Tilley LP, Goodwin J-K (eds): Manual of Canine and Feline Cardiology, 3rd ed. Philadelphia, W.B. Saunders, 2001, pp 371–405.
2. Goodwin J-K: Electrocardiography. In Tilley LP, Goodwin J-K (eds): Manual of Canine and Feline Cardiology, 3rd ed. Philadelphia, W.B. Saunders, 2001, pp 43–70.
3. Haskins SC: Perioperative monitoring. In Paddelford RR (ed): Manual of Small Animal Anesthesia, 2nd ed. Philadelphia, W.B. Saunders, 1999, pp 123–146.
4. Kruse-Elliott KT: Cardiopulmonary resuscitation: Strategies for maximizing success. Vet Med 96:51–59, 2001.
5. Opie LH: Electrophysiology and Electrocardiogram. In The Heart: Physiology, from Cell to Circulation, 3rd ed. Philadelphia, Lippincott Williams & Wilkins, 1998, pp 71–145.

25. HYPOTHERMIA

Ralph C. Harvey, D.V.M., M.S., D.A.C.V.A.

1. What is significant perioperative hypothermia in cats and dogs?

In anesthetized and recovering patients, a decrease in core body temperature of as little as 1°C (or about 2°F) results in adverse challenges for many patients. Healthy patients often compensate quite well for the physiologic challenges presented by mild or moderate perioperative hypothermia. However, patients that are otherwise compromised, and certainly the critically ill patients, suffer increased morbidity and mortality secondary to avoidable perioperative hypothermia.

2. What effect does general anesthesia have on thermoregulation?

Anesthetics alter one or more of the three components of heat balance in the body: the afferent pathway, the central control mechanism, and the efferent responses. General anesthetics, particularly the volatile anesthetics, reset the threshold for thermoregulation, so that a broader range of body temperatures is tolerated without response. Once a response is triggered, the magnitude of that response may be near normal yet incapable of restoring normal body temperature.

3. How does body temperature decrease during anesthesia?

Three phases of heat loss are observed. There is an initial and precipitous decrease in body temperature due to vasodilation and a redistribution of core body heat to the periphery. Thereafter, a progressive linear decline in temperature continues until a vasoconstrictive response occurs. This thermoregulatory response partially limits further decreases in body temperature by reducing blood flow to peripheral tissues.

4. What physiologic mechanisms act to maintain or restore body temperature?

Behavioral responses (e.g., seeking warm places, curling to minimize exposed surface) are blocked by sedatives, anesthetics, and even by physical constraints of caging or hospitalization without a sunny rock available. Piloerection increases the thermal barrier of warmed insulating air surrounding the body. This barrier helps reduce further heat loss. Shivering thermogenesis is very effective in generating body heat. Shivering may even occur during light anesthesia. Nonshivering thermogenesis is the generation of body heat through increased muscle tone. This may also be blocked, although perhaps to a lesser extent, by anesthesia. There is a significant vasoconstriction, induced by hypothermia, that limits delivery of blood and heat from the core to the periphery and is relatively well maintained during anesthesia.

5. What are the adverse circulatory effects of hypothermia in anesthetized patients?

A significant stress response is elicited by hypothermia. Moderate hypothermia, 35°C (95°F), triggers a two- to sevenfold increase in release of catecholamines, with resulting vasoconstriction, tachycardia, and hypertension. The morbidity associated with these stress responses typically occurs during the postoperative period, rather than during anesthesia and surgery. More severe hypothermia, in the range of 30°C (86°F), is associated with increased risk of atrial fibrillation. Profound hypothermia, between 24°C (75.2°F) and 28°C (82.4°F), induces refractory ventricular fibrillation and death.

6. What are the effects of hypothermia on coagulation and bleeding?

Hypothermia has been shown to cause deficiencies in coagulation in many species, including dogs. Hypothermia impairs platelet function, decreases activity of the coagulation pathways, and increases fibrinolysis.

7. Does hypothermia increase the risk of operative infection or delay wound healing?

In a retrospective study of dogs and cats with clean surgical wounds, mild perioperative hypothermia was not a significant risk factor for postoperative wound infection. In human patients undergoing colon surgery, the incidence of infection is increased threefold, from 6% if the patient is normothermic, to 19% if moderate hypothermia occurs. Similar increases in the risk of surgical infection have been confirmed in hypothermic animal research models. This increased risk of infection is attributed to impairment of macrophage function and reduced tissue oxygen tension secondary to thermoregulatory vasoconstriction. Compared to normothermic patients, patients that are hypothermic during anesthesia and surgery have impaired wound healing that has been attributed to decreased collagen deposition.

8. What are the metabolic consequences of hypothermia?

The catabolic postoperative stress response, with muscle protein breakdown and a negative nitrogen balance, is increased by even slight hypothermia. Patients who developed as little as a 2°C loss of body temperature developed a doubling of urea nitrogen excretion, compared with normothermic patients. Heat conservation with maintenance of normothermia has been shown to reduce muscle protein breakdown in geriatric patients undergoing major gastrointestinal surgery.

9. What changes in anesthetic requirement occur with hypothermia?

Hypothermia decreases the requirement for general anesthetics by several mechanisms. There is a 5% decrease in the MAC requirement for volatile anesthetics with each 1°C decrease in body temperature. Hypothermia increases the solubility of volatile anesthetics in the body, thereby increasing the effective dose delivered. Decreases in the clearance of anesthetic drugs are also attributed to hypothermia. The combined result of these processes can be a significant potential for anesthetic overdose in hypothermic patients. Monitoring patients' body temperature in the perioperative period is simple and inexpensive. Temperature monitoring should lead to recognition of hypothermia, and the anesthetic doses or vaporizer settings should be appropriately reduced to minimize anesthetic complications.

10. Why does body temperature decrease so rapidly under anesthesia?

All anesthetics impair thermoregulation. At the induction of anesthesia, initial vasodilation allows for a redistribution of core heat to the skin and extremities. The loss of thermal units from the core is irreversible. Subsequent vasoconstriction, as hypothermia proceeds, does not restore core temperature.

11. How much is body temperature decreased by anesthesia?

While under anesthesia, patients practically become poikilothermic. After the initial decline due to vasodilatation, temperature continues to fall until vasoconstriction reduces blood flow, and heat distribution, to the periphery. This lower plateau is reported to be about 34°C (about 93°F). Decreases in body temperature are somewhat dose-dependent and are relatively linear over time. Many factors influence the extent of hypothermia in the anesthetized patient.

12. Other than by application of active warming, what can be done to reduce the loss of body heat during anesthesia?

Heat loss may be reduced by covering or insulation to control radiant heat loss, prevention of contact with cool surfaces and prep solutions, and use of lower flow gas circuits and techniques. Covering or wrapping the patient helps to maintain the crucial layer of warm air surrounding the body, thereby minimizing convective losses. The choice of material seems to be of relatively little importance in maintaining this envelope of warm air. Exposure of large areas of skin for surgical procedures, or particularly the opening of large body cavities, greatly increases cooling through both radiation and evaporation.

13. What active heating strategies can be employed during the perioperative period to maintain or restore body temperature?

Active heating can be pursued, with acceptable safety, by use of warmer operating room and recovery area ambient temperatures, warm air blankets, circulating warm water blankets, radiant heat sources above the patient and surgical field, and warmed intravenous and surgical irrigation fluids, and perhaps by use of devices to warm and humidify inspired anesthetic gases. The effectiveness of these techniques varies tremendously. By far the most effective is the convective warm air device, delivering controlled warm air through porous blankets to surround the patient with an envelope of warm air. While less effective, the circulating warm water blankets can help prevent, or minimize, severe hypothermia when used optimally. Heating devices and strategies should be applied early, to prevent hypothermia, and with monitoring of body temperature.

14. How safe are these methods for warming patients?

There is a risk of thermal injury with all active heating systems. The broad distribution of heat, to avoid localized hot spots, tissue drying, and burning, is important for patient safety. Warmed intravenous fluids may cool to near room temperature in the fluid delivery tubing. Only very high fluid flow rates are significant in patient warming (or cooling). Overheated intravenous or irrigation fluids can be very damaging. Temperature monitoring should be considered mandatory whenever active heating is used. Radiant heat in surgical and recovery settings can overheat tissues. Heated and humidified anesthetic gases may burn or dry the airway, if too hot, and may increase fluid load by delivery of excessive airway moisture. Recumbent pressure may limit blood flow to skin areas in direct contact with warmed surfaces, thereby facilitating tissue burning. Anesthesia, as well as any residual anesthesia or sedation during recovery, obviously interferes with the possibility for a patient to sense overheating and interferes with the patient's ability to move away from heat sources to escaping injury. Control and monitoring are of paramount importance in the use of all active heating systems.

15. Why are conventional electric heating pads not acceptable?

The use of resistance wire electric heating pads is not acceptable in anesthesia or recovery. There is extreme risk of iatrogenic thermal injury due to unacceptably high temperatures of these electric heating pads. These pads are designed for use on awake humans having both the mental faculty and physical capability to recognize excess heat and to make the appropriate responses to remove the device or alter the heat. There is an uneven distribution of delivered heat and focal delivery of excess heat. Tissue burns are very frequently seen in patients that have been placed on electric heating pads during anesthesia or recovery.

16. Are hot water bottles reasonable for patient warming?

Hot water bottles or surgical gloves filled with warm or hot water are also potentially quite dangerous for any anesthetized, sedated, or stuporous patient. Burns from hot water bottles can result by the same mechanisms as with electric heating pads. If the warm or hot water bottles or gloves are kept at acceptably moderate temperatures, to avoid the potential for burns, the effectiveness for heating is lost. An inordinate number of gloves or bottles would be needed to effect any patient warming. Once gloves or bottles of warmed water cool to the temperature of the patient, and then continue to cool, they contribute to loss, rather than gain, of body heat.

17. Does shivering occur during anesthesia?

Yes, patients under light levels of anesthesia may be observed to shiver. The shivering activity can range from very fine fibrillary contractions of the facial muscles to more generalized and intense contractions of the trunk or limbs. Much more common is the development of gross shivering upon recovery from anesthesia. When necessary, postoperative opioid analgesics can be used to suppress shivering. Meperidine is commonly used for this purpose in human patients.

18. What are the consequences of shivering?

Postoperative shivering can range from subtle to severe. Although shivering can be very effective in restoring body temperature, it substantially increases metabolic oxygen requirements. Early studies indicated that postoperative shivering could increase metabolic rates as much as

400%. More recent research suggests that there is typically a doubling of the oxygen requirement (reported range of 40% to 200% increase) during postoperative shivering. This can result in an oxygen debt, since there is often residual reduction in ventilation, residual pulmonary atalectasis, or other respiratory insufficiency during the immediate postoperative period. Even when there is a fourfold increase in minute ventilation, shivering patients can still have arterial oxygenation values well below baseline and inadequate oxygen delivery to tissues. In spite of the potential cooling effect of increased oxygen flow from loose-fitting facemasks, patients shivering during recovery should be supplied with supplemental oxygen.

BIBLIOGRAPHY

1. Beal MW, Brown DC, Shofer FS: The effects of perioperative hypothermia and the duration of anesthesia on postoperative wound infection rate in clean wounds: A retrospective study. Vet Surg 29(2):123–127, 2000.
2. Ben-Eliyahu S, Shakhar G, Rosenne E, et al: Hypothermia in barbiturate-anesthetized rats suppresses natural killer cell activity and compromises resistance to tumor metastasis: A role for adrenergic mechanisms. Anesthesiology 91(3):732–740, 1999.
3. Collins VJ: Temperature regulation and heat problems. In Collins VJ (ed): Physiologic and Pharmacologic Bases of Anesthesia. Baltimore, Williams & Wilkins, 1996, pp 316–343.
4. Frank SM: Thermoregulation. In Foundations of Anesthesia Basic and Clinical Sciences. London, Mosby, 2000, pp 665–673.
5. Haskins SC: Hypothermia and its prevention during general anesthesia in cats. Am J Vet Res 42(5):856–861, 1981.
6. Machon RG, Raffe MR, Robinson EP: Warming with a forced air warming blanket minimizes anesthetic-induced hypothermia in cats. Vet Surg 28(4):301–310, 1999.
7. Meyer RE, Gleed RD, Harvey HJ: Isoflurane anesthesia as an adjunct to hypothermia for surgery in a dog. J Am Vet Med Assoc 184(11):1387–1389, 1984.
8. Sessler DI. Perioperative thermoregulation and heat balance. Ann NY Acad Sci 813:757–777, 1997.
9. Sessler DI. Perioperative heat balance. Anesthesiology 92(2):578–596, 2000.
10. Tomasic M. Temporal changes in core body temperature in anesthetized adult horses. Am J Vet Res 60(5):556–562, 1999.
11. Yamakage M, Kamada Y, Honma Y, et al: Predictive variables of hypothermia in the early phase of general anesthesia. Anesth Analg 90(2):456–459, 2000.

26. HYPERTHERMIA

Ralph C. Harvey, D.V.M., M.S., D.A.C.V.A.

1. How do patients become hyperthermic under anesthesia?
Body temperature is usually balanced between metabolic generation of heat and the processes of heat loss. Patient warming during anesthesia and surgery is almost always necessary to avoid hypothermia. Accidental hyperthermia most often arises during warm ambient temperatures, in larger animals with thick hair coats, and with the use of active external warming devices. Excessive external heating is the most common contributory cause of perioperative hyperthermia. Increased body temperature is far less common in the context of anesthesia and surgery than is decreased body temperature, particularly for small patients. Body temperature may rise to above normal levels by three mechanisms: (1) decreased loss of body heat through increased insulation, particularly in larger patients with extensive insulating hair coats plus added insulation or padding; (2) excessive or poorly controlled exogenous heating, often in combination with increased insulation or other environmental factors; and (3) increased metabolic production of heat, including stress-related hyperthermia, increased muscle tone, resetting of thermoregulatory processes, and rarely malignant hyperthermia or related syndromes.

2. How is heat lost from the body?
Heat loss occurs by radiation, convection, conduction, evaporation of moisture from the skin and respiratory tract, and excretion of urine and feces. Most significant losses are normally by radiation and evaporation. There is considerable species variability in strategies for evaporative heat loss. Panting is a remarkably effective mechanism for heat dispersion in dogs, whereas sweating is remarkably effective in horses and even more so in humans. In normal awake subjects, the relative contribution of each mechanism varies also with ambient temperature, humidity, and windspeed. At high ambient temperatures, severe and sustained exercise can generate heat through metabolic work in excess of the capacity of heat loss mechanisms. Although anesthetic hypothermia is much more common than hyperthermia, disruption of the normal processes for heat loss may also lead to abnormal increases in body temperature during anesthesia.

3. How does fever differ from other forms of hyperthermia?
Fever specifically refers to a regulated increase in core body temperature. Hyperthermia is the more general term and refers to an increase in body temperature, based on any etiology.

4. What is significant perioperative hyperthermia in cats and dogs?
Adverse effects of hyperthermia vary with the causative factors. Hyperthermia of even a degree or two increases circulatory work. More extreme increases in body temperature, above 42° C (108° F) increase metabolic rate, consume energy substrate, and increase oxygen utilization beyond oxygen supply. Cellular hypoxia results with potential damage to the brain, liver, kidneys, and blood. Relatively moderate hyperthermia, with temperatures below 42°, requires active cooling and dedicated monitoring of organ function, but specific therapy for organ damage may not be needed unless patients are otherwise compromised. Thorough patient evaluation is necessary to identify complications and to evaluate the success of management of the hyperthermia and any related consequences.

5. How should moderate hyperthermia be managed?
Upon recognition of hyperthermia, the underlying cause or causes should be identified (usually excessive external heating) and corrected. Supplemental oxygen should be administered in such a manner as to avoid rebreathing and carbon dioxide retention. Increases in convective and conductive heat loss often suffice to reduce body temperature. Evaporative cooling can be

increased by the application of alcohol or water to the skin and by the use of a fan to increase air-flow across the skin. Conductive heat loss can be increased by contact with cold packs, with caution to avoid tissue damage. Administration of cool intravenous fluids increases cooling and increases peripheral perfusion and peripheral heat loss. More aggressive methods of cooling include cool or cold water immersion, cool enemas, and gastric or abdominal lavage. It is important to discontinue active cooling before the return of body temperature to normal. "Afterdrop" is the continued decrease in body temperature after the removal of cooling methods. It may be difficult to anticipate the extent of continued decrease in body temperature. Cooling should be discontinued once body temperature decreases below 40° C (104° F).

6. What additional steps should be taken when hyperthermia is more severe, with body temperature above roughly 42°?

Continued monitoring of body temperature should be accompanied by repeated evaluation of multiple organ systems for signs of compromise or failure. Of particular importance are significant acidosis, renal and hepatic function, evidence of disseminated intravascular coagulation or other coagulopathy, neurologic function, and cardiac function. Patients treated for moderate or severe hyperthermia should be observed and monitored closely for adverse sequelae. Specific therapy must be based on identification of dysfunction.

7. Should antipyretics be used in treating hyperthermia?

Dipyrone or other antipyretics may lower hypothalamic thermostatic control of body temperature but are rarely, if ever, indicated for control of hyperthermia.

8. What is malignant hyperthermia?

Malignant hyperthermia (MH) is a rare syndrome, most fully described in human patients and in several strains of purebred swine, in which susceptible individuals may develop a syndrome of progressive and potentially fatal hyperthermia that is "triggered" by commonly used general anesthetics. Classical MH in human patients was originally described as a syndrome including progressive muscle rigidity, tachycardia, and fever. MH has been suspected in several other species, including dogs, cats, and horses. Classical MH is considered a "pharmacogenetic" disorder, in that genetically susceptible individuals may develop the syndrome upon exposure to a specific "triggering" drug. The signs of MH include greatly increased body metabolism, muscle rigidity and eventual hyperthermia, which may exceed 110° F. Death can result from cardiac arrest, brain damage, internal hemorrhaging or failure of other body systems. Closely related syndromes, which bear similarities to MH, have been described in humans, swine, dogs, and other animal species. The Malignant Hyperthermia Association of the United States (MHAUS) is an informative and useful source of support, information, and referral network dedicated to MH and related syndromes in human patients.

9. What is the underlying pathophysiology of the MH syndrome?

This complex disorder is based on an abnormal mechanism for release of calcium from the sarcoplasmic reticulum and abnormal calcium channel function. The calcium excess is thought to represent the functional defect in classical MH. The excess concentration of calcium in the myoplasm induces extraordinary catabolic anerobic and anerobic metabolic reactions. The genetic component of classical MH is well supported by data in humans, pigs, and most recently dogs. MH susceptibility in humans has an autosomal dominant mode of inheritance. The rate of occurrence in humans has been estimated to be as frequent as one in 5,000 or as rare as one in 65,000 administrations of anesthesia.

10. How does the presentation of the classical MH syndrome in dogs differ from the signs described for the MH syndrome in humans and swine?

The syndrome of MH in dogs typically includes rapid increases in temperature and increased end-tidal carbon dioxide. Muscle rigidity and acidosis are more marked in the MH syndrome in humans and swine.

11. Which anesthetics are recognized as potential triggering agents for malignant hyperthermia?

All of the volatile anesthetics and succinylcholine are the classically recognized anesthetic drugs that may initiate an episode of MH in susceptible individuals. MH, or closely related syndromes, may occur in apparent absence of specific triggering agents.

There is controversy regarding whether these nonclassic episodes are mechanistically identical to MH. Nonclassic episodes, like many syndromes symptomatically resembling MH, may respond differently to therapy and may also have considerably more favorable prognosis.

12. How is malignant hyperthermia treated?

Suspected cases of MH are treated aggressively with immediate removal of possible triggering agents, aggressive intravenous fluid therapy, treatment for hypoxia, administration of dextrose as a substrate for brain metabolism, active cooling, administration of dantrolene sodium, management of acidosis (if present), and other therapies as indicated by intensive monitoring and patient evaluation.

13. How does dantrolene sodium work in the treatment of malignant hyperthermia?

After initiation of the classic MH syndrome, intracellular calcium levels become abnormally elevated. Dantrolene counteracts this abnormality by preventing the ongoing release of calcium from the sarcoplasmic reticulum storage sites in muscle tissue. Through control of calcium release, dantrolene is thought to reduce muscle tone and metabolism. Dantrolene is recognized as an essential and life-saving component of the immediate treatment of MH in human patients. Although it is a fairly expensive medication, supplies of dantrolene are commonly stocked in the immediate area where human patients are anesthetized. Muscle weakness and other side effects are possible with dantrolene therapy. Dantrolene has been used with variable success in the treatment of MH and MH-like syndromes in animals.

14. What are the syndromes related to MH?

A malignant neuroleptic syndrome has been documented in dogs and humans. Key features include an underlying (presumably inherited) susceptibility and exposure to a triggering pharmaceutical, typically a major tranquilizer. Substantial exercise, excitement, or psychological or physiologic stresses are recognized as common contributing factors as well. MH-like syndromes have been suggested as causes of mortality in exercise-induced heat stroke. Postoperative and postanesthetic myopathies in horses have been compared to classical MH.

15. What anesthetics and anesthetic techniques are recommended as relatively safe for patients with medical histories suggesting a susceptibility to MH-like syndromes?

The most current recommendations include the avoidance of triggering agents, particularly inhalants and succinylcholine. Accepted medications include tranquilizer and opioid preanesthetics, propofol induction and infusions for the maintenance of anesthesia, plus fentanyl administered as a constant-rate infusion for added pain management if necessary.

16. What are other causes of postoperative hyperthermia?

Dramatic increases in postoperative body temperature can result from increased muscle activity and inappropriate thermoregulation. Relatively marked hyperthermia is occasionally a problem in excited or stressed cats recovering from dissociative anesthetics. Early recognition by routine monitoring of body temperature is important in avoiding damaging increases in body temperature. Upon recognition of excessive or inappropriate increases in body temperature, removal of external heating (such as circulating warm air blankets or warm water blankets), administration of tranquilizers, intravenous fluids, and other therapies based on clinical signs and ongoing evaluation of the patient usually prevent further progression of hyperthermia.

17. Can local anesthetics cause hyperthermia that is distinct from the classical MH syndrome?
In excessive and toxic doses, local anesthetics can cause inappropriate increases in body temperature through cortical stimulation and increased muscle tone. Seizure activity, as a toxic side effect of local anesthetic overdose, can further increase body temperature.

BIBLIOGRAPHY

1. Amsterdam JT, Syverud SA, Barker WJ, et al: Dantrolene sodium for treatment of heatstroke victims: Lack of efficacy in a canine model. Am J Emerg Med 4:399–405, 1986.
2. Bagshaw RJ, Cox RH, Knight DH, Detweiler DK. Malignant hyperthermia in a Greyhound. J Am Vet Med Assoc 172:61–62, 1978.
3. Bailey JE, Pablo L, Hubbell JAE: Hyperkalemic periodic paralysis episode during halothane anesthesia in a horse. J Am Vet Med Assoc 208:1859–1865, 1996.
4. Cabell LW, Perkowski SZ, Gregor T, Smith GK: The effects of active peripheral skin warming on perioperative hypothermia in dogs. Vet Surg 26:79–85, 1997.
5. Claxton-Gill MS, Cornick-Seahorn JL, Gamboa JC, Boatright BS: Suspected malignant hyperthermia syndrome in a miniature pot-bellied pig anesthetized with isoflurane. J Am Vet Med Assoc 203: 1434–1436, 1993.
6. Cosgrove SB, Eisele PH, Martucci RW, Gronert GA: Evaluation of greyhound susceptibility to malignant hyperthermia using halothane-succinylcholine anesthesia and caffeine-halothane muscle contractures. Lab Anim Sci 42:482–485, 1992.
7. Court MH: Anesthesia of the sighthound. Clin Tech Small Anim Pract 14:38-43, 1999.
8. de las Alas V, Voorhees WD, Geddes LA, et al: End-tidal carbon dioxide concentration, carbon dioxide production, heart rate, and blood pressure as indicators of induced hyperthermia. J Clin Monit 6:183–185, 1990.
9. Eshel G, Safar P, Sassano J, Stezoski W: Hyperthermia-induced cardiac arrest in dogs and monkeys. Resuscitation 20:129–143, 1990.
10. Kirmayer AH, Klide AM, Purvance JE: Malignant hyperthermia in a dog: Case report and review of the syndrome. J Am Vet Med Assoc 185:978–982, 1984.
11. Morgan JG, Gatz EE. Facilitation by oxygen of an induced hyperpyrexia during general anesthesia in dogs. J Oral Surg 32:823–828, 1974.
12. Negishi C, Lenhardt R, Ozaki M, et al: Opioids inhibit febrile responses in humans, whereas epidural analgesia does not: An explanation for hyperthermia during epidural analgesia. Anesthesiology 94: 218–222, 2001.
13. Sessler DI: Perioperative heat balance. Anesthesiology 92:578-596, 2000.
14. Short CE, Paddleford RR: Letter: Malignant hyperthermia in the dog. Anesthesiology 39:462–463, 1973.
15. Sladky KK, Kelly BT, Loomis MR, et al: Cardiorespiratory effects of four alpha-2-adrenoceptor agonist-ketamine combinations in captive red wolves. J Am Vet Med Assoc 217:1366–1371, 2000.
16. Steffey EP, Eger EI II: Hyperthermia and halothane MAC in the dog. Anesthesiology 41:392–396, 1974.
17. Stephen CR: Fulminant hyperthermia during anesthesia and surgery. JAMA 202:178–182, 1967.

VI. Anesthesia and Systemic Disease

27. ANESTHESIA OF PATIENTS WITH CARDIAC DISEASE

Thomas K. Day, D.V.M., M.S., D.A.C.V.A., D.A.C.V.E.C.C.

1. Can one anesthetic agent or protocol be used safely in all dogs and cats with cardiac disease?

The complexity of the pathophysiologic changes that occur with cardiovascular disease, the differences between dogs and cats, and the specific types of cardiac disease make it impossible for one anesthetic agent or one anesthetic protocol to be safe and effective for all patients with cardiac disease. Activation of the renin-angiotensin-aldosterone system and the sympathetic nervous system and increases in myocardial oxygen consumption are a few of the changes that can occur at various levels of cardiac disease. The decision to use individual anesthetic agents can be based on the specific cardiac diseases that occur in dogs and cats with the primary goal of preventing further compromise to the cardiovascular system and other body systems (renal and hepatic). Common cardiac diseases in dogs that may require sedation or general anesthesia include congenital cardiac defects such as patent ductus arteriosus (PDA) and stenotic lesions (pulmonic and subaortic stenosis), valvular disease (mitral insufficiency, and primary muscle dysfunction (dilated cardiomyopathy [DCM]). Common cardiac diseases in cats that may require sedation or general anesthesia include congenital defects (ventricular septal defect), valvular disease (mitral insufficiency), and primary cardiac muscle disorders (hypertrophic cardiomyopathy [HCM]).

2. What important physiologic changes that occur with heart disease make anesthesia more of a concern?

A decrease in intravascular volume for any reason, including cardiac disease, activates a complex series of events. The renin-angiotensin-aldosterone system causes retention of sodium and water and arterial vasoconstriction, which serves to maintain intravascular volume and return to the heart. Early in cardiac disease, this is a very beneficial system. Late in cardiac disease, however, this system can be detrimental to cardiac output. The sympathetic nervous system is also activated to maintain heart rate and contractility. Concentric ventricular hypertrophy results from increased pressure (stenotic valve), and eccentric hypertrophy occurs in response to increases in volume (mitral insufficiency and PDA). Changes in ventricular size and volume can result in increased myocardial oxygen consumption, which can predispose to production of arrhythmias. The goal of selecting anesthetic drugs for sedation or general anesthesia is to minimize further cardiovascular changes due to drug effects.

3. How do I know if I should sedate or anesthetize a patient with cardiac disease?

The International Small Animal Cardiac Health Council has provided guidelines for three functional classifications of heart disease that are based on clinical signs. This classification does not differentiate the type of heart disease but provides decision-making guidelines based on the clinical presentation. This classification is combined with the classification of physical status for anesthetized patients (Table 1) adopted by the American Society of Anesthesiologists (ASA) to assess anesthetic risk to aid in choosing the safest anesthetic protocol. The first decision, whether to sedate or anesthetize the patient with cardiac disease, should be made based on these guidelines.

*TABLE 1. Classification of Physical Status for Anesthetized Patients
with Emphasis on Cardiac Disease*

CATEGORY	DESCRIPTION	EXAMPLES
I	Normal healthy	No discernible disease
II	Mild systemic disease	Compensated cardiac disease (no cardiac medications)
III	Severe systemic disease	Compensated cardiac disease (cardiac medications)
IV	Severe systemic disease (constant threat to life)	Decompensated heart disease
V	Moribund, not expected to live 24 hours	Terminal heart disease, refractory to cardiac medications

*Adapted from the American Society of Anesthesiologists.

Class I patients have confirmed cardiac disease based on radiographs and echocardiography, yet do not show any signs of cardiac failure (pulmonary edema, exercise intolerance, pleural effusion). Such patients may have radiographic cardiac changes and may be receiving cardiac drugs but show no signs of congestive heart failure.

The ASA classification of patients with cardiac disease not receiving cardiac drugs is class II, and the ASA classification in patients with cardiac disease that are receiving cardiac drugs is class III. Such patients can be safely sedated or anesthetized without further stabilization.

Class II patients have mild-to-moderate signs of heart failure at rest or with mild exertion. Such patients are considered ASA class IV and are at much higher risk for debilitation or death in the perioperative period. They require further stabilization with cardiac drugs and should be free of signs of heart failure for several days prior to sedation or anesthesia. Drug therapy should continue throughout anesthesia and surgery.

Class III patients have signs of fulminate cardiac failure and can present in cardiogenic shock. Intense and aggressive stabilization are required before sedation or anesthesia. Patients on presentation are considered ASA class V, and general anesthesia is not indicated. After appropriate stabilization, such patients are considered ASA **class IV or V**, and anesthesia can cause debilitation or death in the perioperative period.

4. What important diagnostic tests should be considered in a patient with heart disease?

A complete physical examination is required in every patient with cardiac disease with increased attention to thoracic auscultation, examination of the jugular size, presence of jugular pulses, and palpation of the femoral pulses. Three important tests required for each patient with cardiac disease are thoracic radiographs to asses cardiac size and any changes in the pulmonary vascular or parenchyma, electrocardiography, and echocardiography, which can provide the definitive diagnosis and quantification of chamber size and ventricular wall thickness. Serum chemistries are also important to assess renal and hepatic systems and a packed cell volume and total solids.

5. Which cardiovascular drugs affect anesthetic management the most?

Diuretics such as furosemide can have effects on intravascular and interstitial volume, predisposing to the possibility of dehydration and hypovolemia. Close attention should be paid to clinical signs and laboratory values that indicate dehydration. Angiotensin-converting enzyme (ACE) inhibitors such as enalapril can cause vasodilation, hypotension, and decreased renal perfusion. Digitalis glycosides can cause arrhythmias including ventricular arrhythmias, and bradyarrhythmias, and changes in the QRS complex. Calcium channel antagonists can cause bradycardia, vasodilation predisposing to hypotension, and decreased contractility. Interactions between cardiac drugs and anesthetic drugs are discussed later.

6. Are any commonly used anesthetic drugs contraindicated in patients with underlying heart disease?

Any anesthetic drug used for sedation or general anesthesia that causes severe effects on cardiovascular function should not be used in cardiac patients. The alpha-2 agonists (medetomidine and xylazine) should not be used because they produce bradycardia, decreased contractility, increased cardiac work, vasoconstriction and arrhythmias. The inhalation anesthetic halothane should not be used because it produces a decrease in contractility and predisposes the myocardium to arrhythmias. Ketamine should not be used as the primary restraint drug alone or in combination in cats with HCM. The increase in contractility and heart can be very detrimental in cats with HCM and cause fulminate cardiac failure. Mask or box induction with isoflurane or sevoflurane without proper sedation causes extreme stress and activation of the sympathetic nervous system and should not be considered as an appropriate technique to induce anesthesia. The phenothiazine tranquilizer acepromazine produces vasodilation that can lead to hypotension, is long-acting, and does not have antagonists. Acepromazine should not be used in patients with cardiac disease.

7. Which commonly used anesthetic drugs should be used with caution in patients with cardiac disease?

The combination of tiletamine and zolazepam should be used with caution in dogs and cats, primarily because of dose-dependent prolonged recoveries. Small doses used as an induction agent can be safe. The same precaution for ketamine use in cats applies to tiletamine-zolazepam, because increases in contractility and heart rate can predispose to cardiac failure in cats with HCM. Tiletamine-zolazepam should be reserved for the most stable dogs and cats and should be used as an induction agent only to minimize the length of recovery. The ultrashort-acting barbiturate thiopental should also be used with caution. Decreased contractility, hypotension, apnea, and arrhythmias are known effects of thiopental. Thiopental can be used safely in dogs and cats with very mild cardiac disease at low doses as an induction agent. Avoid use of thiopental as an induction agent without use of a preanesthetic medication. Propofol is a nonbarbiturate, nonopioid induction agent that can cause similar cardiovascular effects as thiopental, minus arrhythmia production. Propofol is very short-acting, as opposed to thiopental, and is very safe and effective in low doses after preanesthetic medication.

8. Does the fact that an anesthetic drug has a reversal agent make it a safe anesthetic choice?

No, because the deleterious effects of drugs such as the alpha-2 antagonists still occur and can potentially be very detrimental to cardiovascular function. Caution should also be applied to reversal of useful anesthetic drugs such as the opioids. Reversal of sedative and analgesic effects of opioids can result in excitement, anxiety, and stress that can be potentially harmful to the known effects of cardiovascular disease. Benzodiazepines have reversal agents as well. However, drugs such as flumazenil are expensive, and benzodiazepines cause minimal-to-no deleterious effects on cardiovascular function, rarely requiring reversal.

9. What are the most useful anesthetic drugs in patients with cardiac disease?

Opioids are useful and safe anesthetic agents for patients with cardiac disease (Table 2). Examples include butorphanol, oxymorphone, hydromorphone, morphine, buprenorphine, and fentanyl. The mu agonists (oxymorphone, hydromorphone, morphine and fentanyl) produce the most reliable sedation and analgesia. Fentanyl, oxymorphone, and hydromorphone can be used as induction agents in compromised and depressed patients. Butorphanol produces less reliable sedation and analgesia because it is considered a mu antagonist and a kappa receptor agonist. Buprenorphine is a partial mu agonist with limited sedation properties but excellent analgesia. The benzodiazepines diazepam and midazolam produce limited sedation but have little-to-no deleterious effects on the cardiovascular system. The effect produced by the combination of an opioid and tranquilizer or sedative such as the benzodiazepines is called neuroleptanalgesia. Neuroleptanalgesia is an effective method of preanesthetic medication in dogs and cats with cardiac disease. Useful and safe induction agents include ketamine-diazepam, propofol, and etomidate. Ketamine-diazepam provides an effective induction characterized by maintenance or increase in contractility and heart rate. Propofol induces a smooth induction of anesthesia. There can be transient decreases in blood pressure and contractility based on the dose and rate of administration.

TABLE 2. *Useful Anesthetic Drugs for Patient with Cardiac Disease*

DRUG	DOSE (MG/KG)
Diazepam or midazolam	0.2–0.4, IV, IM
Butorphanol	0.2–0.8, SC, IV, IM
Oxymorphone	0.05–0.1 IV, IM
Hydromorphone	0.1–0.2, IV (lower dose), IM (higher dose)
Buprenorphine	0.05–0.1, IV, IM
Morphine	0.5–1, IM
Propofol	1–6, IV (lower dose with more potent preanesthetic)
Etomidate	1–2, IV, no more than 2 IV boluses
Ketamine-diazepam	1 ml or 50:50 mixture, IV
Ketamine	2–5, IM, after neuroleptanalgesia in cats

IV = intravenously, IM = intramuscularly, SC = subcutaneously.

Apnea can be a prominent feature of propofol induction, and the extent is highly dependent on rate of administration with slow administration (30–45 seconds), resulting in less severe and less prolonged apnea. Etomidate is an intravenous induction drug that produces minimal-to-no effect on heart rate, rhythm, contractility, blood pressure, or cardiac output. Etomidate is considered the ideal induction agent for patients with cardiac disease, especially those with severe cardiac disease. Etomidate is in a hypertonic solution, and more than one- or two-bolus administrations should not be used because of fear of red blood cell lysis. Isoflurane and sevoflurane are inhalation anesthetic agents that have minimal effects on contractility and cardiac output. Both agents can cause vasodilation and hypotension and are potent respiratory depressants. Ventilatory support is highly recommended during inhalation anesthesia. Sevoflurane has a slightly faster onset of action and return to recovery.

10. How are cats with heart disease different than dogs?

Cats respond to anesthetic drugs in a different manner from dogs. The prime example is the response to neuroleptanalgesia. Dogs can become heavily sedated with neuroleptanalgesia, whereas cats do not have as prominent an effect. Another primary difference is that the primary restraint drug in cats is ketamine and combinations including ketamine. Therefore, using drug combinations without ketamine usually results in less of a response. The number-one cardiac disease in cats is hypertrophic cardiomyopathy. Dogs rarely have this type of cardiac disorder. Hypertrophic cardiomyopathy is a diastolic dysfunction resulting in inadequate filling of the ventricle. The heart is very thick, and the heart rate can be very high. Dogs can develop dilated cardiomyopathy, which is a systolic dysfunction with almost the opposite effects compared to HCM; it requires the use of very different anesthetic agents.

11. What noninvasive monitoring techniques can be used during anesthesia of patients with cardiac disease?

Indirect blood pressure monitoring is important during anesthesia and some sedation protocols. Doppler blood pressure gives systolic blood pressure and produces an audible heart rate. Oscillometric blood pressure monitoring gives systolic, diastolic, and mean arterial blood pressure as well as heart rate. Both types of indirect blood pressure monitoring require following of trends in blood pressures and not necessarily the actual numbers. The smaller the patient, the more difficult it is to have reliable actual numbers. End-tidal carbon dioxide monitoring offers breath-by-breath analysis of the respiratory system and is valuable during anesthesia when opioids and inhalation anesthetics are used, because the combination can produce severe respiratory depression. Pulse oximetry can also be used but does not provide as much information about respiratory depression as end-tidal carbon dioxide monitoring. Monitoring heart rate and rhythm with the ECG is also important during anesthesia and some sedation protocols. An esophageal stethoscope can provide audible information about heart rate and can be very useful with the

Doppler during periods of hypotension in accessing heart rate. No one noninvasive monitoring device can provide all important information. Therefore, use of all of the listed noninvasive monitoring devices is highly recommended during anesthesia of patients with cardiac disease.

12. What are the indications for using invasive monitoring techniques?

The most critically ill dogs and cats with heart disease may require invasive cardiovascular monitoring to provide the most accurate information about intravascular volume and blood pressure. A catheter can be placed in a peripheral artery (dorsal pedal or femoral) to monitor blood pressure directly. More expensive equipment is required, including a pressure transducer and monitor capable of providing blood pressure information. Direct blood pressure monitoring provides the most accurate assessment of arterial blood pressure. Monitoring central venous pressure via the jugular vein is the best clinical method of proving information about venous volume, especially venous overload secondary to fluid administration. An alternative is to place a catheter in the lateral or medial saphenous vein and pass a catheter to the caudal vena cava. Any central venous measurement of volume requires normal right heart function. Therefore, trends in the central venous pressure are more important than actual numbers. Normal central venous pressure (CVP) ranges form 0 to +2 cmH$_2$O. Pulmonary edema usually occurs when the CVP is over 20–25 cm H$_2$O. Many cardiac patients that present for emergency surgeries require measurement of CVP, and some also require direct arterial blood pressure monitoring.

13. What are the anesthetic options for an ASA class II dog undergoing surgical repair of a patent ductus arteriosis?

Most of these patients are very stable before surgery, and there are no special requirements besides avoidance of contraindicated anesthetic drugs. Neuroleptanalgesia with diazepam or midazolam, combined with hydromorphone or oxymorphone administered intramuscularly should provide adequate preanesthetic sedation for catheterization of the cephalic vein. Epidural injection of morphine and placement of a fentanyl patch provide excellent postoperative analgesia. The fentanyl patch can be placed the day prior to anesthesia. A good choice for induction is ketamine-diazepam, with the animal placed on isoflurane or sevoflurane. Use of the lowest effective amount of inhalation helps minimize hypotension. Atropine should be administered if the heart rate drops below that appropriate for the size of the patient. Prophylactic administration of atropine or glycopyrrolate with the preanesthetic medication should be used with caution, because tachycardia can increase myocardial requirements. Intraoperative monitoring of direct blood pressure is ideal, although indirect monitoring is also adequate. Measurement of CVP is not considered necessary. Postoperative analgesia with intrapleural administration of bupivacaine (1.5 mg/kg) also helps with analgesia.

14. What are the anesthetic options for an ASA class III or IV dog undergoing surgical repair of a patent ductus arteriosis?

The anesthetic options are similar to those for ASA class II patients with some exceptions. Neuroleptanalgesia can be provided in a manner similar to that described for the previous patient. Placement of a direct arterial blood pressure catheter and a jugular catheter for measurement of CVP is considered mandatory. Induction of anesthesia with etomidate is ideal. Use of low dose isoflurane or sevoflurane with opioid supplementation helps prevent inhalation agent-induced hypotension. The analgesia plan is similar to that for the previous patient.

15. Is the commonly used induction agent ketamine-diazepam a safe option for cats that have hypertrophic cardiomyopathy?

Ketamine is the number-one chemical restraint for use in cats, either alone or combined with diazepam or acepromazine. However, cats with HCM should not receive ketamine as the primary restraint drug. The increase in heart rate and contractility produced by ketamine can potentially exacerbate HCM by causing dynamic outflow obstruction that results in fulminate heart failure. A neuroleptanalgesic is the preanesthetic medication of choice in cats with HCM. If the sedation is inadequate, a decreased dose of ketamine can be administered following the neuroleptanalgesic without the deleterious effects on the thickened myocardium.

16. What are the anesthetic options for a cat that requires an ovariohysterectomy and has asymptomatic hypertrophic cardiomyopathy?

The combination of diazepam or midazolam and hydromorphone or oxymorphone intramuscularly is the preanesthetic medication of choice. If sedation is inadequate, a lower dose of intramuscular ketamine can be administered. Induction with propofol is adequate, with avoidance of intravenous ketamine as discussed in the previous question. Inhalation anesthesia can be accomplished using low doses of either isoflurane or sevoflurane.

17. Which anesthetic protocol is most effective in an older dog that requires surgery to repair a ruptured cruciate ligament and has mitral valvular insufficiency?

Mitral insufficiency is common in small and medium breeds of dogs. The incompetent mitral valves allow blood to go back to the atrium with less ejected out the ventricle. The goals for anesthesia of patients with mitral insufficiency include maintenance of heart rate and contractility and prevention of arterial vasoconstriction. Neuroleptanalgesia with diazepam or midazolam and butorphanol is adequate preanesthetic medication. Induction with ketamine-diazepam or propofol is adequate. Isoflurane or sevoflurane results in arterial vasodilation and can actually promote cardiac output, unless the vasodilation is excessive enough to cause hypotension.

18. A dog diagnosed with DCM 6 months ago and receiving furosemide, digitalis, and enalapril requires injectable anesthesia to biopsy a mass near the eye. What are the sedative options for the procedure, which will last less than 10 minutes?

Dilated cardiomyopathy results in poor myocardial contraction. Therefore, maintaining heart rate without decreasing contractility is imperative. Sedation with a combination of diazepam or midazolam and butorphanol is adequate for preanesthetic medication, followed by one bolus of etomidate. Local anesthesia around the lesion can also be helpful. Prophylactic use of atropine is not recommended.

19. Describe general anesthesia options for a Beagle puppy with pulmonic stenosis that requires repair of a laceration on the ear.

The key to stenotic valvular or subvalvular lesions is understanding that maintainance of output through the lesion is a factor more of heart rate than contractility. Sedation with a neuroleptanalgesic combination of diazepam or midazolam and butorphanol should provide sedation enough for catheter placement and administration of a local anesthetic around the laceration. Use of a mu agonist (oxymorphone, hydromorphone) can result in bradycardia. Use of atropine may result in tachycardia that increases myocardial oxygen consumption of the ventricle. One bolus of ketamine-diazepam or propofol should provide adequate maintenance of heart rate and contractility to allow the procedure to be completed.

20. What is the anesthetic protocol of choice for a 2-year-old Golden Retriever with asymptomatic subaortic stenosis that requires surgery to remove an intestinal foreign body?

Subaortic stenosis is a much more difficult defect to manage under anesthesia. The results of bradycardia, hypotension, or decreases in volume can be detrimental to cardiac output. On the other hand, overzealous administration of fluids, arrhythmias, and tachycardia can result in fulminate left-sided heart failure. Therefore, vigilant and aggressive monitoring should be considered. The use of a neuroleptanalgesic combination with butorphanol instead of a mu agonist may result in less chance of bradycardia but may not provide adequate sedation or analgesia. Therefore, diazepam or midazolam plus hydromorphone or oxymorphone is preferred. Heart rate should be maintained in the normal range and low doses of atropine (0.01–0.02 mg/kg, IV) may be required. Induction with etomidate is preferred. Isoflurane or sevoflurane used at the lowest effective vaporizer setting with opioid supplementation is indicated. Invasive monitoring of CVP and direct blood pressure monitoring are ideal.

21. What are the most important interactions between commonly used anesthetic and cardiac drugs?

The interaction of isoflurane and sevoflurane with enalapril can cause severe vasodilation and hypotension. Treatment is reduction of the inhalation anesthetic. Ventricular arrhythmias caused by digitalis can be exacerbated with halothane anesthesia. The bradycardia that can occur with digitalis can be potentiated by opioids. Calcium channel antagonists combined with inhalation agents can also result in vasodilation and hypotension. Opioids can potentiate the potential for bradycardia with calcium channel antagonists.

22. Which arrhythmias are the most likely to occur with cardiac disease?

Many dogs that have atrial enlargement can present with atrial fibrillation (AF). Rarely, AF can occur during or after anesthesia of dogs with large left atriums. The most common arrhythmias are ventricular in origin because the ventricle usually has increased oxygen consumption and increased work. Any decrease in blood pressure or oxygen delivery to the cardiac muscle as a result of anesthesia may result in the development of ischemic foci and ventricular arrhythmias. Arrhythmias can occur at any time during the perioperative period. Continuous ECG monitoring is highly recommended.

23. How do arrhythmias affect anesthetic management?

Most arrhythmias are rapid in origin and can affect ventricular filling. Decreased ventricular filling combined with the specific heart disease can result in tremendous decreases in cardiac output and blood pressure. Severe ventricular arrhythmias can result in sudden death secondary to ventricular fibrillation

24. What are the most commonly used oral antiarrhythmic drugs?

Most dogs with ventricular arrhythmias associated with heart disease receive procainamide as an oral antiarrhythmic agent. Some dogs receive digitalis to control heart rate associated with atrial fibrillation, and some receive oral beta blockers such as propranolol or atenolol. The most common oral antiarrhythmic in cats is a beta blocker, either propranolol or atenolol.

25. How do oral antiarrhythmic drugs interact with commonly used anesthetic drugs?

Procainamide can produce bradycardia and hypotension that can be exacerbated by opioids and inhalation agents (isoflurane and sevoflurane). Procainamide interacts with ranitidine to produce extremely high and sometimes lethal levels of procainamide. The most common side effect of beta blockers is bradycardia that is not responsive to atropine or sympathomimetics. Therefore, opioids may potentiate bradycardia induced by beta blockers.

26. How does cardiac disease affect administration of fluids during anesthesia?

Fluid therapy should be limited in rate in patients with heart disease. The usual anesthetic rate of fluids (10 ml/kg/hr) should be reduced 50–75% in most patients. Regardless of the disease process (systolic, diastolic or valvular incompetence), excessive fluid administration can result in signs of congestive heart failure.

27. What are the recommended types and rates of fluid administration during anesthesia?

The type of fluid is not as important as the rate of administration. Most patients can handle lactated Ringer's solution, Normosol and other fluids. However, the rate should be 2–5 ml/kg/hr based on the specific cardiac disease and ASA status. Close monitoring for signs of congestion are imperative. In some instances, placement of a central venous catheter is the only method to confidently assess the status of fluid administration.

BIBLIOGRAPHY

1. Cornick-Seahorn JL: Anesthetic management of patients with cardiovascular disease. Comp Cont Educ 16:1121, 1994.

2. Day TK: Anesthesia of the cardiac patient. In Goodwin JK, Tilley LP (eds): Manual of Canine and Feline Cardiology, 3rd ed. Philadelphia, WB Saunders, 2001, pp 437–456.
3. Day TK: Intravenous anesthetic techniques for emergency and critical care procedures. In Bonagura JD (ed): Kirk's Current Veterinary Therapy XIII. Small Animal Practice. Philadelphia, WB Saunders, 2000, pp 122–125.
4. Hellyer PW: Anesthesia of the patient with cardiovascular disease. In Kirk RW, Bonagura JD (eds): Kirk's Current Veterinary Therapy XI. Small Animal Practice. Philadelphia, WB Saunders, 1992, pp 655-659.
5. Mason DE, Hubbell JAE: Anesthesia and the heart. In Fox PR, Sisson D. Moise NS (eds): Textbook of Canine and Feline Cardiology. Philadelphia, WB Saunders, 1999, pp 853–865.
6. Paddleford RR, Harvey RC: Anesthesia for selected disease: Cardiovascular dysfunction. In Thurmon JC, Tranquilli WJ, Benson GL (eds): Lumb and Jones' Veterinary Anesthesia, 3rd ed. Baltimore, Williams & Wilkins, 1996, pp 183–209.

28. ASPIRATION

Lynne I. Kushner, D.V.M., D.A.C.V.A.

1. What is the difference between gastric reflux, or regurgitation, and vomiting?

Vomiting is the forceful expulsion of gastric contents into the pharynx and involves diaphragmatic and abdominal muscular contractions. Reflux, or regurgitation, is a passive action that results in gastric contents entering the esophagus and oropharynx.

2. How does gastroesophageal reflux occur?

The lower esophageal sphincter (LES) acts as a barrier in preventing regurgitation of stomach contents into the esophagus. Barrier pressure, the difference between esophageal sphincter pressure and gastric pressure, may be reduced when gastric pressure increases (increased abdominal pressure, straining against the endotracheal tube, coughing) or when LES pressure decreases (drug-induced).

Ruminants are predisposed to regurgitation owing to large volumes of gastrointestinal tract contents and excessive gas production. Withholding food and water in sheep and cattle does not eliminate the incidence of regurgitation. Positions of recumbency, particularly dorsal or head-down positions, and restrictive tight bellybands predispose these animals to regurgitation.

Endotracheal intubation attempts during light planes of anesthesia may initiate regurgitation, particularly in ruminants.

3. What are the consequences of gastroesophageal reflux?

Certainly, pulmonary aspiration of gastric contents is a consequence that may result in significant morbidity and possible mortality. However, lack of aspiration may still lead to morbidity such as esophageal mucosal damage, esophagitis, and, in severe cases, stricture. More often there are no serious consequences.

4. How can anesthesia affect lower esophageal sphincter and barrier pressure?

Many drugs—probably all drugs—administered during the anesthetic period lower LES pressure, making reflux more likely. Various studies in dogs and cats have found statistically significant decreases in LES tone after administration of oxymorphone, acepromazine, diazepam, anticholinergics, xylazine, fentanyl-droperidol, propofol, and thiopental. Opioids delay gastric emptying and contribute to the risk of regurgitation.

5. How common is gastroesophageal reflux in the anesthetic period?

It certainly does occur. There are few clinical veterinary studies, but two similar studies in dogs reported an incidence of reflux during anesthesia as 16.3% and 17.4%. Reflux was defined by documenting esophageal pH as being less than 4.0 or greater than 7.5. No reflux was reported in one other study of 40 dogs. In a study of 100 humans scheduled for elective surgery, the incidence of gastric reflux was zero.

In ruminants, it is quite common to observe rumen and gastric contents passively draining from the pharynx during general anesthesia. The incidence in anesthetized, non-fasted sheep was 60% to 80%. Hence, these animals are at greater risk of aspiration in the anesthetic period.

6. How common is pulmonary aspiration of gastric contents?

Several human population studies have found the incidence to be minimal—an incidence of around 0.01% with low mortality. In small veterinary patients, the specific incidence is unknown but appears to be low. Because of the high incidence of reflux in anesthetized ruminants, pulmonary aspiration is likely to be higher.

7. What are the pulmonary consequences of aspiration?

This will depend on the amounts and contents aspirated, which can be liquid acid, liquid non-acid, particle-related, or combinations. Pulmonary complications from aspiration of small amounts of food and liquid are often well tolerated and may not cause significant complications.

Acidic fluid aspirates generally have a pH less than 2.5 and, in high enough volumes, can immediately result in a chemical pneumonitis resulting in hypoxia, interstitial edema, intra-alveolar hemorrhage and atelectasis. An inflammatory phase occurs a few hours later that could lead to respiratory failure. Non-acidic fluid aspirates may produce hypoxia, alveolar collapse, and atelectasis, but the late inflammatory response is not as severe as with acidic aspirates.

Aspiration of particulate matter can lead to hypoxemia, atelectasis, acute airway obstruction, and immediate death. Signs may appear several hours after the event and include coughing, tachypnea, and dyspnea. Later, an inflammatory response occurs similar to foreign body reactions. The regurgitant material in ruminants is more particulate, as would be the contents of a stomach after recently ingested food. However, the pH of ruminant ingesta is not as acidic as in small animals.

8. Name some of the risk factors for aspiration.

Not protecting the airway with endotracheal intubation is an obvious risk. An uncuffed or inadequately inflated endotracheal tube also will not protect from aspiration if regurgitation occurs. Inadequate fasting of solid food will increase the risk of aspiration if regurgitation occurs, as will premature extubation, before protective laryngeal reflexes have returned.

9. List some diseases or physiologic conditions that place a patient at risk for aspiration.

Patients that:
- Have been vomiting
- Are undergoing esophageal, gastric, or intestinal surgery
- Are recumbent or mentally depressed
- Are heavily pregnant or severely obese
- Have laryngeal paralysis
- Have esophageal motility disease
- Are ruminants

10. Will increasing the duration of fasting minimize the incidence of regurgitation in small animals?

No. A study in dogs examined the effects of various fasting times and various premedication on the incidence of gastroesophageal reflux. Increasing the duration of fasting was associated with increased incidence of reflux and lower gastric pH. Recent studies in humans have found that allowing coffee or orange juice 2 to 3 hours prior to induction had no effect on residual gastric volume or pH, so residual gastric volume and pH are not good predictors of regurgitation.

11. What are the current recommendations concerning fasting?

The recommendations for withholding solid food for dogs and cats range from 6 to 12 hours. Water should be allowed up to 3 hours prior to anesthesia (some do not advocate withholding water). In human medicine, the recommendations for fasting have been relaxed and some advocate unrestricted clear liquids up to 2 to 3 hours prior to anesthesia and no solid food the day of surgery.

It has been advised to fast large ruminants of food for 18 to 24 hours and of water for 12 to 18 hours. Small ruminants should be fasted of food for 12 to 18 hours and water 8 to 12 hours.

12. How do you recognize reflux or regurgitation and aspiration in an anesthetized dog or cat?

If the material does not reach the oropharynx, reflux may go unrecognized. When the material enters the pharynx, it is often noticed as fluid in the mouth or on the table. Typically the fluid is brown or yellow. Clinical signs from aspiration depend on the volume and composition of the material aspirated. Small amounts may not produce clinical signs. Typical clinical signs include bronchospasm, abnormal breath sounds, increased respiratory rate and/or effort, hypoxia, or cyanosis.

13. Some brown fluid is noticed under a dog's mouth on the surgery table. More fluid along with pieces of partially digested food can be seen in the mouth. It is obvious that the dog has refluxed. What should be done?

Verify that the cuff on the endotracheal tube is adequately inflated. If possible, position the head so the nose is pointing downward. Lavage the mouth and esophagus with water and suction as much as possible until it is clear. Leaving gastric fluid in the esophagus can lead to esophagitis and stricture. If aspiration is suspected, suction down the endotracheal tube into the trachea. If it appears dry and clean, significant aspiration is unlikely. Extubate with the cuff slightly inflated to remove any material that may be left around the laryngeal opening.

14. If it appears that the dog has aspirated what should be done?

Controversies exist concerning prophylactic antibiotic administration if aspiration occurs. Ideally, antibiotics should be started after a positive culture is obtained from an endotracheal wash. What is advocated is good supportive care including immediate suctioning and careful physical evaluation of lung sounds, respiratory rate and character. The patient should be watched carefully over the next several hours. Thoracic radiographs may not always reflect clinical signs. An arterial blood gas or pulse oximetry measurement will identify patients that are hypoxemic and require oxygen support. In severe cases, ventilator support may be necessary.

15. Should gastrokinetic medications such as metoclopramide and H_2 blockers such as cimetidine be used routinely to prevent regurgitation and minimize the consequences of aspiration?

Metoclopramide increases LES tone and promotes gastric emptying. H_2 blockers such as cimetidine and ranitidine decrease the production of gastric acid. Current recommendations in human medicine do not support the routine administration of these drugs to patients not at risk for aspiration. However, there may be rational use for them in patients who are at risk.

16. A golden retriever is believed to have a polyneuropathy and requires anesthesia for electromyography, nerve conduction velocities, and possible muscle and nerve biopsies. The history includes episodes of vomiting or regurgitation. Thoracic radiographs show a dilated esophagus. Describe how you would minimize the risk of aspiration in this dog during the anesthetic period.

Avoid premedication if possible so somnolence can be avoided before the airway can be secured. If the dog's temperament requires premedication, avoid drugs that may result in vomiting, such as full agonist-opioids. If opioids are needed, they may be administered intravenously after intubation. Use a rapid induction technique (see Chapter 29) to secure the airway quickly. Intubate the dog in sternal position and inflate the cuff before laying the head down. If possible, as permitted by the procedure, elevating the neck may impede regurgitant material from passing to the pharynx while material that has entered the oropharynx can drain from the mouth. Pay careful attention that the endotracheal tube cuff remains adequately inflated. Suctioning the esophagus may help if the esophagus contains a large amount of fluid.

Try to keep the endotracheal tube in place for as long as possible before extubation. Try to keep the dog sternal with the head elevated until the dog can maintain sternal recumbency and protective laryngeal reflexes have returned. If possible, reverse any residual depressant drug effects unless analgesia is warranted. Use the lowest dosage necessary that provides analgesia without heavy sedation. Always try to use regional analgesic techniques when possible.

BIBILIOGRAPHY

1. Blaze CA, LeBlanc PH, Robinson NE: Effect of witholding feed on ventilation and the incidence of regurgitation during halothane anesthesia of adult cattle. Am J Vet Res 49:2126–2129, 1988.
2. Engelhardt T, Webster NR: Pulmonary aspiration of gastric contents in anaesthesia. Br J Anaesth 83:453–60, 1999.
3. Galatos AD, Raptopoulos D: Gastro-oesophageal reflux during anaesthesia in the dog: The effect of pre-operative fasting and premedication. Vet Rec 137:479–483, 1995.

4. Gibbs CP, Modell JH: Management of aspiration pneumonitis. In Miller RD (ed): Anesthesia, 3rd ed. New York, Churchill Livingstone, 1990, pp 1293–1319.
5. Hall JA, Magne ML, Twedt DC: Effect of acepromazine, diazepam, fentanyl-droperidol, and oxymorphone on gastroesophageal sphincter pressure in healthy dogs. Am J Vet Res 48:556–557, 1987.
6. Hardy JF, Lepage Y, Bonneville-Chouinard N: Occurrence of gastroesophageal reflux on induction of anaesthesia does not correlate with the volume of gastric contents. Can J Anaesth 37:502–508, 1990.
7. Riebold TW: Ruminants. In Thurmon JC, Tranquilli WJ, Benson GJ (eds): Lumb and Jones' Veterinary Anesthesia, 3rd ed. Baltimore,Williams & Wilkins, 1996, pp 610–626.
8. Strombeck DR, Harrold D: Effects of atropine, acepromazine, meperidine and xylazine on gastroesophageal sphincter pressure in the dog. Am J Vet Res 46:963–965, 1985.
9. Tams TR: Pneumonia. In Kirk, RW (ed): Current Veterinary Therapy X, Philadelphia, W.B. Saunders,1989, pp 376–384.
10. Waterman AE, Hashim MA: Effects of thiopentone and propofol on lower oesophageal sphincter and barrier pressure in the dog. J Small Anim Prac 33:530–533, 1992.

29. RESPIRATORY DISEASES

Lynne I. Kushner, D.V.M., D.A.C.V.A.

1. What kinds of respiratory diseases are frequently encountered in dogs and cats?

Lower airway diseases (bronchitis, asthma [feline], pulmonary parenchymal diseases such as pulmonary edema, pulmonary hemorrhages or contusions, pneumonias) and pulmonary space-occupying lesions. Extrapulmonary diseases produce restriction to adequate lung inflation and include pneumothorax, pleural effusion, diaphragmatic hernia and intrathoracic space-occupying lesions. Upper airway disease leads to increased airway resistance, and includes collapsed trachea, laryngeal paralysis, and brachycephalic syndrome.

2. What important information should be obtained before anesthetizing a patient with respiratory disease?

Obviously, it is important to know what kind of respiratory disease is present, and knowing the history (chronic vs acute; traumatic) can help. Understanding the severity of the disease will allow you to determine an appropriate anesthetic plan for that particular patient. An animal demonstrating increased respiratory efforts at rest would have more severe disease than one who is dyspneic only on exertion. However, mild signs may become severe when the patient is compromised with recumbency or respiratory depressant drugs. Inspiratory noises such as honking or snoring suggest upper airway disease or obstruction. Auscultation of lung fields as well as the heart along with the assessment of hydration is paramount. Assessment of blood chemistries and hematology should be done, as with any other anesthetic patient. Any other concurrent abnormalities should be addressed.

Chest radiographs should be taken to assess severity and ascertain a more specific cause. However, radiography should be delayed in those patients who are in acute respiratory distress.

3. How would an arterial blood gas measurement be helpful in assessing the severity of respiratory disease?

Patients who have lower than expected arterial oxygen tensions (PaO_2) have severe respiratory disease usually from inadequate pulmonary gas exchange. Because CO_2 is more diffusible than O_2, most hypoxemic patients have low to normal $PaCO_2$. However, patients in ventilatory failure often are hypercarbic and may also have low PaO_2. Arterial blood gas analysis will identify those patients with abnormalities in PaO_2 and $PaCO_2$.

4. What if blood gases are not available or an arterial sample cannot be obtained?

It may be difficult to collect an arterial blood sample without stress to the patient (especially in cats). A venous sample is not useful in assessing oxygenation. Pulse oximetry is a noninvasive method to determine whether hypoxemia is present; however, mechanical difficulties may result in inaccurate readings in conscious patients. Patients with hemoglobin saturation (SpO_2) less than 93% or PaO_2 less than 75 mmHg while breathing room air are at risk for severe hypoxemia. Capnometry (measurement of end-tidal CO_2) is a noninvasive way of assessing ventilation, as the end-tidal CO_2 closely approximates the $PaCO_2$ when ventilation and perfusion is well matched. Increases in $PaCO_2$ (> 50–55 mm Hg) may suggest restrictive or obstructive pulmonary disease.

5. How does anesthesia affect the respiratory system in a healthy patient without respiratory disease?

In the conscious animal, central medullary chemoreceptors respond to increases in H^+ and $PaCO_2$, by activating respiratory control centers in the brain stem. This response is blunted by volatile anesthetics, opioids, and most hypnotics in a dose-dependant manner. Most inhalants cause an increase in respiratory frequency that does not compensate for the decrease in tidal volume resulting in dose dependant increases in $PaCO_2$. Peripheral carotid body chemoreceptors respond to critically low PaO_2 to increase respiration (hypoxic response). This response is also blunted by general anesthetics.

Motor neurons of the intercostal muscles and diaphragm can be depressed by general anesthetics, with the diaphragm being more resistant. Patient positioning, restrictive bandages, or weights (surgeons' hands and equipment) on the patient during surgery can mechanically impede the muscles of respiration. Functional residual capacity (FRC) is the volume of gas remaining in the lung after normal exhalation. In general, FRC is reduced during recumbency, in obese animals, and in conditions with increased respiratory muscle tone. Airway closure can occur at volumes approaching low FRC, thus contributing to larger alveolar-arterial oxygen differences $(P(A-a)O_2)$ and lower PaO_2 in susceptible animals. Although this may be a typical finding in large animal species, as well as in humans, in small animals this decrease in FRC may be minimal.

Hypoxia induces pulmonary vasoconstriction to divert blood away from poorly oxygenated areas of lung in order to optimize ventilation/perfusion relationships (hypoxic pulmonary vasoconstriction [HPV]). When HPV is hindered, PaO_2 is decreased. Inhaled, but not injectable, anesthetics inhibit HPV.

It should be realized that patients with preexisting respiratory diseases may lack the pulmonary reserves needed to compensate for all of the above effects.

6. What effects do sedatives and tranquilizers have on the respiratory system? Describe the advantages and disadvantages of the commonly used sedatives in dogs and cats as they relate to a patient with respiratory disease (see table for dosages).

- Phenothiazines
  Acepromazine causes minimal respiratory depression. Provided that these patients are hemodynamically stable, most dogs or cats can benefit from its sedative effects. However, adequate sedation may not be accomplished in aggressive or excitable dogs and cats. Synergistic sedative effects can be accomplished when they are combined with other agents such as opioids.
- Benzodiazepines (diazepam, midazolam)
  These agents, when administered alone, usually cause little respiratory depression and sedation. However, they will potentiate the sedative effects of opioids; thus, a marked synergism in sedative and side effects between opioids and benzodiazepines has been demonstrated. Midazolam, in particular, has been associated with life-threatening cardiopulmonary depression in people when combined with potent opioids such as fentanyl.
- α_2-agonists (xylazine, medetomidine)
  These drugs have marked cardiovascular effects and may be contraindicated in these patients; thus, they should be avoided in ill patients. The respiratory depressive effects are variable and can be minimal or marked, particularly when used with other central nervous system depressant drugs.
- Opioids (full agonists such as morphine, oxymorphone; hydromorphone)
  These drugs may be used for their sedative effects, but they depress the central medullary responses to $PaCO_2$ in a dose-dependent manner. Low dosages, especially when administered with a tranquilizer, may be acceptable in some cases. In the patient with severe respiratory disease, however, modest respiratory depression could be detrimental. Patients who rely on respiratory drive to maintain oxygenation would be most negatively affected; therefore, these drugs should be used with caution or not at all in these patients. In addition, some dogs may pant after its administration and some dogs may vomit, which would be undesirable in the dyspneic patient.
- Mixed agonists (butorphanol, buprenorphine)
  Butorphanol is an antagonist at the μ-receptor. Therefore, a ceiling effect on respiratory depression is attained with high dosages. Panting is less likely, as is vomiting. Buprenorphine is a partial agonist with high affinity at the μ-receptor. The respiratory depressant effects may

also be less severe, but it has a longer onset time and duration and may not be reversed as readily if needed. Its use may not be advantageous in the acute setting. Intramuscular administration of butorphanol with acepromazine or diazepam could be a good choice for a dog with mild to moderate respiratory disease. If intravenous access is available, a low dosage of butorphanol with or without diazepam may produce adequate sedation with little cardiovascular or pulmonary depression.

The above drug combinations may not be effective in cats, although sedation may be achieved in aged or very depressed cats. The addition of very small amounts of ketamine (1–4 mg/kg) to tranquilizer-opioid combinations administered intramuscularly may produce excellent restraint. However, it must be stressed that combined effects may result in significant respiratory depression in certain patients.

- Dissociatives (ketamine, Telazol)
- Dissociatives cannot be specifically reversed.

In small animal species, ketamine in low to moderate dosages have minimal respiratory depressant effects. The response to increased $PaCO_2$ and low PaO_2 is well maintained. However, when combined with other drugs, respiratory depression may be more marked. With high dosages, an apneustic pattern of breathing (that of holding breath on inspiration) is typical. Thus, it cannot be overemphasized that oxygen supplementation should be administered and tracheal intubation performed if necessary.

In experimental animals, ketamine had significant pulmonary vasodilatory activity, particularly under conditions of increased pulmonary vascular tone. Ketamine has been demonstrated to be an effective bronchodilator, particularly in the presence of increased airway resistance, and may be the induction agent of choice in asthmatic cats or dogs with increased bronchomotor tone.

Ketamine, however, can produce seizures in dogs if used without adequate sedation. Ketamine and diazepam in a ratio of 1:1 or 1:2 may be used in small amounts intravenously if immobilization is necessary. However, supplemental oxygen should always be administered and intubation is highly recommended.

Telazol, similar to ketamine-diazepam combination, may result in longer durations of action and thus not recommended for short procedures.

Suggested Opioid/Sedative Combinations for Patients with Respiratory Disease*

DRUG(S)	DOSAGE, MG/KG	ROUTE	SPECIES	ADVANTAGES	DISADVANTAGES
Acepromazine Oxymorphone	0.02–0.04 0.025–0.05	IM	dog, cat	Excellent sedation	Hypotension possible in cases of cardiovascular instability. Dogs may pant or vomit. Respiratory depression possible.
Diazepam Oxymorphone	0.3–0.5 0.025–0.05	IM	dog, cat	Good sedation Minimal cardiovascular depression	Dogs may pant or vomit. May not be effective in cats. Respiratory depression possible.
Diazepam Oxymorphone	0.25–0.4 0.015–0.25	IV	dog, cat	Excellent sedation Minimal cardiovascular depression.	May not be effective in cats. Significant respiratory depression possible.
Acepromazine Butorphanol	0.02–0.04 0.2–0.4	IM	dog, cat	Good sedation Minimal respiratory depression	Hypotension possible in cases of cardiovascular instability.

Continued on next page

Suggested Opioid/Sedative Combinations for Patients with Respiratory Disease* (continued)

DRUG(S)	DOSAGE, MG/KG	ROUTE	SPECIES	ADVANTAGES	DISADVANTAGES
Diazepam Butorphanol	0.25–0.4 0.1-0.3	IV	dog, cat	Good to excellent sedation Usually minimal respiratory depression	May not be effective in cats. Moderate respiratory depression possible.
Oxymorphone Midazolam Ketamine	0.025–0.05 0.2–0.3 1-5	IM	cat	Excellent sedation/ restraint	Moderate respiratory depression possible. Ketamine not reversible.
Ketamine Diazepam	2.5–5 0.25-0.5	IV	dog, cat	Excellent sedation/ restraint Usually minimal respiratory depression	Ketamine not reversible. Moderate respiratory depression possible.
Ketamine Butorphanol Midazolam	1–5 0.1–0.3 0.2–0.4	IM	cat	Excellent sedation/ restraint Usually minimal respiratory depression	Ketamine not reversible. Moderate respiratory depression possible.

*Dosage and route should depend on the patients' needs. Anticholinergics may be added to avoid bradycardia.

7. How can thoracic radiographs safely be taken in a patient who is having breathing difficulties?

If a chest radiograph is to be taken, it should be carried out after thought and preparation so it can be accomplished as quickly and safely as possible. Stressing the animal further with handling can be life-threatening, and therefore should be avoided unless absolutely necessary. If possible, in severe cases, the animal should be allowed to stabilize in an oxygen-enriched environment (oxygen cage or nasal insufflation).

Supplemental oxygen should be readily available and administered via a mask or nasal insufflation during the procedure. In severe cases, it is prudent to have an endotracheal tube and laryngoscope readily available. In some cases, it may be best to sedate the animal to avoid additional stress.

8. What are the advantages and disadvantages to sedating an animal with respiratory disease?

Allowing the animal to struggle leads to increased oxygen demands and consumption by increasing heart rate and respiratory rates in an animal already facing an oxygen debt. Increased sympathetic nervous system activity leads to increased circulating catecholamines, which, in the presence of hypoxia, can lead to tachydysrythmias. In these cases, sedation may be beneficial in that it may reduce oxygen demands and promote deeper breathing and lower respiratory rates (promoting greater alveolar ventilation, less dead space ventilation). Heart rate and rhythm may be more stable. Providing that the animal is not somnolent, some residual sedation may be beneficial. In addition, sedation may facilitate intravenous catheterization, which would be advisable in this kind of patient.

Most, if not all, of the sedatives produce some degree of respiratory depression. In a patient already compromised with respiratory disease, further depression, even mild, may be life-threatening. Also, it may be prudent for the animal to return to full capacity after the procedure, thus residual depression could be undesirable.

The advantages and disadvantages of sedation must be considered for each individual.

9. What precautions should be taken when general anesthesia is planned in a patient with respiratory disease?

If the procedure cannot be postponed, attempts should be made to improve the patient's ability to ventilate and oxygenate. For example, if pleural fluid or air is present, thoracocentesis should be attempted prior to or immediately after induction.

Intubation and oxygen administration are required in any patient with significant respiratory disease, even for short procedures. Ideally, premedication with sedatives should be avoided if intravenous catheterization and induction can be accomplished without added stress to the animal. The animal should be preoxygenated at high flow rates prior to and during induction. The appropriate-sized endotracheal tube should be estimated and prepared prior to induction. If an upper airway obstruction is suspected, smaller than expected endotracheal tubes should also be prepared. If an emergency tracheostomy is even a remote possibility, the necessary preparatory items should be readily available. In any animal with significant respiratory disease, a rapid induction and intubation should be accomplished to gain control of the airway for administration of oxygen and manual ventilation. Nitrous oxide should be used with caution or avoided in patients with abnormalities in gas exchange.

10. What anesthetic techniques are suitable for rapid induction?

Thiopental (6–12 mg/kg) and propofol (4–8 mg/kg), when administered intravenously to effect produce rapid unconsciousness allowing for rapid intubation. Ketamine (5 mg/kg) and diazepam (0.25–0.5 mg/kg) also can be used to secure an airway rapidly. Some techniques are not suitable for rapid induction. Mask or chamber induction would be contraindicated, as this may produce excitement and struggling in the patient and the time required for intubation is prolonged. In general, opioid–tranquilizer inductions are slower inductions that may or may not be suitable, depending on the condition of the animal.

11. What are the respiratory effects of the induction agents?

Thiopental and propofol produce dose-dependant depression of medullary and pontine ventilatory center, decreasing sensitivity to increases in $PaCO_2$. Respiratory depression is potentiated when used concurrently with other agents, such as opioids and, in some cases, the benzodiazepines. Apnea can occur, particularly with propofol, unless the drug is administered slowly. Therefore, these drugs should not be administered if you do not have the ability to provide the patient with oxygen and ventilatory support. As long as the patient is intubated and manual ventilation can be administered, these agents are excellent choices for the patient with respiratory disease.

Etomidate, a nonbarbiturate hypnotic, produces mild to moderate dose-dependent respiratory depression and may actually stimulate ventilation independent of the medullary centers that normally respond to carbon dioxide. However, etomidate can produce retching or gagging and vomiting, which may be undesirable in a patient with respiratory disease.

Ketamine/diazepam induction is less likely to produce apnea, although an apneustic pattern of breathing is not uncommon. Manual ventilation should be provided as needed.

12. How would you define hypoxemia? Would cyanosis always be present?

Hypoxemia may be defined as an arterial oxygen tension less than 80 mm Hg or an SpO_2 less than 93% and severe hypoxemia occurs when the PaO_2 is < 60–65 mm Hg and hemoglobin saturation is less than 90%. Carbon dioxide tensions may or may not be normal. The absence of cyanosis does not rule out the possibility of hypoxemia, as there must be at least 5 g of reduced hemoglobin present and a hypoxemic anemic patient may not have 5 g of reduced hemoglobin.

13. How could you recognize hypoxemia in the anesthetized patient?

When the PaO_2 falls below 40–60 mm Hg receptors in the carotid bodies respond by stimulating respiration. As previously stated, most anesthetics inhibit the response to hypoxia, so this response may not occur until hypoxemia is severe. Patients who are hypoxic may increase respiratory rate or effort ("buck the ventilator"), and this should not be confused with inadequate depth of anesthesia. $PaCO_2$ may or may not be normal. Heart rate may increase due to an attempt to increase cardiac output and oxygen content. Heart rate may drop, however, due to the inability to maintain cardiac output in the face of high oxygen demands. Blood pressure may or may not be low for similar reasons.

Dysrhythmias, specifically extrasystoles such as ventricular premature contractions, and alterations in T wave and Q-T intervals may be a sign of hypoxemia and/or ischemia. Other signs such as increased resistance to ventilation (the generation of increased airway pressures for a given tidal volume when the rebreathing bag is squeezed), although not specific for hypoxemia, indicate that serious problems have developed, such as an obstructive airway disease, (bronchoconstriction; kinked or obstructed endotracheal tube), severe intrapulmonary disease (pulmonary edema), or restrictive disease (pneumothorax, pleural fluid).

14. How should a patient with significant disease in gas exchange be managed under anesthesia?

As stated previously, intubation and oxygen administration should be provided to patients with respiratory diseases. Intermittent positive pressure ventilation (IPPV) should be provided to most patients to overcome and/or prevent atelectasis. Pulse oximetry is an invaluable monitor in these cases to ensure adequate oxygenation. In severe cases, positive pressure ventilation may be necessary to maintain an acceptable SpO_2 (>92%). In some cases of pulmonary contusions or chronic atelectasis (chronic diaphragmatic hernia), airway pressures during IPPV should be minimized (< 15–20 cm H_2O) to avoid alveolar damage or re-expansion pulmonary edema.

In severe cases, positive end-expired pressure (PEEP) may be applied to improve oxygenation. PEEP prevents small airway closure by maintaining some positive pressure (usually 5–10 cm H_2O) in the alveoli after expiration. This can be accomplished with a specific PEEP valve or by subjecting the scavenging hose of the pop-off valve to a resistance (such as placing the end of the hose under 5–10 cm H_2O). However, some intrapulmonary diseases do not respond favorably to PEEP.

Patients with pulmonary disease may have problems oxygenating when placed in unfavorable positions during surgery. Patients with unilateral pulmonary disease should be positioned to favor the better side if possible.

End-tidal CO_2 monitors are invaluable in monitoring ventilation noninvasively. Since anesthetics produce respiratory depression in normal patients, end-tidal CO_2 monitoring is always useful to identify patients who are hypoventilating significantly. Unfortunately, these monitors can be very expensive. It should be realized however, that the end-tidal CO_2 does not always reflect the $PaCO_2$ in cases in which pulmonary perfusion is less than pulmonary ventilation (pulmonary dead space).

As with any other anesthetized patient, blood pressure and electrocardiographic monitoring is highly recommended.

15. What are the concerns for recovering a patient with respiratory disease?

Some patients may be at risk for severe hypoxemia if proper vigilance and supportive measures are not used once the patient is extubated and breathing room air. Patients breathing 100% oxygen should have a PaO_2 of around 500 mm Hg, so the SpO_2 would be 98–100%. If the patient has a PaO_2 of only 120 mm Hg, the SpO_2 would still be 98–100%. If blood gas analysis is not available, these patients can be identified by keeping the pulse oximeter in place while the patient breathes room air prior to extubation. If the SpO_2 drops below 91–93%, the patient requires supplemental oxygen. A nasal catheter for oxygen supplementation can be placed before the animal is too awake to object.

Bandages around the neck, chest, or abdomen can significantly impede ventilation if applied too tightly. Hypercarbia and/or hypoxemia can occur from residual respiratory depressant drug effects and atelectasis due to recumbency in patients with respiratory disease.

Animals with unilateral pulmonary disease should be positioned to favor the better side. For most patients with respiratory disease, sternal recumbency is best to allow optimal expansion of all lung fields.

Reversal of opioids may be necessary to improve alveolar ventilation and oxygenation. Reversal agents, however, should always be administered carefully and to effect, to avoid sudden and excitable awakening.

Excitable recoveries should be avoided in patients with respiratory disease as this increases stress, and oxygen consumption and demands. If anticipated, a low dose of acepromazine (0.005–0.02 mg/kg IV) can prevent delirium and smooth the recovery period with minimal respiratory depression.

16. Should opioid analgesics be avoided in patients with respiratory disease?

Pure agonist opioids should be administered with care to avoid respiratory depression, which can be detrimental in some patients. If analgesia is warranted, opioids with partial or no μ activity (e.g., buprenorphine and butorphanol, respectively) may be more desirable. Regional anesthetic techniques are excellent choices that provide pain relief without significant respiratory compromise (for example: intercostal or interpleural administration of local anesthetics for thoracotomies; epidural opioids with or without local anesthetics for celiotomies or fractures).

17. What effect does shivering have on an animal with respiratory disease?

Shivering is an attempt by the body to generate heat, but it also increases metabolic rate and oxygen consumption, which can be detrimental in hypoxemic patients who have few oxygen reserves. Shivering animals with respiratory disease should be given supplemental oxygen in the recovery room. Forced warm air or radiant warmers help to minimize shivering and hypothermia.

18. List the anatomic abnormalities and clinical signs that occur in dogs with upper airway disease. Which breeds are commonly affected?

Dogs with upper airway disease typically present with noisy breathing and increased inspiratory effort, honking coughs, and, in severe cases, cyanosis, all of which can be exacerbated by excitement. Laryngeal paralysis typically occurs in larger breeds, such as the retrievers. Some of these patients may have underlying neuromuscular disease. Dogs with collapsing trachea usually are small dogs, such as the Yorkshire terrier and Pomeranian, may have an inducible as well as a spontaneous cough, and exhibit honking noises, particularly when excited. These dogs may also have cardiac disease. Dogs with brachycephalic syndrome, particularly the English bulldog, may have marked inspiratory effort, snore, and be noisy at rest. Anatomical abnormalities include stenotic nares, everted laryngeal saccules, elongated soft palate, and hypoplastic trachea. Secondary lower airway disease may also be present in all these patients and should not be overlooked.

19. What precautions should be taken when anesthetizing a patient with upper airway disease?

The precautions are similar to those for any patient with respiratory disease, and choosing an appropriate anesthetic plan is dependent on the specific needs of the patient. However, it is most important to avoid excitement in these patients since this increases respiratory effort and generates greater negative airway pressures, which may lead to exacerbation of airway obstruction. This increased activity may provoke panting that further exacerbates the obstruction. If the patient cannot be managed without causing further stress and excitement, then premedication would be warranted. However, heavy sedation may potentiate an obstruction; hence, sedatives should be used carefully. Neuroleptic combinations such as acepromazine and butorphanol (see table) can be very effective, but the lowest dosage necessary to achieve adequate control of the patient should be used. It is paramount to closely observe these patients after these drugs are administered so as to be ready to intervene with supportive measures (immediate intubation and oxygen) if needed.

Bulldogs have redundant airway tissue that may pose difficulties with intubation, hence another good reason to preoxygenate these patients during induction. Because of hypoplastic tracheas, the tracheal tube size required may be much smaller than that needed for another breed of comparable weight. Brachycephalic breeds tend to have high vagal tone, making them more susceptible to bradyarrhythmias; therefore, anticholinergics are recommended in these patients.

20. What are the concerns for recovering a patient with upper airway disease?

It is very important to avoid emergence delerium or excitement in animals with upper airway disease. Low-dose acepromazine (0.005–0.02 mg/kg IV) administered prior to extubation can be very effective in promoting a quiet, smooth recovery. In brachycephalic breeds, it is advisable to leave the endotracheal tube in place for as long as possible before extubation. After extubation, these patients should be closely observed until fully recovered, and a laryngoscope, clean endotracheal tube, and oxygen should be readily available in case obstruction occurs. If airway surgery was performed, anti-inflammatory agents such as dexamethasone (0.05–0.25 mg/kg IV) may be administered prior to completion of surgery to minimize swelling.

Dogs with laryngeal paralysis have lost their protective laryngeal reflexes, especially after laryngeal tie-back surgery. Therefore, these patients are more susceptible to aspiration if regurgitation or vomiting occurs, and efforts should be made to minimize this risk (see Chapter 28).

21. Diagnostic procedures such as bronchoscopy and endotracheal lavage are often required in patients with pulmonary disease, but these procedures can severely compromise airway patency. How are these procedures performed? How can they be accomplished in these patients safely?

Endotracheal lavage is often performed by injecting and then aspirating saline from a sterile, small-diameter catheter that is passed down the lumen of the endotracheal tube. Ideally, premedication should be avoided so that no residual sedative effects remain after the procedure is terminated. The animal should be preoxygenated and a rapid induction (see previous sections) should be used. The patient must be depressed enough to allow endotracheal intubation, but the anesthetic level must be light enough that the animal retains a cough reflex.

After the sterile sample is collected, further suctioning of the airway should be done if heavy secretions are still present. Oxygen should be administered via the endotracheal tube if needed until extubation and then insufflated at the nares if necessary. The pulse oximeter is an invaluable aide in identifying those patients who become hypoxemic.

For bronchoscopy, anesthesia is induced rapidly, and the patient is intubated and well oxygenated. Inhalation anesthesia, without nitrous oxide, may be used to achieve anesthetic depth sufficient to allow passage of the bronchoscope. Propofol and oxygen may be more desirable than inhalation anesthesia, as this will avoid pollution of anesthetic gases that will escape from around the bronchoscope. However, propofol should be delivered in small, slow boluses (0.25–1.0 mg/kg) or infusions (0.2–0.4 mg/kg/min) to avoid apnea. Whether the bronchoscope is passed directly down the trachea (cats and small dogs) or through the lumen of the endotracheal tube, the ability of the animal to ventilate is impeded and oxygenation of the patient is greatly compromised.

Pulse oximetry can be an invaluable monitor during bronchoscopy, as visual inspection of mucous membrane color is an insensitive measure of adequate oxygenation. When the oxygen-hemoglobin saturation falls below 91%, the bronchoscope should be removed and the animal should be ventilated with 100% oxygen until saturation is restored. In addition, oxygen can be insufflated through the bronchoscope or directly into the oral cavity via a cannula, which may prevent or delay desaturation during the procedure. The ECG should be monitored, because developing arrhythmias could signal a developing hypoxemia. When the procedure is completed, pulse oximetry can be employed to ensure that the patient is adequately oxygenated and to determine whether oxygen supplementation is necessary in the recovery period.

22. What is asthma? What are some concerns of anesthetizing a cat with asthma?

Asthma is a disease of the small airways resulting in airflow obstruction from smooth muscle constriction, bronchial wall edema, and inflammation. Clinical signs result in increased respiratory effort (inspiratory and expiratory effort), coughing, and, in severe severe cases, open-mouth breathing and cyanosis. Cats with severe signs should be stabilized with medical treatment before anesthesia is attempted. Cats with mild or moderate signs may need anesthesia or sedation for diagnostic studies such as bronchoscopy or endotracheal lavage.

As with any other patient, the anesthetic protocol should be tailored specifically to the patient's needs. Although there may be no specific contraindication to any anesthetic or analgesic agents, as stated previously, ketamine is a good choice for the asthmatic cat because of its bronchodilatory effects. Propofol has been demonstrated to decrease airway resistance in the presence of histamine-induced bronchoconstriction. The potent volatile anesthetics such as halothane and isoflurane also relax bronchial smooth muscle.

Deep bronchoscopic washings in asthmatic cats may induce severe bronchospasm and constriction secondary to release of inflammatory mediators. This can result in a marked increase in resistance to manual ventilation. In these situations, administration of bronchodilators (terbutaline 0.01 mg/kg IV or aminophylline 4–6 mg/kg diluted *slowly*) and corticosteroids (prednisolone succinate 1 mg/kg IV; dexamethasone Na phosphate 0.25 mg/kg) may be warranted.

For human asthmatic patients, extubation of the trachea before laryngeal responses return has been recommended, so as to avoid laryngeal spasms that may be initiated by coughing in response to the endotracheal tube. In the asthmatic cat, it may be prudent to follow a similar recommendation.

Cats with a history of asthma who have little or no clinical signs at the time of anesthesia may not necessarily require any specific anesthetic protocol. However, unnecessary stress and excessive attempts at intubation should be avoided if possible to prevent coughing and airway reactivity.

BIBLIOGRAPHY

1. Bjorling DE: Laryngeal paralysis. In Bonagura JD (ed): Kirk's Current Veterinary Therapy XII. Small Animal Practice, Philadelphia, WB Saunders, 1995, pp 901–905.
2. Conti G, Dell'Utri D, Vilardi V, et al: Propofol induces bronchodilation in mechanically ventilated chronic obstructive pulmonary disease (COPD) patients. Acta Anaesth Scand 37:105–109, 1993.
3. Corssen G, Gutierrez J, Reves JG, Huber FC: Ketamine in the anesthetic management of asthmatic patients. Anesth Analg 51:588, 1972.
4. Hendricks JC: Recognition and treatment of congenital respiratory tract defects in brachycephalics. In Bonagura JD (ed): Kirk's Current Veterinary Therapy XII. Small Animal Practice. Philadelphia, WB Saunders, 1995, pp 892–894.
5. Hirshman CA: Ketamine block of bronchospasm in experimental canine asthma. Br J Anaesth 51:713, 1979.
6. McDonell, W: Respiratory system. In Thurmon JC, Tranquilli WJ, Benson GJ (eds): Lumb and Jones' Veterinary Anesthesia, 3rd ed. Baltimore, Williams & Wilkins, 1996, pp 115–147.
7. Mecca RS: Postoperative Recovery. In Barash PG, Cullen BF, Stoelting RK (eds): Clinical Anesthesia, 3rd ed. Philadelphia, Lippincott-Raven, 1997, pp 1279–1303.
8. Paddleford, RR: Preanesthetic agents: Anesthetic agents. In Paddleford, RR (ed): Manual of Small Animal Anesthesia, 2nd ed. Philadelphia, WB Saunders, 1999, pp 12–77.
9. Stock MC: Respiratory function in anesthesia. In Barash PG, Cullen BF, Stoelting RK (eds): Clinical Anesthesia, 3rd ed. Philadelphia, Lippincott-Raven, 1997, pp 747–768.
10. Thurmon JC, Tranquilli WJ, Benson GJ: Preanesthetics and anesthetic adjuncts. In Thurmon JC, Tranquilli WJ, Benson GJ (eds): Lumb and Jones' Veterinary Anesthesia, 3rd ed. Baltimore, Williams & Wilkins, 1996, pp 183–209.

30. PERIOPERATIVE MANAGEMENT OF PATIENTS WITH LIVER DISEASE

Jana L. Jones, D.V.M., D.A.C.V.A., D.A.C.V.E.C.C.

The patient with moderate to severe liver disease constitutes a high risk for anesthesia and surgery. The clinician should develop a plan to (1) be thorough in the preoperative assessment of the cause and severity of the liver problem through evaluation of the patient's history, physical examination, and diagnostic studies, (2) preoperatively optimize the patient's hepatic function, and (3) avoid perioperative factors known to cause deterioration of liver function.

1. Rational management of anesthesia in the presence of liver disease requires an understanding of the physiologic function of the liver. What are the basic physiologic functions of the liver?

Physiologic functions of hepatocytes, the principal cells of the liver, include glucose homeostasis, fat metabolism, protein synthesis, drug and hormone metabolism and bilirubin formation and excretion, with further functions as follows:

- Glucose homeostasis: Gluconeogensis, glycogenolysis and glycogenesis.
- Fat metabolism
- Protein synthesis: All proteins except gamma globulins and factor VIII.
  - Drug binding
  - Coagulation
  - Hydrolysis of ester linkages (plasma cholinesterase)
  - Albumin production: albumin provides 80% of the colloid oncotic pressure of plasma
- Drug and hormone metabolism
- Bilirubin formation and excretion: conjugation of bilirubin with glucuronic acid in the liver, rendering bilirubin water soluble.

Hepatic sinuses are lined by Kupffer cells, which are capable of phagocytosing bacteria in portal venous blood. This is an important function as well, since portal venous blood drains the gastrointestinal tract and usually contains bacteria from the colon.

2. What are some common clinical signs of hepatobiliary disease in dogs and cats?

Symptoms of liver disease can be extremely variable. General nonspecific clinical signs may include anorexia, depression, weight loss, small body stature, vomiting, diarrhea, and dehydration. More specific, although not pathognomonic, signs may include abdominal enlargement secondary to organomegaly or effusion (ascites), hyperbilirubinuria, jaundice, acholic feces, behavioral changes, trembling, seizures, hypersalivation, coagulopathy, polydipsia, and polyuria.

3. Why do some animals with serious hepatic disease develop signs of abnormal mentation and neurologic dysfunction?

Hepatic encephalopathy may develop as a result of exposure of the cerebral cortex to absorbed intestinal toxins that are not removed properly by the liver. Some encephalotoxins may include substances such as ammonia, aromatic amino acids, short-chain fatty acids, indoles, tryptophan, and serotonin. Abnormal detoxification by the liver may be due to marked reduction in functional hepatic mass (affects intrinsic metabolism), alterations in hepatic blood flow such as portal blood flow diversion by development of portosystemic venous anastomoses, or shunts (congenital or acquired in response to sustained portal hypertension). Multiple factors are involved in the pathogenesis of hepatic encephalopathy, including the accumulation of encephalotoxins, shifts in amino acid composition, and increased cerebral sensitivity secondary to biochemical changes in the brain such as altered neurotransmitters and membrane physiology.

4. What is the role of the inhibitory neurotransmitter gamma-aminobutyric acid (GABA) in the pathogenesis of hepatic encephalopathy? How does this affect your choice of an anesthetic agent?

Evidence exists to support the theory that the normally small amounts of GABA present as a neurotransmitter in the brain may combine with substances with GABA-like activity in the intestine and portal blood and result in the disruption of the normal balance of excitatory and inhibitory neurotransmitters. GABA receptors may also be increased in patients with hepatic disease. GABA receptors have sites for benzodiazepines and barbiturates. Animals with severe liver disease and portosytemic shunting often have increased sensitivity to these agents.

5. What diagnostic tests should be performed in your preoperative evaluation of a patient with suspected liver dysfunction?

The common battery of tests should include determinations of serum bilirubin, aminotransferases (transaminases), alkaline phosphatase, albumin, total protein, prothrombin time, hematocrit and hemoglobin, creatinine and blood urea nitrogen, platelet count, glucose, electrolytes, and arterial/venous blood gases and pH. Of these tests, increased serum bilirubin and prothrombin time and decreased albumin concentration are considered to be the most reliable for identification of anesthetic and surgical risk in human patients.

Hepatic dysfunction is seldom quantified in clinical practice. Conventional liver tests do not measure liver function. Hepatic metabolism normally occurs at a small fraction of capacity, making detectable increases in serum concentrations of hepatic enzymes a very late occurrence.

In younger patients, causes of hepatic insufficiency are likely to be congenital anomalies such as in intrahepatic or extrahepatic portosystemic shunt. In these patients, a definitive diagnosis may be made through the measurement of blood ammonia levels in the ammonia tolerance test (ATT), fasting and post-prandial serum bile acid concentrations, and imaging techniques such as angiography, ultrasonography, and nuclear scintigraphy.

6. What clotting abnormalities are commonly present in the patient with liver disease?

Coagulopathies are extremely common in patients with liver disease and involve qualitative as well as quantitative changes in clotting regulation. Most of the factors involved in coagulation are primarily or exclusively formed by the liver, with the exception of factor VIII, which is produced extrahepatically. Important coagulation inhibitory factors (antithrombin-III, protein C, protein S, and α_2-antitrypsin and the procoagulant fibrinogen) are also produced by the liver.

Clotting abnormalities in patients with liver disease include the following:
- Decreased synthesis of coagulation factors:
  - Reduced vitamin K–dependent factors (II, VII, IX, X)
  - Reduced non- vitamin K–dependent factors (V, XIII, fibrinogen)
- Shortened circulating half-lives of coagulation factors:
  - Increased utilization (disseminated intravascular coagulation)
  - Loss from bleeding
- Platelet abnormalities:
  - Decreased platelet count (hypersplenism)
  - Impairment of platelet function

7. What are the vitamin K–dependent factors?

The Vitamin K-dependent factors include prothrombin (II), factors VII, IX, and X, protein C, and protein S.

8. Why is Vitamin K necessary in the coagulation process?

The six factors listed in question 6 require carboxylation after release from the liver for proper function. Vitamin K is necessary for this process to occur. When vitamin K is deficient, these vitamin K–dependent factors are no longer able to bind calcium or adhere to lipids correctly, resulting in a coagulopathy.

9. Does liver disease contribute to vitamin K deficiency? Would vitamin K administration be of benefit in patients with liver disease?

Extrahepatic or intrahepatic cholestasis, malabsorption, dietary deficiency, biliary fistulas, toxins such as anticoagulant rodenticides, and cholestyramine use typically result in vitamin K deficiency and parental therapy should correct this deficiency. In severe liver disease, however, there are additional qualitative changes such as platelet function and impaired carboxylation. Vitamin K, even if deficient, would not be expected to be of much value in these patients.

10. What can be done preoperatively to help with clotting regulation?

Treatment of coagulation abnormalities should be aggressive and begin before incision if possible. Administration of fresh frozen plasma (FFP) can correct all plasma protein deficiencies for clotting except fibrinogen and platelets. Platelet deficiencies of less than 50,000/mm^3 should be treated by infusion of platelet-rich supplements, and decreased fibrinogen can be treated with cryoprecipitate. Prothrombin time should be remeasured after FFP replacement and should be no greater than 2 seconds over control. Bleeding time should be determined even in the presence of sufficient platelets to ascertain qualitative platelet function.

11. What is the significance of hypoalbuminemia in a patient with liver disease?

The presence of any of the four pathologic variables in a patient with liver disease in human medicine constitutes a high anesthetic and surgical risk and decreased prognosis (Child's classification with the Pugh modification): elevated prothrombin time, elevated plasma bilirubin, decreased plasma albumin, or ascites.

Secondly, the decreased levels of albumin seen in liver disease may affect protein binding of many drugs given during anesthesia and result in greater than expected levels of free or active agents. The binding properties of albumin allow it to serve as a carrier protein for many substances such as drugs, hormones, enzymes, ions, amino and fatty acids, and bilirubin. Because liver disease often impairs metabolism as well, drug toxicity can be potentiated. Narcotics, diazepam, and barbiturates are highly protein (albumin) bound, and a decrease in serum albumin can be associated with an increased incidence of side effects. These considerations may partially explain the increased susceptibility of patients with severe liver disease to sedatives and tranquilizers. As a general rule in anesthesia, drug dose should be titrated to effect.

A third concern is that of maintenance of plasma colloid osmotic pressure (COP). Albumin, a natural blood colloid with a molecular weight of 69,000 daltons, accounts for 70–80% of the plasma COP. Albumin is the most oncotically active plasma protein and is responsible for a major portion of intravascular fluid retention. Hepatocytes are responsible for albumin synthesis, with production regulated by perihepatic interstitial osmoreceptors and influenced by many hormones. Major abdominal surgical procedures (even without major blood loss) are associated with redistribution of albumin from the intravascular space to abnormal extracellular sites with a resultant decrease in plasma COP, an increase in interstitial fluid, and a reduction in plasma volume. In a healthy patient, the decrement in extracellular fluid volume and plasma COP may be offset by acceleration in the rate of albumin synthesis. A patient with liver disease, however, may be unable to compensate owing to impaired ability to synthesize and/or secrete albumin.

12. In a patient with liver disease, many drugs may contribute to intraoperative complications such as hypotension, as well as effect postoperative speed of emergence from anesthesia. Some drugs used in anesthesia are of particular concern in patients with liver disease as drug handling and response can be profoundly altered. What is the pathophysiology thought to explain the increased susceptibility of patients with liver disease to many drugs used as part of an anesthetic protocol?

First, the decreased levels of albumin seen in many patients with liver disease may affect protein binding of many commonly used anesthetic drugs. The result of decreased protein binding may be *increased free or active agent*s. For example, narcotics and barbiturates are highly protein bound, and a decrease in serum albumin may be associated with an increased incidence of side effects secondary to more active agent available and increased effects.

Second, as the liver plays a critical role in the kinetics and dynamics of most pharmacologic agents, impaired ability for *drug metabolism* (intrinsic clearance ability of the liver) may result in potentiated drug effect and toxicity.

Third, *increased sensitivity of the central nervous system (CNS)* to actions of sedatives, narcotics, and hypnotics may occur in patients with liver disease. The exact mechanism is unknown but may be due to altered CNS receptor kinetics, altered blood-brain barrier, or undefined circulating amine. It is well known that patients with severe liver disease cannot tolerate injectable opioids, sedatives, or hypnotics and that use of these drugs should be minimal. The role of gamma-aminobutyric acid (GABA) and GABA receptors in the pathogenesis of hepatic encephalopathy and susceptibility to increased sedation is being investigated. The benzodiazepine antagonist, flumazenil, has been shown to reverse hepatic encephalopathy and coma to a certain degree

Fourth, *hepatic blood flow* may be altered. In patients with portal hypertension, portal blood flow may be reduced and the effects of drugs that depend on high hepatic clearance rates may be prolonged. In addition, for highly extracted drugs, any form of intra- or extrahepatic *shunting* around the liver may result in increased drug availability.

13. What are the basic pathways of drug metabolism?

The four basic pathways of drug metabolism are oxidation, reduction, hydrolysis, and conjugation (to glucuronic acid). The liver is the main organ involved in drug metabolism; other sites of drug metabolism include plasma, lungs, kidneys, and the gastrointestinal tract.

14. What are hepatic microsomal enzymes?

Hepatic microsomal enzymes participate in the metabolism of many drugs and are located in the hepatic smooth endoplasmic reticulum. The term "microsomal enzyme" is derived from the fact that centrifugation of hepatocytes concentrates fragments of the disrupted smooth endoplasmic retculum in what is designated as the microsomal fraction. This fraction includes an iron-containing family of proteins termed cytochrome P-450, which is also known as the "mixed function oxidase system," since it involves oxidation and reduction steps. Cytochrome P-450 functions as the terminal oxidase in the electron transport scheme. Microsomal enzymes catalyze most of the oxidation, reduction, and conjugation (with glucuronic acid) reactions that lead to metabolism of drugs.

15. What are non-microsomal enzymes?

Non-microsomal enzymes are present in liver but are also found in plasma and in the gastrointestinal tract. All conjugation reactions, except for conjugation with glucuronic acid, are catalyzed by non-microsomal enzymes. They also catalyze hydrolysis reactions and some oxidation and reduction reactions. Non-microsomal enzyme reactions conjugate substances with acetic acid, glycine, and glutathione. Nonspecific esterases in the liver, plasma, and gastrointestinal tract are examples of non-microsomal enzymes responsible for hydrolysis of drugs that contain ester bonds, such as some local anesthetics.

16. Which biotransformation pathways are most altered in liver dysfunction? How does this apply to drugs commonly used in the anesthetic protocol?

The cytochrome P-450 oxidative pathways seem most susceptible. Drugs that are substrates for cytochrome P-450, such as barbiturates, diazepam, midazolam, fentanyl, and meperidine, have prolonged effects in patients with liver dysfunction. On the other hand, the conjugation biotransformation pathways (involving glucuronide conjugation) are more rugged and may continue to function until the very late stages of liver disease. Drugs dependent on conjugation mechanisms for metabolic inactivation, such as the injectable hypnotic agent propofol may be handled better. However, biotransformation deficiency (intrinsic clearance) is not the only problem of drug handling in these patients (consider also hepatic blood flow and decreased protein binding), thus drug administration to patients with liver dysfunction or disease should always be approached with caution.

17. What is the blood supply to the liver?

Blood supply to the liver is via the hepatic artery and the portal vein. Approximately 25% of the total cardiac output courses through the liver, which is about 100 mL of blood flow per 100 g of tissue.

18. How are blood and oxygen (O_2) supplied to the liver?

Blood supply to the liver is unique among the major organs. Both the hepatic artery and the portal vein are responsible for total liver blood flow. Actually, more flow and more oxygen are delivered by the portal vein than by the artery.

The hepatic artery distributes about 25% of total blood flow and supplies approximately 45 to 50% of hepatic O_2. The portal vein delivers about 75% of hepatic blood flow and, although partially deoxygenated from transit through the stomach, pancreas, spleen, and intestines, provides the remaining 50% to 55% of hepatic O_2 requirements.

19. How is hepatic blood flow regulated?

Portal flow is regulated by arterioles in the preportal splanchnic organs and to a limited extent by resistance in the liver. The major site of venous resistance within the liver is thought to be the post-sinusoidal sphincters. Smooth muscles in the wall of the venules regulate venous compliance and blood volume. Both resistance and compliance are predominantly controlled by the sympathetic innervation mediated through α-adrenergic receptors. Thus the primary regulating mechanism of hepatic venous resistance is mediated via sympathetic α-adrenergic receptors.

The major site of resistance in the hepatic arterial vasculature is the arterioles. Regulation of the hepatic arteriolar tone is mainly achieved by local and intrinsic mechanisms that adjust hepatic arterial flow to compensate for changes in portal blood flow. This buffer response results in an increase in hepatic arterial flow when portal flow decreases in an attempt to maintain hepatic O_2 supply and total blood flow. Hepatic arterial autoregulation is complex, because neural, metabolic and myogenic factors are important, as are the effects of substances within portal blood. A decrease in portal O_2 content or pH is associated with an increase in hepatic arterial blood flow, even if portal flow is experimentally maintained.

20. How do volatile anesthetics affect hepatic blood flow?

As described in questions 18 and 19, under normal circumstances the portal vein and the hepatic artery engage in a reciprocity or buffer response to maintain hepatic blood flow and oxygen delivery. When portal venous blood flow drops, the hepatic artery decreases resistance and increases flow. On the other hand, when portal flow increases, hepatic artery resistance increases and its flow decreases. Total liver blood flow is therefore maintained within narrow limits. All of the potent inhalation anesthetics are capable of causing hepatocellular injury by reducing liver blood flow and oxygen delivery. However, isoflurane is most likely to better maintain tissue oxygen supply and thus is the agent least likely to produce liver injury even when administered for prolonged periods. Sevoflurane and desflurane are similar to isoflurane whereas halothane produces the most striking adverse changes. The general anesthetic halothane attenuates the reciprocity of flow status and thus produces greater decrements of hepatic blood flow than other anesthetic agents. Halothane should therefore not be used in patients with liver disease. It should also be remembered that decreases in total hepatic blood flow are proportional to decreases in systemic blood pressure and many factors may reduce hepatic blood flow in surgery.

21. What other factors encountered during general anesthesia may negatively affect hepatic blood flow?

Many factors may ultimately reduce hepatic blood flow during anesthesia and surgery and include low arterial carbon dioxide partial pressure ($PaCO_2$) and pH, low blood volume (hypovolemia), hypotension, position of the patient during surgery, surgical traction or packing, trauma to splanchnic nerves, the use of vasoconstrictors, positive pressure ventilation with high inspiratory pressures, positive end-expiratory pressure (PEEP), portal hypertension, and anything that may contribute to a decrease in systemic blood pressure (e.g., epidural with local anesthetic, blood loss).

22. Why is it important to maintain hepatic blood flow, especially in individuals with hepatocellular disease?

Underlying liver disease will make hepatocytes more vulnerable to adverse affects of reductions in hepatic blood flow. Reduction in hepatic blood flow may lead to decreased extraction of drugs, prolonged clearance of drugs, increased drug availability (increased free drug concentration), and ultimately more adverse drug side effects. The clearance of a drug that has a high extraction ratio (i.e., extraction ratio approaches 1) is "flow-limited" and thus very affected by a decrease in hepatic blood flow. In contrast, the disposition of a drug with a low extraction ratio may be less affected by a decrease in hepatic blood flow but more affected by intrinsic metabolic pathways ("capacity-limited").

23. What is your choice for analgesia during the surgical time and postoperatively?

Systemic morphine may be used, but only in small incremental doses and titrated to effect. The pharmacokinetics of morphine are different from those of other opioids; morphine is the least lipophillic of all the opioids, thus less likely to accumulate in lipid and fatty tissue. It is also minimally protein bound. Hepatic clearance for morphine is high (about 70% hepatic extraction), so elimination is flow dependent. Most opioids are metabolized by the liver via n-dealkylation catalyzed by the cytochrome oxidase P-450 enzyme system. However, morphine is metabolized by glucuronidation, which is often preserved in liver failure. Cats do not possess the amount of glucuronyl transferase that other species do. Therefore, morphine undergoes a different type of conjugation reaction in the cat. Many patients with liver disease do not tolerate systemic morphine because of increased CNS sensitivity in addition to alteration of basic factors of drug distribution and biotransformation; thus, the administration of epidural morphine is very effective for analgesia with fewer CNS effects. An epidural should be administered only if clotting abnormalities have been ruled out or corrected through administration of plasma and/or platelets (check bleeding time, prothrombin time (PT), partial thromboplastin time (PTT), and platelet count). Regional anesthetic techniques should also be considered for perioperative analgesia.

24. How would your patient with liver disease be monitored under general anesthesia?

Electrocardiogram, pulse oximeter, capnogram, central venous catheter, arterial line for direct blood pressure and blood gas measurement, urine output, packed cell volume (PCV)/total plasma (TP), and electrolytes should be monitored. Coagulation factors such as PT, PTT, and platelet count should also be determined during surgery and assumes more importance as the duration of surgery increases, blood loss is greater, and blood replacement is given.

25. What concerns do you have in regard to ventilation and positive pressure ventilation of the patient with liver disease under anesthesia?

These patients may have ventilation to perfusion (V/Q) mismatches (due to mechanical causes such as ascites), which contribute to hypoxemia, so a high FiO_2 is recommended. It is wise to avoid hyperventilation, hypocarbia, and high levels of PEEP in patients with liver disease. It is recommended that the ideal $PaCO_2$ be kept between 40 and 42 mm Hg intraoperatively. The reasons for this are as follows: (1) The increased mean intrathoracic pressure occurring with hyperventilation and positive pressure ventilation can reduce hepatic blood flow by as much as 35% through decreased cardiac output secondary to decreased venous return and preload to the heart. (2) Decreased $PaCO_2$ can decrease portal venous blood flow. (3) Low $PaCO_2$ and alkalosis favors ammonium conversion to ammonia, the non-polar species that crosses the blood-brain barrier and generates hepatic encephalopathy. (4) Respiratory alkalosis increases the urinary potassium loss in patients who are sensitive to and may already be hypokalemic. (5) Hypocarbia may cause a withdrawal of sympathetic tone, decreasing the inotropic state of the heart. (6) Hypocarbia and alkalosis may decrease ionized calcium. (7) Hypocarbia and alkalosis may shift the oxygen-hemoglobin dissociation curve to the left, increase hemoglobin affinity for oxygen, and ultimately impede delivery of oxygen to tissue.

26. In summary, what would be an ideal anesthetic protocol in a patient that has liver dysfunction and is undergoing surgery?

After optimizing patient status, guidelines for anesthetic management of a patient with liver disease include the following:

- Little or no premedication. Morphine or butorphanol in small, titrated doses. Avoid diazepam and tranquilizers such as acepromazine.
- Preoxygenate the patient. Induction with small amounts of propofol, or mask induction with isoflurane or sevoflurane.
- Administration of an epidural for perioperative analgesia (if blood clotting parameters are normal or have been corrected).
- Maintenance of anesthesia with isoflurane or sevoflurane in oxygen.
- Effective monitoring
- Avoid detrimental effects on hepatic blood flow
  - Maintain volume status and blood pressure
  - Avoid hyperventilation
  - Avoid halothane

27. What are the effects of halothane on the liver? Can they lead to hepatocellular damage?

Studies have shown that halothane inhibits the drug-metabolizing capacity of the liver (reduction in intrinsic drug clearance). This, taken together with the alteration of other pharmacokinetically important variables such as reduced hepatic blood flow during halothane administration, will lead to delayed drug removal and/or an increase in plasma drug concentration during anesthesia. Prolonged or increased plasma concentrations of many drugs have important toxic implications, especially in a patient with underlying liver disease or other major physiologic compromise. Hepatocelluar injury (centrilobular necrosis) may occur with halothane administration. The etiology is a topic of much debate. Localized hypoxia secondary to reductions in hepatic blood flow may damage the hepatocyte directly. In humans, the "halothane hepatitis syndrome" (severe necrosis with fulminant liver failure) is due to antigen formation to the oxidative metabolite (trifluoroacetate) of halothane. Hepatocellular damage occurs via an autoimmune-mediated reaction. Diagnosis is confirmed through measurement of trifluoroacetyl antigen-antibody complex titers (TFA). The cause of sensitivity to this halothane metabolite is unknown, but certain risk factors have been identified, such as increased age and obesity.

28. Which newer opioid analgesic agents may be appropriate for patients with liver dysfunction?

The opioid remifentanil has an ester linkage in its molecule and can be broken down by blood and tissue nonspecific esterases rather than by liver enzymes. It is structurally similar to and related to the phenylpiperidine derivatives fentanyl and sufentanil. This drug has not yet been fully evaluated in the veterinary literature; however, one study in dogs demonstrated it to be about half as potent as fentanyl. Remifentanil also has the advantage of rapid recovery because of its short elimation time, but it must be given as a constant infusion.

BIBLIOGRAPHY

1. Brown BR, Frink EJ: Anesthesia considerations in patients with liver disease. Anesthesiol Rev 20(6):213-220, 1993.
2. Brown BR: The newest thoughts on management of patients with liver disease: Anesthesia for the patient with hepatic disease. Proceedings of the California Society of Anesthesiologists: What's New in Clinical Anesthesia 1995, pp 117–124.
3. Merritt WT, Gelman S: Anesthesia for liver surgery. In Rogers MC, Tinker JH, Covino BG, Longnecker DE (eds): Principles and Practice of Anesthesiology, St. Louis, Mosby, 1993, pp 1991–2034.
4. Michelsen LG, Salmenpera M, Hug CC, et al: Anesthetic potency of remifentanil in dogs. Anesthesiology 84:865–872, 1996.
5. Nelson RW, Couto CG: Diagnostic tests for the hepatobiliary system. In Nelson RW, Couto CB (eds): Essentials of Small Animal Internal Medicine, St. Louis, Mosby, 1992, pp 379–397.
6. Rogers EL: Evaluation of the patient with liver disease. In Rogers MC, Tinker JH, Covino BG, Longnecker DE (eds): Principles and Practice of Anesthesiology, 1992, pp 311–340.

31. RENAL DISEASE

Robert E. Meyer, D.V.M., D.A.C.V.A.

1. What are the main factors to be considered when faced with anesthetizing a patient with renal or urinary tract disease?

Perioperative considerations include the effect of anesthetic drugs on renal function, the effect of renal disease on anesthetic drug metabolism, and the effect of renal disease on fluid and electrolyte balance.

2. What is the principal function of the kidneys?

Some might argue, with tongue planted firmly in cheek, that the renal system principally creates employment for veterinary behaviorists. However, the principal function of the kidneys is to maintain a constant extracellular milieu by regulating water and electrolyte balance and excreting hydrogen ions and nitrogenous waste. To do this, the kidneys receive about 25% of the total cardiac output. The glomerular filtration rate (GFR) is about 20% of the renal plasma flow. One milliliter of urine is produced for every 100 ml of glomerular filtrate. In normal dogs, urine is produced at the rate of 0.5 to 1.0 ml/kg/hr.

3. What else does the kidney do besides make urine?

The kidneys also serve as a target organ for various hormones (parathyroid hormone, aldosterone, and antidiuretic hormone or ADH). In addition, the kidneys can metabolize and secrete regulatory substances, such as insulin, renin, prostaglandins, and erythropoietin.

4. How do anesthesia and surgery affect glomerular filtration?

Surgical stress and anesthetic agents influence physiologic factors and cause release of neurohumoral substances that can subsequently affect glomerular filtration and reabsorption of filtered water and solutes. These factors include changes in arterial blood pressure, release of catecholamines, production of ADH, endothelin, nitric oxide, prostaglandins, and the aldosterone-renin-angiotensin system.

5. How is renal blood flow regulated?

Renal blood flow (RBF) is autoregulated between 60 to 160 mm Hg, such that renal perfusion is held constant within this range of mean arterial pressures (MAPs). Glomerular capillary hydrostatic pressure, and therefore glomerular filtration, is held constant when blood pressure is maintained within this range. RBF generally becomes pressure-dependent should the MAPs fall outside this range.

6. How are perfusion pressure and renal output related?

Decreased perfusion pressure during anesthesia reduces hydrostatic pressure in the glomerular capillaries, and outward filtration is predictably reduced. Sympathetic nervous system stimulation associated with surgery results in renal artery vasoconstriction, with reduction of RBF and glomerular filtration rate despite maintenance of perfusion pressure within the range of autoregulation. Hemorrhage, hypovolemia, or dehydration all reduce filtration pressure through increased plasma oncotic pressure. Any decrease in RBF will initiate renin release, which, combined with release of catecholamines, can further reduce RBF and alter the distribution of blood flow within the kidney.

7. Are anesthetics nephrotoxic?

In a sense, *all* anesthetics are functional nephrotoxins, in that they produce generalized reduction of measureable renal function. The exception to this is the fluoride-containing anesthetic methoxyflurane (see delayed toxicity discussion in question 11). In addition, renal ischemia may occur secondary to anesthetic-induced systemic hypotension and reduced cardiac output, or secondary to drug- or stress-induced renal vasoconstriction.

8. How do injectable anesthetic agents acutely affect renal function?

Most injectable anesthetics do not directly affect the kidney; however, systemic hypotension associated with injectable anesthetics may reduce RBF and GFR. Pre-existing hypovolemia will exacerbate these effects. It is best to avoid drugs with primary renal excretion, such as the muscle relaxant pancuronium, or highly protein-bound drugs, such as barbiturates. The effects of some common injectable anesthetics on renal function are listed in the table.

Effect of Injectable Anesthetics on the Kidney

DRUG	DIRECT EFFECTS	INDIRECT EFFECTS	NOTES
Phenothiazines	None	Systemic hypotension may lead to reduced RBF and GFR	Prolonged sedation noted in uremic patients
Benzodiazepines	None	None	Renal excretion of active metabolite (oxazepam) may result in prolonged effect in uremic or oliguric patients
α_2-agonists	None	RBF reduced due to vasoconstriction; pronounced hyperglycemia may lead to glucosuria; polyuria; may potentiate hyperkalemic bradycardia and other dysrhythmias	Avoid or use cautiously in patients with urinary tract obstruction
Opioids	None	None	Surgical stimulation in presence of high-dose morphine can lead to ADH release and oliguria; renal excretion of active metabolite (morphine-6-glucuronide) may result in prolonged effect in uremic or oliguric patients
Barbiturates	None	Reduction in blood pressure and cardiac output may reduce RBF, GFR	Increased sensitivity noted in uremic patients due to increased blood levels of active unbound nonionized drug
Cyclohexamine dissociatives (ketamine, Telazol)	None	RBF reduced due to increased sympathetic tone, vasoconstriction	Renal excretion of drug or active metabolite (e.g., norketamine) may result in prolonged effect in uremic or oliguric patients
Etomidate	None	None	None noted
Propofol	None	Systemic hypotension may lead to reduced RBF, GFR	None noted

9. How do inhalant anesthetic agents acutely affect renal function?

Inhalant anesthetics themselves have no direct effect on autoregulation of GFR or RBF. They can, however, indirectly reduce GFR and RBF through their depressant effects on cardiac function and blood pressure. The effect of inhaled anesthetic agents on RBF and GFR can be attenuated by perioperative fluid administration and reduction of the inhaled anesthetic concentration.

10. How long do anesthetic agents affect renal function?

The renal effects of most anesthetic agents are generally transient, limited to the anesthetic period, and usually clinically insignificant as long as their metabolites are inactive. Anesthetic effects on RBF and GFR are generally attenuated by perioperative fluid administration.

11. Can anesthetic agents cause delayed nephrotoxicity?

Delayed nephrotoxicity occurs secondary to biotransformation of the fluoride-containing inhalant anesthetic methoxyflurane (and possibly enflurane) to oxalate and free fluoride ion. Methoxyflurane may enhance the nephrotoxic effect of other drugs administered during anesthesia, including *flunixin meglumine* and the *aminoglycoside antibiotics* (see table). Although dogs appear to be more resistant to fluoride-induced nephrotoxicity than humans, it is prudent to *avoid* methoxyflurane in patients with renal disease.

Potential Perioperative Nephrotoxins

Aminoglycoside antibiotics	Inorganic fluoride ion
Amphotericin B	Oxalate
Hemoglobin	Iodinated contrast agents
Myoglobin	Nonsteroidal anti-inflammatory agents
Bilirubin	Flunixin meglumine (when combined with methoxyflurane)

12. Is there a risk of nephrotoxicity with other fluoride-containing inhaled anesthetics?

Sevoflurane is transformed in the presence of soda lime or Baralyme in the CO_2 absorber of the anesthetic circuit to the fluoride-containing substance known as compound A. Compound A is nephrotoxic to rats but is unlikely to build to toxic concentrations during routine semiclosed administration of sevoflurane. Defluorination of halothane and isoflurane is insufficient to result in plasma fluoride levels high enough to cause nephrotoxicity.

13. What kinds of renal failure patients am I likely to anesthetize?

Generally, these kinds of cases fall into two groups: animals with an *acute* post-renal problem for which anesthesia and surgery are emergently required, such as traumatic injury to the urinary tract or obstruction of outflow, and animals with *chronic* renal disease, for which anesthesia is required to facilitate an unrelated problem. Animals with primary drug- or toxin-induced renal tubular damage are rarely presented for anesthesia. Unless surgery is life-saving, renal disease patients should be stabilized prior to anesthesia.

14. What is the best laboratory test for clinical evaluation of renal function?

Most renal function tests are insensitive measurements, and no single test is ideal. Clinical evidence of renal failure occurs only after more than 70% of nephrons are nonfunctional and, therefore, significant renal disease can be present despite normal laboratory values. A combination of tests to evaluate GFR and renal tubular function is best (see table). Trends are more useful in evaluating renal function than isolated measurements. In addition, you should ideally assess hematocrit (remember, the kidney produces erythropoietin), acid-base status, and circulating sodium and potassium levels.

Tests for Evaluation of Renal Function

GLOMERULAR FILTRATION RATE TESTS	RENAL TUBULAR FUNCTION TESTS
Blood urea nitrogen	Urine specific gravity
Plasma creatinine	Urine osmolarity
Creatinine clearance	

15. What is the best way to anesthetize a patient in acute postrenal failure?

These cases include trauma to the ureters, bladder, or urethra and outflow obstruction secondary to urethral calculi. Several metabolic derangements can be present in these patients, including dehydration secondary to vomiting and fluid shifts into the peritoneal cavity, hyperkalemia, hyponatremia, hypochloremia, metabolic acidosis, and uremia. The abdomen may be quite distended, with reduced diaphragmatic movement and hypoxemia. Excessively rapid removal of free peritoneal urine can result in severe systemic hypotension. The kidneys may or may not have normal function.

The key to managing these cases is presurgical stabilization, including peritoneal dialysis and treatment of electrolyte and acid-base disturbances. Isotonic saline can be administered intravenously at rates up to 10 ml/kg/hr, although lactated Ringer's solution (which contains only 4 mEq/L of K+) can be safely administered to these patients. In trauma patients, a colloid (Dextran 70 or Hetastarch, 5–10 ml/kg IV) can also be quite useful in restoring circulating blood volume. Acute postrenal failure patients can be safely anesthetized once the metabolic derangements are resolved, taking into account the effect of individual anesthetic agents on renal function (see tables at questions 8 and 11).

16. Can I use the electrocardiogram to estimate plasma potassium concentration?

Yes! Although patients with serum K+ levels greater than 5.5-6.0 mEq/L should not be anesthetized for elective procedures, characteristic electrocardiographic changes can be quite useful in the diagnosis and treatment of hyperkalemia in the absence of laboratory data. Mild elevations in serum potassium level (6.0–6.5 mEq/L) cause T waves to become tall and peaked, but heart rate and the P waves usually remain normal. The heart rate begins to slow at moderate elevations (6.5–7.0 mEq/L), and the P waves begin to flatten. At high elevations (≥7.5 mEq/L), the heart rate becomes very slow, atrial standstill may occur, and the T wave may or may not be large. Cardiac arrest may occur at any time, even without anesthesia, when serum potassium reaches 9.5 mEq/L or greater.

17. What is the treatment for acute hyperkalemia?

Ideally, hyperkalemia should be treated prior to anesthesia. Calcium salts are initially administered to counteract hyperkalemic bradycardia. Once a stable heart rate is achieved, therapy is subsequently directed to drive extracellular potassium intracellularly. Common treatments for hyperkalemia are listed in the table.

Treatment for Acute Hyperkalemia

TREATMENT	COMMENTS
1.5–2.0 ml 10% Ca++ chloride 2 or 2–10 ml 10% Ca++ gluconate per 15 kg body weight	Lasts 15–120 min, works immediately; increased inotropic effect counteracts negative cardiac effects of increased K+ only
Hyperventilation	Every 10 mm Hg decrease in PaCO2 will decrease K+ 0.5 mEq/L
5–10 % dextrose-containing fluids or 1–2 ml/kg of 50% dextrose IV	Stimulates endogenous insulin release and drives K+ intracellularly. Effects start within 1 hr and last several hours
1.0–2.0 mEq/kg Na HCO₃ – infusion IV	Drives K+ intracellularly in exchange for H+ ions. Effects start within 1 hr and last several hours

18. What is the best way to anesthetize a patient in chronic renal failure?

Animals with chronic renal disease have pre-existing renal impairment but can show varying degrees of compensation. Maintenance of renal blood flow and avoidance of hypovolemia, hypotension, and renal vasoconstriction are necessary to the successful anesthetic management of these patients. Fluid administration is likely the most important management factor. In the absence of congestive heart failure, pulmonary edema, or anuria, an isotonic crystalloid solution such as lactated Ringer's (10–20 ml/kg/hr) can be administered to promote diuresis. Continuation of fluids may be necessary in the postanesthetic period as well. Chronic renal failure patients can be safely anesthetized, taking into account the effect of individual anesthetic agents on renal function (see tables at questions 8 and 11).

19. My anesthetized patient is oliguric. What should I do to restore urine production?

Cases in which acute perioperative renal failure is due to hypovolemia (prerenal) can usually be resolved with intravenous fluid therapy. If the patient does not have pulmonary edema or congestive heart failure, first try an isotonic crystalloid fluid bolus challenge of 5–10 ml/kg IV (lactated Ringer's solution works well for this purpose). If urine production improves, the animal was likely hypovolemic and intravenous fluids should be continued while you monitor urine production. In cases in which low cardiac output is the reason for perioperative oliguria, inotropes such as dobutamine 2–10 μg/kg, or dopamine 5–10 μg/kg/min, can be given following restoration of circulating volume. Diuretics, such as furosemide or mannitol (0.25–0.5 g/kg IV), can be administered to promote diuresis in oliguric, normovolemic patients but should not be administered to hypovolemic patients.

20. Can a low-dose dopamine infusion be used to stimulate renal dopaminergic receptors and improve renal output?

This is controversial. Dopamine, at low intravenous doses of 1–3 μg/kg/min, has been advocated to increase renal blood flow and glomerular filtration rate, urine output, and sodium excretion and to decrease renal vascular resistance. However, recent evidence in human volunteers has shown 10- to 75-fold intersubject variability following constant rate dopamine infusion (MacGregor et al, 2000). Based on the unpredictability of dopamine pharmacokinetics, the effectiveness of low-dose dopamine infusion to selectively improve renal function is questionable at best.

21. Can I safely administer a nonsteroidal anti-inflammatory drug such as carprofen or ketoprofen for analgesia during anesthesia and surgery?

Ketoprofen and carprofen are nonsteroidal anti-inflammatory drugs (NSAIDs) that are used for perioperative pain control (Grisneaux et al, 1999). Both drugs are cyclooxygenase inhibitors and have adverse effects similar to other NSAIDs, including gastric ulcers, renal failure, and hemorrhage. Lobetti and Joubert (2000) recently reported transient azotemia, increased renal tubular epithelial cells and sediment, and decreased urine specific gravity following the use of NSAIDs but concluded that the use of these agents was not contraindicated in clinically normal dogs undergoing anesthesia and surgery. Nonetheless, it would be prudent to limit use of these agents to well-hydrated patients with normal renal function and to give supplemental intravenous fluids during anesthesia and surgery.

22. I know mean arterial pressure should be maintained above 60 mm Hg to maintain renal perfusion and urine production in adults. Should mean arterial pressure be similarly maintained above 60 mm Hg in neonatal or pediatric patients?

Probably not. The MAP range for renal blood flow autoregulation in neonatal and pediatric patients is not well described. Mean arterial pressure generally increases with physiologic age and does not approach adult values in dogs until 6–9 months of age. In mongrel puppies, awake MAP rises from 49 mm Hg at 4 weeks of age to adult pressures by 28–36 weeks (Adelman and Wright, 1985; Magrini, 1978). Thus, it is inappropriate to expect adult blood pressure values in pediatric patients. It is probably reasonable during anesthesia in pediatric patients to target blood pressure at 80% of the awake baseline pressure.

BIBLIOGRAPHY

1. Adelman RD, Wright J: Systolic blood pressure and heart rate in the growing beagle puppy. Dev Pharmacol Ther 8:396–401, 1985.
2. Greene SA: Renal disease. In Thurmon JC, Tranquilli WJ, Benson GJ (eds): Essentials of Small Animal Anesthesia and Analgesia. Philidelphia, Lippincott Williams & Wilkins, 1999, pp 450–459.
3. Grisneaux E, Pibarot P, Dupuis J, Blais D: Comparison of ketoprofen and carprofen administered prior to orthopedic surgery for control of postoperative pain in dogs. J Am Vet Med Assoc 215:1105–1110, 1999.
4. Lobetti RG, Joubert KE: Effect of administration of nonsteroidal anti-inflammatory drugs before surgery on renal function in clinically normal dogs. Am J Vet Res 61:1501–1507, 2000.
5. MacGregor DA, Smith TE, Prielipp RC, et al: Pharmacokinetics of dopamine in healthy male subjects. Anesthesiology 92:338–346, 2000.
6. Magrini F: Haemodynamic determinants of the arterial blood pressure rise during growth in conscious puppies. Cardiovascular Res 12:422–428, 1978.
7. Paddleford RR: Manual of Small Animal Anesthesia, 2nd ed. Philadelphia, WB Saunders, 1999, pp 292–297.
8. Waterman-Pearson AE: Urogenital disease. In Seymour C, Gleed R (eds): Manual of Small Animal Anaesthesia and Analgesia. Cheltonham, British Small Animal Veterinary Association, 1999, pp 211–215.

32. ANESTHESIA FOR THE PATIENT WITH NEUROLOGIC DISEASE

Stephen A. Greene, D.V.M., M.S., D.A.C.V.A.

1. What are the anesthetic considerations for animals with a history of seizures?

There is evidence that phenothiazine tranquilizers may lower the seizure threshold in animals. Therefore, acepromazine is generally contraindicated in animals with a history of seizures. It is less clear whether acepromazine or other phenothiazine tranquilizers pose a risk of increased seizure activity in animals with seizures due to factors other than idiopathic epilepsy. Although some anesthetics (e.g., ketamine, tiletamine, or methohexital) can induce seizures in otherwise normal animals, coadministration of phenothiazine tranquilizers is not likely to increase their incidence. As a rule, if other anesthetic agents are available, their use is preferred over the use of seizure-related anesthetics when performing procedures known to result in seizure activity (i.e., cervical myelography).

2. Describe autoregulation of cerebral blood flow.

Autoregulation of cerebral blood flow refers to the intrinsic vasodilation or vasoconstriction of cerebral blood vessels that maintain relatively constant blood flow to brain tissue even though the systemic arterial blood pressure varies significantly. The typical range of systemic blood pressure over which cerebral autoregulation of blood flow occurs is between mean arterial pressures of 60 and 140 mm Hg.

3. What is the effect of elevated arterial carbon dioxide tension on cerebral blood flow?

Elevated arterial carbon dioxide tension and the accompanying acidemia are disruptive of the normal mechanisms associated with cerebral blood flow autoregulation. During hypercapnia, cerebral blood vessels are dilated, allowing increased blood flow and therefore increased cerebral blood volume.

4. What is the effect of decreased arterial carbon dioxide tension on cerebral blood flow?

Alteration of the normal arterial carbon dioxide tension in either direction will interfere with cerebral blood flow autoregulation. The relationship between arterial carbon dioxide tension and cerebral blood flow is linear. When arterial carbon dioxide tension is decreased by means such as hyperventilation, the cerebral blood flow will decrease. This is believed to be due to cerebral vessel vasoconstriction that overrides autoregulatory mechanisms during hypocapnia.

5. What effect does hypoxia have on cerebral blood flow?

Hypoxia is also associated with a disruption of cerebral blood flow autoregulation. At arterial oxygen tensions of less than 60 mm Hg, cerebral blood flow will increase dramatically. This represents a protective effect for the brain when threatened by low oxygenation. On the other hand, when arterial oxygen tension increases above normal, cerebral blood flow autoregulation remains intact for up to 12 hours. Patients breathing concentrations of oxygen greater than 40% to 50% for periods longer than 12 hours are at risk for development of pulmonary edema due to damage from free radicals of oxygen (oxygen toxicity).

6. What is the relationship between cerebral blood flow and intracranial pressure?

The relationship between cerebral blood flow and intracranial pressure (ICP) is linear. That is, when cerebral blood flow increases, the ICP will increase, and vice versa. As blood flow into the noncompliant cranial vault is increased, the pressure within will increase. Likewise, in patients with elevated ICP, cerebral blood flow can be therapeutically decreased to concurrently decrease ICP.

7. What is the Monro-Kellie doctrine?

The intracranial compartment is composed of cerebrospinal fluid (10%), blood (10%), and parenchymal tissue including interstitial water (80%). The Monro-Kellie doctrine states that any change in one of the components of the intracranial compartment will result in an opposing change in the other components in an attempt to maintain constant ICP. In general, when there is an increase in the parenchymal component, cerebrospinal fluid diversion occurs early. During chronically raised ICP, cerebrospinal fluid production is decreased. A later compensatory change would be decreased intracranial blood volume. When compensatory mechanisms are overcome by a pathologic condition, ICP will dramatically increase, leading to brain herniation.

8. What are the determinants of cerebral perfusion pressure?

The cerebral perfusion pressure (CPP) is the difference between the mean systemic arterial pressure (MAP) and the ICP (CPP = MAP – ICP). Thus, when ICP is increased, the cerebral perfusion pressure is decreased. Extreme elevations of ICP are associated with increased neurologic morbidity due to poor perfusion of brain tissue. For this reason, it is important to monitor the arterial blood pressure during anesthesia of patients with raised ICP. Mean arterial blood pressure should be maintained above 75 mm Hg to prevent loss of cerebral perfusion in these patients.

9. How is intracranial pressure measured in the clinical setting?

Intracranial pressure can be measured using invasive techniques that involve placement of a pressure transducer into intraventricular, subarachnoid, or epidural sites. The oldest technique involves the intraventricular placement of a probe using a strain-gauge transducer. This technique requires perforation of brain tissue. Subarachnoid devices avoid insertion through the brain and require drilling a burr hole in the skull. For epidural placement, there are fiberoptic and pneumatic transducers available. Recently, fiberoptic measurement devices have become available for measuring ICP through a burr hole in the skull as well. Some of these devices are tolerated by animals relatively well after they recover from anesthesia, thereby allowing continuous monitoring of the ICP during the recovery and early convalescent periods.

10. What are the most common causes of increased ICP in dogs?

Cerebral disease and trauma constitute most of the cases of increased ICP in dogs. Brain tumors may increase the mass of the intracranial tissues, produce cerebral edema fluid, and may disrupt cerebral blood flow autoregulation. Trauma to the head may result in intracranial hemorrhage and cerebral edema. Less common causes of raised ICP include severe systemic hypertension, stroke, or obstruction of cerebrospinal fluid outflow from the head. Increased intracranial blood volume and ICP may also result from hypoxia, hypercapnia, acidosis, or acute respiratory failure.

11. Which anesthetics are associated with increased ICP?

Anesthetics that are known to increase the ICP include ketamine, tiletamine, and the inhaled halogenated agents. In normal animals, modest increases in ICP occur during anesthesia and are not associated with neurologic morbidity. However, patients with intracranial masses or cerebral trauma are predisposed to life-threatening increases in ICP when these anesthetics are used. Special precautions such as controlled hyperventilation must be used during anesthesia to prevent neurologic morbidity during anesthesia.

12. How does controlled hyperventilation prevent neurologic morbidity in patients with brain tumors during inhalant anesthesia?

By decreasing the arterial tension of carbon dioxide, controlled hyperventilation effectively counteracts the effects of inhaled anesthetics on ICP. A typical end-expired or arterial carbon dioxide tension target during hyperventilation is 25 to 30 mm Hg. Positive pressure ventilation is associated with decreased venous return to the heart due to increased intrathoracic pressure. Decreased venous return may lead to decreased cardiac output and mean arterial pressure. The hyperventilation technique must carefully balance the benefit associated with respiratory alkalosis against the concomitant reduction in cardiac output and arterial blood pressure. Excessive hyperventilation may result in carbon dioxide tension less than 25 mm Hg and ensuing vasoconstriction of cerebral vasculature. Although this consequence may decrease cerebral blood flow and ICP to some degree, the net effect on cerebral perfusion pressure is likely detrimental to patient survival. If blood pressure is severely decreased by positive pressure ventilation, the presence of raised ICP will dramatically decrease the cerebral perfusion pressure, thereby increasing neurologic morbidity.

13. How do opioid analgesics affect ICP?

The direct effects of opioids on cerebral blood flow and ICP are negligible. However, if respiratory depression associated with administration of opioids causes a significant increase in the arterial carbon dioxide tension, the vasodilatory effects of carbon dioxide will disrupt cerebral blood flow autoregulation, allowing increased ICP. Clinical experience in dogs and cats dictates that for commonly used doses of opioids in the perianesthetic period, respiratory depression is not of significant concern to warrant elimination of opioids from the anesthetic protocol.

14. How do tranquilizers affect ICP?

Benzodiazepine tranquilizers such as diazepam, midazolam, or zolazepam have no direct effect on ICP. Controversy exists as to whether co-administration of these agents with dissociative anesthetics negates the increase in ICP observed following administration of dissociative anesthetics alone. Currently, it is recommended that dissociative anesthetics be avoided in patients with raised ICP. Phenothiazine and butyrophenone tranquilizers (e.g., acepromazine and droperidol, respectively) also demonstrate no effect or decreased intracranial pressure in spite of their α-adrenoceptor blocking activity that may cause systemic vasodilation.

15. What is the effect of nitrous oxide on ICP?

Nitrous oxide has no direct effect on ICP when used at concentrations of 50–70 % in oxygen. However, nitrous oxide will equilibrate in closed gas spaces to increase the volume and/or pressure within the space. Thus, in patients undergoing pneumoencephalography, the addition of nitrous oxide to the breathing mixture can increase the gas volume in the cranium, resulting in increased ICP.

16. How do neuromuscular blocking agents affect ICP?

The effect of neuromuscular blocking agents on ICP depends on which agent is used. Most of the nondepolarizing neuromuscular blockers (e.g., atracurium, pancuronium, vecuronium, or mivacurium) have no effect on ICP. Agents that cause a significant release of histamine after administration (e.g., *d*-tubocurarine) may increase ICP secondarily via histamine-mediated cerebral vasodilation. Succinylcholine causes a direct increase in ICP, but this effect may be attenuated by the common practice (in human medicine) of preadministering a nondepolarizing agent. There is no compelling reason to justify use of succinylcholine in animals with intracranial disease.

17. Which anesthetics are considered best for induction of anesthesia in patients with raised ICP?

Animals with raised ICP can be premedicated with opioids alone or opioids combined with α_2-agonists or benzodiazepine tranquilizers. For example, hydromorphone (0.2 mg/kg IM) and atropine (0.04 mg/kg IM) can be given as premedicants. Then, induction of anesthesia is readily accomplished by intravenous administration of thiopental or propofol, given to effect. The trachea is intubated and the animal maintained using isoflurane with controlled ventilation. End-tidal carbon dioxide is monitored, and the ventilator is adjusted to maintain CO_2 at about 25 mm Hg.

18. What is the "Cushing reflex"?

The Cushing reflex is the physiologic response to increased ICP characterized by systemic hypertension. In late stages, the reflex may include profound bradycardia. If the hypertension is treated medically prior to relief of raised ICP, a deleterious decrease in systemic blood pressure may occur following craniotomy. Thus, the hypertension should not be aggressively treated in patients with intracranial disease. Instead, the underlying causes of raised ICP should be addressed.

BIBLIOGRAPHY

1. Greene SA, Harvey RC, Sims MH: Neurologic disease. In Thurmon JC, Tranquilli WJ, Benson GJ (eds): Essentials of Small Animal Anesthesia and Analgesia. Baltimore, Lippincott, Williams & Wilkins, 1999, pp 437–450.
2. Marshall WK, Arancibia CU, Williams CL: Monitoring intracranial pressure. In Lake, Hines, and Blitt (eds): Clinical Monitoring: Practical Applications for Anesthesia and Critical Care, Philadelphia, W.B. Saunders, 2001, pp 659–686.
3. Schell RM, Cole DJ: Cerebral protection and neuroanesthesia. Anesthesiol Clin North Am 10:453–469, 1992.

33. ENDOCRINE DISEASE

Julie A. Smith, D.V.M., D.A.C.V.A.

1. What common guidelines assist in the management of animals with endocrine disorders?

- A complete and thorough physical examination should be performed on all patients prior to anesthesia.
- A complete preanesthetic laboratory workup should be performed, including a complete blood count (CBC), serum chemistry panel, and urinalysis.
- A preanesthetic electrocardiogram (ECG), thoracic radiographs, and echocardiography should be obtained before induction in patients with a high risk of cardiac complications.
- Every effort should be made to stabilize any abnormalities prior to anesthesia.
- To avoid potentially fatal complications, anesthesia should be postponed in any animal that is not in a stable or controlled condition.
- No specific anesthetic protocols are recommended for any of the endocrine disorders. Instead, each animal is evaluated separately, and a protocol is formulated based on their condition and the procedure performed.
- Use drugs that are short-acting or readily reversible.
- Rapid recovery and return to normal function are desirable in all situations to avoid decompensation and potential problems.
- All patients should be closely monitored in the recovery period.

2. What should I be monitoring during recovery in patients with endocrine disease?

As with all patients, the extent of monitoring during recovery is determined by the underlying disease and the condition of the patient. In some situations, patients that have done well during anesthesia may decompensate and have problems during the recovery period. Therefore, postanesthetic monitoring is especially critical in animals with underlying endocrine disease. Minimal postanesthesia monitoring should include evaluation of the pulse rate and quality, respiratory rate and rhythm, mucous membrane color, capillary refill time, and body temperature. Additional monitoring may be indicated, such as intermittent or continuous evaluation of the ECG, direct or indirect measurement of blood pressure, and intermittent determination of the central venous pressure. Intravenous fluid support and oxygen supplementation should be provided when indicated.

3. What short-acting anesthetic agents can be used in animals with endocrine disorders?

Propofol, thiopental, ketamine, and etomidate are acceptable injectable anesthetic agents for use in patients with endocrine disorders. Isoflurane and sevoflurane are the inhalation anesthetics of choice because of minimal metabolism and rapid induction and recovery.

4. Should a diabetic patient fast before being anesthetized?

Yes. Animals with preexisting diabetes mellitus should fast overnight on the evening prior to anesthesia. It is important to withhold food in the preanesthetic period to prevent regurgitation and possible aspiration. The animal should be fed and insulin administered in the routine manner on the evening before. On the morning of anesthesia, one-half of the morning dose of insulin should be given and food withheld. Surgery should be scheduled first thing in the morning in an effort to have the animal recovered and back on schedule in time for the evening meal.

5. How often should you monitor serum glucose levels during anesthesia of the diabetic patient?

Hypoglycemia is the most important and most common complication associated with the anesthetic management of diabetic patients. Blood glucose should be measured before induction of anesthesia, every 60 minutes during anesthesia, and throughout recovery. A second venous catheter—not the one used to administer the intraoperative fluids—should be placed for the collection of blood for serial glucose levels.

6. What is an acceptable blood glucose concentration during anesthesia?

Blood glucose levels should be maintained between 150 and 250 mg/dl. If hypoglycemia occurs, a balanced electrolyte solution with 2.5–5.0% dextrose should be administered at a rate of 10–15 ml/kg/hr. The rate and concentration should be adjusted based on sequential glucose levels. If glucose levels are within the normal range, a balanced electrolyte, non–dextrose-containing solution is used for fluid maintenance during anesthesia.

7. Is decompensation a concern after anesthesia in diabetic animals?

In addition to the change in the patient's feeding routine, the stress of hospitalization and surgery may cause well-controlled diabetic animals to decompensate and become unregulated. Decompensation may also follow corticosteroid administration.

8. Are there any anesthetic agents I should avoid in diabetic patients?

Xylazine and other alpha-2 agonists cause a dose-dependent transient hypoinsulinemia and hyperglycemia and should be avoided in diabetic patients.

9. What if I have to anesthetize a ketoacidotic animal?

Every effort should be made to stabilize the decompensated or ketoacidotic animal before administration of anesthetic agents. The ketoacidotic animal is hyperglycemic, has metabolic acidosis, and is dehydrated and in circulatory collapse. Rehydration and correction of the acidosis and electrolyte abnormalities are critical to decreasing the risk of intraoperative cardiac arrhythmias and hypotension. Sufficient correction of potentially life-threatening fluid and electrolyte disturbances can often be accomplished in just a few hours. Few emergent situations do not allow stabilization for a few hours prior to anesthesia.

Stabilization should include insulin therapy (use regular insulin with either the low-dose IV or the low-dose IM method) and volume deficit replacement with sodium chloride or balanced electrolyte solutions (maximum rate: 70 ml/kg/hr). Acid–base abnormalities often resolve with rehydration and decreased glucose levels. The most important electrolyte disturbance is depletion of total body potassium. Aggressive replacement therapy is often required (not to exceed 40 mEq/L) because, as acidosis and volume deficits are corrected, potassium moves into the intracellular space and is excreted in the urine.

10. What are the considerations for a patient with an insulinoma?

Blood glucose levels with insulinomas are generally below 70 mg/dl. When blood glucose levels are between 35 and 60 mg/dl, bradycardia and hypotension may be seen. An adrenergic excess, resulting in tachycardia, hypertension, and tachypnea occurs when glucose concentrations drop to 20–35 mg/dl. Levels less than 20 mg/dl lead to seizures, coma, and death.

Animals with insulinomas should be hospitalized on the evening before surgery for removal of the tumor. When the patient is admitted, the blood glucose levels should be evaluated and the patient placed on a 5–20% dextrose infusion overnight to regulate levels. Fasting should be minimal (4–8 hours), and surgery should be performed first thing in the morning. Evaluate blood glucose levels frequently (every 30 minutes), and adjust the dextrose infusion to prevent hypoglycemia. Manipulation of the tumor itself can cause massive insulin release and profound hypoglycemia.

11. What intraoperative monitoring is recommended for patients with insulinoma?

Intraoperative monitoring should include routine multisystem evaluation with special attention to the cardiovascular system. A continuous ECG should be monitored to identify cardiac rhythm abnormalities. An arterial catheter should be placed for the measurement of arterial blood pressure and the collection of blood samples for evaluation of pH and acid–base status. A second venous catheter—not the one used to administer the intraoperative fluids—should be placed for the collection of blood for serial glucose levels.

12. What are the major concerns when anesthetizing an animal with hyperthyroidism?

Animals with hyperthyroidism (most common in cats) have varying degrees of cardiac compromise, usually related to hypertrophic cardiomyopathy. A full cardiac workup should be done to evaluate the degree of cardiac changes. This workup should include an ECG, thoracic radiographs, and echocardiogram. Risk of cardiac compromise or failure is much less after therapy for hyperthyroidism and establishment of the euthyroid condition.

Adequate ventilation and oxygenation are also important in hyperthyroid animals. The increased metabolic rate associated with hyperthyroidism causes an increased oxygen demand and an increased sensitivity to hypoxemia. Preoxygenation by mask prior to induction is recommended. Carbon dioxide (CO_2) production is increased in hypermetabolic conditions. Elevations in CO_2 increase sympathetic tone, which further elevates heart rate and blood pressure and may contribute to the development of cardiac arrhythmias

13. What anesthetic drugs should I avoid when anesthetizing a hyperthyroid cat?

The choice of anesthetic agents for use in cats for thyroidectomy depends on the condition of the cat at the time of surgery. It is best to avoid agents that increase the heart rate, such as anticholinergics. Agents that sensitize the myocardium to catecholamine-induced arrhythmias, such as xylazine and halothane, should also be avoided. Small doses of ketamine can be used safely in euthyroid cats. Ketamine increases sympathetic tone, heart rate, and blood pressure and should be used sparingly.

14. What is thyroid storm?

Thyroid storm is the sudden release of excessive levels of thyroid hormone into the circulation. This life-threatening syndrome is precipitated by catecholamine release, which may be triggered by the stress of illness or surgery. The signs of thyroid storm include tachycardia, tachyarrhythmias, hypertension, hyperthermia, hyperglycemia, and shock.

15. How do I treat intraoperative tachycardia and tachyarrhythmias in a hyperthyroid cat?

A heart rate greater than 240 bpm in the cat with hyperthyroidism can be treated with propanolol (0.04–0.06 mg/kg IV), esmolol (100–200 µg/kg IV), or lidocaine (0.25–0.5 mg/kg IV).

16. What are the postoperative concerns following thyroidectomy?

A thyroidectomy may cause damage to the recurrent laryngeal nerve and result in layrngeal paralysis or tracheomalacia. If a hemotoma develops at the site of surgery, there is also the possibility of tracheal collapse. Vigilant monitoring of the respiratory system is necessary in the postoperative period, even beyond the immediate recovery period.

Body temperature should also be monitored closely and thermal support provided as needed. Animals with hyperthyroidism are generally very thin with little body fat. and hypothermia is commonly seen during the postoperative period. The inability to maintain normothermia is further exacerbated by the combined effects of anesthetic drugs and decreased metabolic rate.

17. Are there any anesthetic concerns in the hypothyroid patient?

Patients with mild to moderate hypothyroidism generally tolerate anesthesia well. Slow recoveries and hypothermia are the most common problems. Efforts should be made to prevent hypothermia by providing external thermal support throughout the anesthetic period. Preanesthetic warming and intraoperative warming have been shown to decrease the incidence of postoperative hypothermia. Recoveries may be prolonged due to slowed metabolism of the anesthetic agents. Use conservative doses and avoid potent, nonreversible tranquilizers.

Animals with severe hypothyroidism should be stabilized and treated with replacement thyroid hormone therapy until a euthyroid state is reached prior to anesthesia. In an emergency, when pretreatment is not possible, close attention should be paid to the cardiovascular system. Untreated, severe hypothyroidism results in a decrease in myocardial β-adrenergic receptors and decreased myosin ATP-ase activity. This results in potentially life-threatening cardiac depression with bradycardia, hypotension, decreased myocardial contractility, and decreased stroke volume.

Avoid potent cardiac depressants and dose injectable agents "to effect." Isoflurane is the inhalant anesthetic of choice, but should be used in a balanced anesthetic protocol so as not to exceed 1.5 MAC ($\approx$ 1.75 – 2.0%).

Muscle weakness, in conjunction with anesthetic agents, leads to hypoventilation in patients with hypothyroidism. Many of these patients are also obese, which further limits their ability to ventilate well during anesthesia. Ventilation should be assisted or controlled to prevent hypoventilation and the resulting respiratory acidosis and hypoxemia.

18. What should I think about when anesthetizing an animal with hypoadrenocorticism (Addison's disease)?

Preventing circulatory collapse and adrenal crisis during anesthesia and in the perioperative period. Adequate intravenous fluid volume replacement should be provided (any balanced electrolyte solution at 10 ml/kg/hr) and glucocorticoids should be administered at induction (dexamethasone 1.0–2.0 mg/kg IV) and during recovery (dexamethasone 1.0–2.0 mg/kg IV or IM).

Animals with hypoadrenalcorticism have a decreased tolerance for stress and should be closely monitored for hypotension and shock. Rapid-acting glucocorticoids such as prednisolone sodium succinate (Solu-Delta-Cortef) 2.0–5.0 mg/kg or prednisolone sodium phosphate (Cortisate-20) 2.5 mg/kg can be administered as needed during anesthesia maintenance.

Patients with hypoadrenocorticism may present varying degrees of dehydration, bradycardia, hypovolemia, hypotension, hyponatremia, hyperkalemia, hypothermia and circulatory shock. It is critical to do a thorough physical examination and a complete baseline laboratory workup to identify any underlying problems and correct any abnormalities before administering anesthetic agents.

19. Are there any special considerations for anesthetizing the patient with hyperadrenocorticism (Cushing's disease)?

Animals with hyperadrenocorticism, no matter what the cause, may be hypertensive due to excessive cortisol levels. This hypertension, especially when combined with atrioventricular valve insufficiency, may lead to left ventricular hypertrophy and congestive heart failure. In addition to the basic preanesthetic workup, a complete cardiac evaluation, to include thoracic radiographs, echocardiology, and blood pressure measurement, is recommended prior to anesthesia.

Muscle wasting and liver enlargement reduce the ability of these patients to ventilate adequately. Ventilation should be assisted or supported throughout the anesthetic period. Multiple metabolic imbalances may be revealed with the preanesthetic laboratory screen. The most common abnormalities include hyperglycemia and electrolyte and acid-base disturbances. These should be identified and corrected prior to administration of sedative or anesthetic agents.

20. What injectable anesthetics are best for use in patients with hyperadrenocorticism?

Both thiobarbiturates and etomidate decrease circulating cortisol concentrations and should be considered as induction agents in these patients, as long as there are no other contraindications to their use.

21. How should I manage glucocorticoid replacement in the adrenalectomy case?

Glucocorticoid supplementation should begin at induction and continue throughout the intraoperative and perioperative periods, similar to the management of patients with hypoadrenocorticism. Dexamethasone (1.0–2.0 mg/kg IV) should be administered at induction and during recovery (1.0–2.0 mg/kg IV or IM). Rapid-acting glucocorticoids such as prednisolone sodium succinate 2.0–5.0 mg/kg or prednisolone sodium phosphate 2.5 mg/kg can be administered as needed during anesthesia maintenance to prevent adrenal crisis.

BIBLIOGRAPHY

1. Paddleford RR, Harvey RC: Endocrine disease. In Thurman JC, Tranquilli WJ, and Benson GJ (eds): Lumb and Jones' Veterinary Anesthesia, 3rd ed. Baltimore, Williams & Wilkins, 1996, pp 804–806.
2. Peterson ME: Pathophysiological changes in the endocrine system. In Short CE (ed): Principles and Practice of Veterinary Anesthesia. Baltimore, Williams & Wilkins, 1987, pp 251–260.

34. OCULAR DISORDERS

Stephen A. Greene, D.V.M., M.S., D.A.C.V.A.

1. What are anesthetic considerations for the patient with glaucoma?

Selection of anesthetic agents for use in the patient with glaucoma should be directed toward avoidance of drugs that may increase the intraocular pressure (IOP). It is unlikely that most of the anesthetics in common practice will directly result in increased IOP. However, depolarizing neuromuscular blocking agents (e.g., succinylcholine) will initially constrict the extraocular muscles and may dramatically increase IOP. Physiologic responses to tracheal intubation such as choking or coughing may also increase the IOP. Therefore, induction of anesthesia should be rapid and smooth, allowing tracheal intubation with adequate patient immobilization.

2. Which anesthetics should be avoided for patients with penetrating eye wounds?

Penetrating eye wounds dictate similar considerations for anesthetic management as glaucoma does. Judicious use of premedications to sedate the patient, suppress the cough reflex, prevent vomiting, and provide analgesia is advised. Control of pain in animals with penetrating eye wounds is a major distinction from treatment of the patient with glaucoma. The cornea is a well-innervated tissue, and laceration of the cornea is often an underlying cause of self-mutilation in animals. Topical anesthesia can be used for immediate and effective relief of pain. Proparacaine (0.5%) is a topical anesthetic that is commonly used for ocular pain. Analgesia is short (10–20 minutes) but may allow easier handling of the patient as the preparation for general anesthesia progresses.

3. What are common topical ophthalmic solutions?

The topical analgesics specific for ophthalmic administration in animals include proparacaine and benoxinate. Proparacaine (0.5%) is often recommended for use in ocular procedures such as removal of foreign bodies, suture placement, conjunctival scraping, or conjunctival injection. Local instillation of proparacaine, butacaine (2%), piperocaine (2%), or oxybuprocaine (0.4%) into the conjunctival sac will anesthetize the cornea and conjunctiva for short procedures. Phenylephrine or epinephrine may be administered topically to the eye for hemostasis. These drugs may increase or decrease the IOP depending on the dose. A bland ophthalmic ointment for protection of the cornea is recommended during anesthesia. General anesthetics and anticholinergic agents will dramatically decrease tear production in most species. Corneal protection with an ophthalmic ointment will help prevent formation of corneal ulcers associated with loss of tear production and corneal drying during anesthesia. Loss of tear production during anesthesia in horses is less profound and may not be necessary to prevent corneal ulceration. However, when alcohol or other skin preparation solutions are used in the vicinity of the eye, it is a good idea to use an ophthalmic ointment to protect the cornea.

4. Why is atropine avoided in cases of parotid salivary gland duct transposition?

The surgical technique of parotid duct transposition is a procedure for correcting inadequate tear production by re-routing salivary gland secretions to the eye. Atropine decreases salivary gland production, which makes identification and cannulation of the parotid duct difficult.

5. What are common systemic ophthalmic drug therapies that are of interest to the anesthetist?

Systemic medications administered during ophthalmic procedures vary depending on the specific procedure. Acetazolamide may be used to decrease production of aqueous humor. Side effects associated with acetazolamine therapy include metabolic acidosis and compensatory respiratory alkalosis brought on by hyperventilation. Hypertonic solutions such as mannitol may be administered systemically to reduce IOP. Mannitol will increase the plasma oncotic pressure and decrease the formation of aqueous humor. Phenylephrine may be administered to promote vaso-constriction of periorbital structures.

6. How is intraocular pressure measured?

Intraocular pressure can be measured using a tonometer. Use of the tonometer may require physical contact with the cornea. Some tonometers emit a burst of air that transduces the IOP without touching the eye. Normal IOP values for dogs are between 10 and 26 mm Hg. The normal IOP for cats is 12 to 32 mm Hg and for horses is 23 to 28 mm Hg. Factors that increase IOP include drugs, cough, gag, vomiting, abnormal head/neck position, and tracheal intubation. Factors that decrease IOP include decreased arterial blood pressure, deep anesthesia, hyperventilation, and hypocapnia.

7. Which anesthetics raise the intraocular pressure?

Anesthetics agents that raise the IOP include etomidate and possibly the dissociative anesthetics such as ketamine and tiletamine. Etomidate may induce myoclonic activity that can raise IOP. Use of dissociative agents for patients with raised IOP is controversial. Dissociative anesthetics can release catecholamines that may increase IOP. When dissociative anesthetics are used in combination with sedative or tranquilizer premedications, it is likely that little change in IOP will occur. The depolarizing neuromuscular blocking agent succinylcholine will dramatically increase IOP.

8. What are the advantages of using neuromuscular blocking agents for surgeries involving the eye?

Use of nondepolarizing neuromuscular blocking agents will have no effect on IOP in ventilated patients. These agents are useful in many ocular surgeries because the skeletal muscle relaxation they provide will result in a central position of the eye. This position of the eye will facilitate surgical approaches to the lens for cataract surgeries or phacoemulsification.

9. What is the oculocardiac reflex?

Stimulation of the eye or extraocular structures may result in afferent nerve traffic via the trigeminal nerve with efferent activity via the vagal nerve. Cardiac effects of vagal stimulation include dysrhythmias (e.g., bradycardia, bigeminy, and ventricular ectopic beats) and cardiac arrest. Poor relaxation of the extraocular musculature and hypercapnia predispose to occurrence of the oculocardiac reflex. When the reflex occurs, eyeball manipulation should cease. If bradycardia continues, atropine should be administered (0.02 mg/kg IV).

10. What is the Peterson block?

The Peterson block is useful for complete anesthesia of the eye. It is commonly performed in cattle undergoing enucleation. The technique involves placement of a long (12 cm), curved needle caudal to the eyeball to the foramen orbitorotundum. Typically, about 15 ml of 2% lidocaine are deposited at the foramen to effect blockade of the oculomotor, trochlear, abducens, and ophthalmic, maxillary, and mandibular branches of the trigeminal nerve. The needle is inserted at the notch formed by the supraorbital process cranially, the zygomatic arch ventrally, and the coronoid of the mandible caudally. This block anesthetizes sensory and motor function of the eye, but not the eyelid. This block requires more skill to administer than a simple retrobulbar block but is associated with fewer complications.

11. What are potential complications associated with performing a retrobulbar eye block?

The retrobulbar administration of local anesthetic involves injection of local anesthetic behind the eyeball via eyelid penetration with a long, curved needle through points around the orbital rim. Complications from the technique include retrobulbar hemorrhage, penetration of the globe, optic nerve damage, oculocardiac reflex, and injection into the optic nerve meninges. Injection of local anesthetic into the optic nerve meninges may cause anesthesia of the brain and can have disastrous results.

12. Which nerves must be blocked to prevent motor activity of the eyelid in cattle and horses?
The motor block of the eyelid in cattle is performed by injecting local anesthetic to the auriculopalpebral branch of the facial nerve. The nerve is palpable in a notch on the zygomatic arch, anterior to the base of the auricular muscles. For both paralysis and analgesia, local anesthetic can be injected in a ring block around the orbit. The motor block of the eyelid in horses is performed by desensitizing the dorsal and ventral branches of the palpebral nerve (auriculopalpebral block). To also anesthetize the eyelid, four branches of the trigeminal nerve must be blocked: supraorbital, lacrimal, infraorbital, and zygomatic.

13. Can nitrous oxide be used for ocular procedures?
Nitrous oxide should not be used during procedures that involve injection of air into the globe of the eye. Eyes that are surgically incised will also be exposed to air. Nitrous oxide administered in the breathing mixture will equilibrate with air in the globe. In a closed globe, the equilibration of nitrous oxide will increase the IOP. Rupture of the eye may be a complication associated with indiscriminant use of nitrous oxide in such instances.

14. What are causes of post-surgical blindness in dogs and cats?
Recently, the antibiotic enrofloxacin has been implicated in cases of post-surgical blindness in cats. Retinal degeneration has been observed in these cases of irreversible blindness. Cases of reversible blindness following surgery have been anecdotally reported. Explanations for transient post-surgical blindness include brief period of hypoxia or hypotension, severe hypocarbia resulting in cerebral vasoconstriction, hypercarbia in patients at risk from raised intracranial pressure (e.g., brain tumor), and ketamine- or tiletamine-induced increases in intracranial pressure.

15. What steps can be taken to ensure a good recovery from anesthesia and surgery of the eye?
Following eye surgery, animals should be recovered in a semidarkened environment. Preemptive use of opioids as a part of the anesthetic protocol will help to provide a quiet emergence from anesthesia. Many dogs and cats also benefit from a small dose of acepromazine (0.05 mg/kg IM). Postoperative analgesia should be reassessed following removal of the endotracheal tube. Full agonist opioids such as morphine should be used as needed over the next 24-hour period. Observation for tendencies to remove bandages or self-mutilation should be performed. A light wrap around the dewclaws may prevent mishaps with dogs and cats emerging from anesthesia. Large animals such as cows and horses may benefit from a protective hood applied before recovery from anesthesia. Some horses will object to the presence of a hood as they awaken. Knowledge of the individual's disposition prior to anesthesia can help guide the selection of horses suitable for recovery with an eye-protective hood.

BIBLIOGRAPHY

1. Skarda RT: Local and regional anesthetic and analgesic techniques. In Thurmon JC, Tranquilli WJ, Benson GJ (eds): Lumb and Jones' Veterinary Anesthesia, 3rd ed. Baltimore, Williams & Wilkins, 1996, pp 426–514.
2. Thurmon JC, Tranquilli WJ, Benson GJ: Anesthesia for special patients: Ocular patients. In Thurmon JC, Tranquilli WJ, Benson GJ (eds): Lumb and Jones' Veterinary Anesthesia, 3rd ed. Baltimore, Williams & Wilkins, 1996, pp 812–818.

35. APPROACH TO TRAUMA PATIENTS

Sheila McCullough, D.V.M., M.S., D.A.C.V.I.M.

1. What is the pathophysiology of trauma?

Little research has been done concerning canine and feline response to trauma, so much information is drawn from human trauma research and animal laboratory studies. The initial response to trauma is the release of catecholamines, hormones, and local inflammatory mediators. The hypothalamus responds to stimuli (osmolality, pH, arterial oxygen levels, pain, cytokines, changes in arterial/venous pressure and volume) by activating the pituitary gland and sympathetic nervous system. Epinephrine and norepinephrine release causes vasoconstriction, tachycardia, increased minute ventilation, and cardiac contractility. (This response to trauma may not be seen in all cats.) Adrenocorticotropic hormone and epinephrine release signals to the adrenal glands to release cortisol to elevate glucose levels. To compensate for hypovolemia, the body releases catecholamines, cortisol, and vasopressin and activates the renin-angiotensin-aldosterone system to retain sodium and water.

Tissue injury and subsequent hypoxia may lead to activation of the endothelium, arachidonic cascade, and cytokine release. Release of tissue thromboplastin and exposure of subendothelial collagen will activate coagulation and complement cascades and lead to formation of thrombi. Amplified cytokine release from macrophages, neutrophils, endothelium, and monocytes may intensify and result in increased vascular permeability, bronchoconstriction, hypertension, impaired myocardial contractility, and metabolic acidosis.

The metabolic rate of traumatized tissue changes with time and degree of injury. For the first 8 to 12 hours after injury, the tissue exists in a hypometabolic state because of hypotension and hypovolemia. After the hypometabolic phase, healing tissues will enter a hypermetabolic phase, exhibiting a marked increase in energy consumption and protein catabolism. Excessive protein catabolism and hypermetabolic state may lead to impaired wound healing, sepsis, and organ failure.

2. Discuss the significance and differences between *primary* and *secondary survey.*

Primary survey is the initial examination of the trauma patient. In this initial survey, you should address the most immediate concerns of the patient while completing a full evaluation of the patient. Secondary survey is a more in-depth evaluation of the patient, using a systems assessment approach, and includes further testing such as blood sampling and radiographs.

3. What is meant by *systems assessment* (tip of the nose to the tip of the tail examination)?

Trauma patients should be examined in a systematic fashion starting with the facial examination and progressing caudally. This allows the examiner to thoroughly evaluate the neurologic, respiratory, abdominal, and musculoskeletal systems.

4. What is the basic approach to treatment of the trauma patient?

- (Have the technician obtain a complete history and record of the traumatic incident.)
- Complete the primary survey and full systems assessment; note lung sounds, temperature, heart rate, and respiratory effort.
- Establish patent airway and supply 100% oxygen (intubation, flow-by, face mask, intranasal, p.o.d., clear plastic bag, tracheostomy, intratracheal oxygen tube, oxygen cage) and place a pulse oximeter on the patient (tongue, lip, toe web, ear pinnae, skinfold, prepuce, vulva).
- Secure venous access with a minimum of two peripheral lines; determine whether a central line is indicated; cut-down to access veins may be needed.
- Monitor heart rate and rhythm with continuous electrocardiography.

- Initiate crystalloid fluid infusion and assess whether colloids (natural or synthetic) are needed.
- Evaluate blood pressure via noninvasive (Doppler or Dinamap) or invasive (arterial line) methods.
- Measure central venous pressure (CVP) if central line is available and assess trend.
- Perform initial packed cell volume (PCV), total plasma (TP), blood urea nitrogen (BUN), and glucose evaluations and progressively monitor these test results
- Evaluate complete blood count (CBC) with platelet count, chemistry panel, coagulation panel, arterial blood gas analysis, and urinalysis.
- Keep patient warm (warm fluids?), dry, and in a padded cage to prevent bedsores and excessive trauma.
- Perform an initial neurologic examination and reassess the patient in the next few hours post-stabilization.
- Re-evaluate the patient continually and establish a plan for pain relief.

5. What are the "CABDs"? Why are they important in evaluation of the trauma patient?
Immediate assessment of the trauma victim should begin with assessment of circulation, airway, breathing, and disabilities.

Circulation is assessed by evaluating the patient's perfusion parameters, such as mucous membrane color, capillary refill time, temperature, pulse (character, strength, and tone), mental status, and coolness of extremities.

Airway patency should be secured and supplementation of 100% oxygen started.

Breathing can be evaluated by thorough auscultation of the thorax and observation of breathing. Note any respiratory effort (inspiratory vs. expiratory or both). Gentle palpation of the thorax for subcutaneous emphysema and rib fractures should be performed.

Disabilities can be observed in the mental status of the patient. If possible, a full neurologic examination should be performed when the patient is stabilized.

6. What are the immediate vs. delayed concerns for the trauma patient undergoing anesthesia?
- Immediate concerns:
  - Hypothermia, hypovolemia, and acidosis from ongoing blood loss (perfusion deficits)
  - Pain, creating a patient that is difficult to restrain
  - Depressed level of conciousness, leading to hypoventilation or loss of protective airway reflexes
  - Flail chest, pulmonary contusions, hemothorax, pneumothoraces, diaphragmatic hernia, contributing to hypoventilation and/or hypoxemia
  - Patient actively seizuring from head injuries
  - Aspiration under anesthesia

- Delayed concerns (12–48 hours post-trauma):
  - Traumatic myocarditis (cardiac arrhythmias)
  - Pulmonary contusions
  - Progressive neurologic deterioration (depressed mentation and seizures)
  - Stabilization of fractures
  - Depressed urine output from poor perfusion or uroabdomen
  - On-going hemorrhage

7. What is the "triad of death" ? How do we prevent it?
The triad of death is the combination of acidosis, hypothermia, and coagulopathy. Regaining effective perfusion in the patient by volume replacement with crystalloid and colloid fluid therapy is the most important step toward preventing this event. Continual reassessment of blood pH with venous or arterial blood gases will guide your therapy. Increased levels of lactate, a product of anaerobic metabolism and a risk factor for multiple organ failure, would indicate the need for improved resuscitation. Aggressive rewarming of the patient with warm crystalloids or colloids,

water-circulating heating pads, blankets (Bear Huggers), and warming of the immediate environment may be warranted. Finally, dilutional or disseminated intravascular coagulation (DIC)–induced coagulopathy needs to be addressed immediately and may play the most important role in survival. Monitoring of coagulopathy may include progressive measurement of activated coagulation time (ACT), prothrombin time (PT), partial thromboplastin time (PTT), platelets and antithrombin III (AT-III).

8. Define *pneumothorax, tension pneumothorax,* and *flail chest.*

Pneumothorax is the result of the introduction of air into the pleural cavity, causing a loss of negative intrathoracic pressure and collapsed lungs. Pneumothoraces can be categorized as closed, open, spontaneous, traumatic, and tension.

Tension pneumothorax is created when air continues to leak through a one-way valve mechanism, resulting in lung collapse and increasing intrapleural pressure that exceeds atmospheric pressure.

Flail chest is defined as multiple adjacent ribs fractured in two places, creating a free-floating section of chest wall.

9. How may a pulmonary contusion manifest during general anesthesia?

Parenchymal hematomas and edema result in poorly compliant lungs, increased airway pressures, and impaired gas exchange. Pulmonary contusions are often associated with multiple rib fractures, pneumothorax, subcutaneous emphysema, and ecchymosis.

10. How is tension pneumothorax differentiated from pulmonary contusion?

Sign	Pulmonary Contusion	Tension Pneumothorax
Hypoxemia	+	+
Increased airway pressure	+	+
Tympany on percussion	–	+
Differential chest rise on inspiration	–	+
Tracheal shift	–	+
Bilateral breath sounds	+	–
Pulmonary edema, rales	+	–

11. How may cardiac contusion be differentiated from cardiac tamponade (both a result of chest trauma)?

Sign	Cardiac Contusion	Cardiac Tamponade
Elevated central venous pressure	+	+
Hypotension	+	+
Muffled heart sounds	–	+
Dysrhythmias	Common	Uncommon
Hypotension during positive pressure ventilation	Minimal	+
Pulsus paradoxus	–	+

12. How do you choose the best anesthetic agent for a trauma patient?

Fortunately, a number of anesthetic agents can be employed; however, what may be more important is the dose given. Trauma patients taken to surgery may still be hypovolemic, thus the dose of anesthetic agent may need to be reduced. It is imperative to start with a low dose and carefully titrate upward to avoid unwanted side effects.

13. What is the best analgesic agent?
- Butorphanol 0.05–0.2 mg/kg IV q1–4h
- Oxymorphone 0.025–0.05 mg/kg IV q1–4h
- Morphine 0.1–1 mg/kg/hr CRI

14. What is the best agent for sedation?
- Butorphanol 0.05–0.2 mg/kg IV, alone or with diazepam 0.05–0.2 mg/kg IV
  or
- Midazolam 0.06–0.2 mg/kg IV

15. What is the best agent for rapid induction of anesthesia
- Oxymorphone 0.05–0.2 mg/kg IV, with diazepam 0.5–0.2 mg/kg IV
  or with midazolam 0.06–0.2 mg/kg IV
- Ketamine 5–10 mg/kg IV, with diazepam 0.05–0.2 mg/kg IV
- Etomidate 1.5–3.0 mg/kg

16. What are the recommended assessment parameters in head trauma patients?

After initial stabilization of the head trauma patient, a thorough neurologic assessment should be performed. The patient should be assessed for level of consciousness (LOC), pupil size and symmetry, and pupillary light responses (PLRs). The Small Animal Coma Scale may be used to evaluate the degree of neurologic damage (see question 17).

Initial bloodwork should include serum chemistry profile (with or without bile acids), a CBC, and an arterial blood gas analysis. Sequential monitoring of the patient to maintain cerebral perfusion is highly recommended and should include the following parameters:
- Mean arterial blood pressure (80–100 mm Hg)
- Blood glucose (>60 mg/dl; avoid hyperglycemia)
- Hemoglobin saturation >98%
- PaO_2 >90 mm Hg
- Continual re-evaluation of neurologic status (LOC, PLRs, etc.)
- Electrolyte status
- Urine output (>1 ml/lb/hr)

17. What is the Small Animal Coma Scale?

Variable	Score	Critieria
Motor activity	6	Normal gait and reflexes
	5	Hemiparesis, tetraparesis, or decorticate rigidity
	4	Recumbent with intermittent extensor rigidity
	3	Recumbent with constant extensor rigidity
	2	Recumbent with intermittent extensor rigidity/opisthotonus
	1	Recumbent, hypotonic with depressed to absent spinal reflexes
Brain stem reflexes	6	Normal pupillary light reflex and oculocephalic reflexes
	5	Slow pupillary light reflex and normal to decresed oculocephalic reflexes
	4	Bilateral/unresponsive miosis and normal to decreased oculocephalic reflexes
	3	Pinpoint pupils and reduced to absent oculocephalic reflexes
	2	Unilateral/unresponsive mydriasis and reduced to absent oculocephalic reflexes 2
	1	Bilateral/unresponsive mydriasis and reduce to absent oculocephalic reflexes 1
Level of consciousness	6	Occasionally alert and responsive
	5	Depressed/delerious, but capable of response to stimulus
	4	Obtunded/stupor, but responds to visual stimuli
	3	Obtunded/stupor, but responds to auditory stimuli
	2	Obtunded/stupor, but responds to noxious stimuli
	1	Comatose and unresponsive to noxious stimuli
Total Score	3–8	9–14	15–18
Prognosis	Grave	Poor to Guarded	Good

18. What are the current recommendations for treatment and analgesia in head trauma patients?

Hypertension and tachycardia in a stabilized patient may indicate the need for pain relief. Although controversy exists as to the best analgesic agent for head trauma patients, it is best to avoid agents that will depress respiration (opioids), increase cerebral metabolic rate (ketamine), or cause vasodilation, which will increase intracranial pressure (ICP) or cause large fluctuations in blood pressure (acepromazine). Opioids act centrally to decrease the responsiveness of the ventilatory centers to carbon dioxide and interfere with regulation of respiratory rhythm by the pontine and medullary ventilatory centers. This depressive effect appears to be more important in humans than in animals, so administration in small doses to effect along with intensive monitoring may be appropriate.

Inducing a barbiturate coma (to decrease cerebral metabolic rate and intracranial pressure) has fallen out of favor because of recent reports in human head trauma patients. If this is the only option, it is critical to monitor blood pressure and blood gases. Patients that cannot maintain normal PaO_2 should be considered for ventilator therapy. The use of propofol, a benzodiazepine, or phenobarbitone also may be used to sedate the patient or employed as an induction agent followed by isoflurane for general anesthesia if needed.

Acute decompensation in patients with elevated $PaCO_2$ can be managed with short-term hyperventilation strategies ($PaCO_2$ 30–35 mm Hg); however, excessive hyperventilation may be hazardous. Acute decompensation of the head trauma patient can be managed with mannitol and Lasix (given to blunt the transient increase in ICP from mannitol administration and for its synergism with mannitol) or hypertonic saline/hetastarch combinations.

Parenteral nutrition and/or tube feeding, physical therapy, and avoiding pressure sores are needed for the long-term head trauma patient.

19. What is the current recommendation for antibiotic use in trauma patients?

A study by Fullen concluded that the use of a single preoperative antibiotic therapy was most effective. Studies found that increased duration of antibiotic treatment did not improve patient survival. The current recommended antibiotics of choice are second- and third-generation cephalosporins. Open wounds or fractures should be cultured and treated accordingly. The use of antibiotics indiscriminately should be avoided.

20. What parameters are important to monitor during anesthesia and postoperatively in a trauma patient?

- Blood pressure (systolic, diastolic, and mean)
- Pulse rate and quality
- Arterial blood gases, PCV/TP
- Central venous pressure
- SpO_2
- Temperature
- Respiratory rate, character, and effort
- Mucous membrane color/capillary refill time
- Heart rate and rhythm
- Urine output

21. How do you treat oliguria associated with trauma or shock?

First, determine whether the patient has been volume resuscitated appropriately, using CVP, blood pressure, PCV/TP, body weight, and perfusion parameters previously mentioned. Second, place an in-dwelling urinary catheter and measure urine output. Urine output should be greater than or equal to 2 ml/kg/hr. If the patient has received appropriate volume resuscitation and is oliguric (<0.5 ml/kg/hr), then a test dose of furosemide (1–2 mg/kg IV) may be indicated. If the patient does not respond to furosemide, check the urinary catheter for any mechanical obstructions, then start a dopamine continuous rate infusion (CRI) at 1 to 5 µg/kg/min. The continued therapy of dopamine CRI and intermittent doses of furosemide in the patient should start the flow of urine. If urine production is still very poor, investigate the patient for uroabdomen with abdominal ultrasonography to detect urine within the abdomen or retroperitoneal space. Fluid analysis will reveal an elevated creatinine and potassium level if the patient has uroabdomen.

22. What are the new versus traditional end-points in resuscitation of the trauma patient in shock?

Traditional	New End-Points
Heart rate	MVO_2
Blood pressure	Base deficit, serum HCO_3
Urine output	Lactate
	Gastric intramucosal pH

23. What is abdominal compartment syndrome and how is it treated?

Abdominal compartment syndrome is the development of intra-abdominal hypertension, which creates increased intrathoracic pressure (increasing airway pressure), decreased cardiac output, oliguria/anuria and splanchnic ischemia. This can be monitored by measuring bladder pressure (in humans, > 25 cm H_2O). Fluid resuscitation and decompression of the abdomen are required in the initial treatment plan. In humans, coagulopathy is a common cause of this syndrome.

BIBLIOGRAPHY

1. Devey J: Vehicular trauma: Initial stabilization. Compendium's Standard of Care, vol. 3, 2001.
2. Devey J and Crowe DT: The physiologic response to trauma. Compend Pract Vet 19:962–977, 1997.
3. Otto C, Syring RS: Head Trauma. Compendium's Standard of Care, vol. 3, 2001.
4. Mahonee L, Flaherty M: Anesthesia for trauma. In Anesthesia Secrets, 2nd ed. Philadelphia, Hanley and Belfus, 2000, pp 287–292.
5. Hellyer P, Wagner A: Pain management in emergencies. In Veterinary Emergency Medicine Secrets. Philadelphia, Hanley and Belfus, 1997, pp 85–91.
6. Wingfield W: Treatment priorities in trauma. In Veterinary Emergency Medicine Secrets. Philadelphia, Hanley and Belfus,1997, pp. 44–47.
7. Carli P: Trauma. Curr Opin Crit Car, 5:479–523, 1999.

VII. Special Anesthetic Considerations

36. NEONATAL ANESTHESIA

David C. Rankin, D.V.M., M.S., D.A.C.V.A.

1. What is the definition of a neonate?

Technically, "neonate" refers to a newborn animal up to 6–8 weeks old. Veterinary patients up to 3 months old are considered neonates or pediatric patients. Anesthesia of patients less than 3 months of age is generally considered to be higher risk and requires special attention to the needs of the immature patient.

2. What is special about 3 months of age?

By 12 weeks, the major systems (cardiovascular, pulmonary, thermoregulatory, renal, and hepatic) are relatively well developed. Neonates gradually mature, with the majority of systems developed by 6 or 8 weeks.

3. How does the cardiovascular system in a neonate differ from that in an adult?

Neonates are more dependent on heart rate for cardiac output than adults. They have less functional contractile tissue than adults do, so changes in cardiac output are mediated by changes in rate rather than contractility. Adults can change their contractility up to 300%, in comparison to a neonate's 30%. The resting cardiac index of neonates is higher than that of adults, resulting in very little cardiac reserve. This is compounded by an immature sympathetic nervous system, which leads to decreased baroreceptor reflex and poor vasomotor regulation. Great care and attention need to be directed toward maintaining heart rate in anesthetized neonates.

4. What is different about the respiratory system in a neonate?

Neonates typically have a high resting respiratory rate (and therefore minute volume) secondary to increased oxygen demand. Their small airways are more prone to obstruction, and closing volume (the volume where alveoli collapse) is much smaller than that of adults. These factors lead to an increased potential for hypoxia during apnea or obstruction. The pliable rib cage leads to greater work of breathing, and respiratory fatigue may occur earlier, especially in cases of respiratory disease.

5. Are other systems immature in the neonate?

We mentioned the immature sympathetic nervous system and the decreased ability to respond to the stress of anesthesia. Renal function is not fully developed, which may result in prolonged drug effects. Hepatic microsomal enzymes are deficient, also leading to prolonged elimination and effect of drugs.

6. Are neonates more susceptible to hypothermia?

Yes, they are. They typically have less body fat compared to an adult, immature thermoregulatory control, and a large ratio of surface area to mass. Warm-water circulating blankets, increased room temperature, warmed fluids, and expeditious surgical and anesthesia times are critical to maintaining body temperature.

7. Do neonates feel pain?

The common opinion among physician neonatologists is that they do. Research supports this supposition, and that pathologic pain is detrimental to development. There is no reason to suggest or infer that our veterinary neonatal patients do not sense pain. The use of local anesthetics and/or opioids is indicated in patients undergoing procedures considered painful in mature animals (e.g., tail docking, dew claw amputation). Care must be taken in dosing, and dilution of drugs may be necessary to obtain an appropriate volume to be administered.

8. How do neonates react to preanesthetic and anesthetic drugs?

The blood-brain barrier of neonates is typically not mature, and exaggerated responses to medications may be seen if adult doses are given. Neonates have a high volume of distribution, because of their large extracellular fluid volume compared to adults. Decreased protein binding of drugs and decreased metabolism also lead to exaggerated responses. It is prudent to reduce doses of sedatives and tranquilizers and to administer anesthetics to effect in the neonatal patient.

9. What are common premedications for neonates?

Low-dose opioids and/or benzodiazepines are commonly used when it is deemed necessary to premedicate these patients. Opioids have very little effect on contractility but may reduce the heart rate and should be given with atropine or glycopyrrolate. In the very young patient, opioids and/or benzodiazepines can produce excellent sedation, unlike older animals. Diazepam or midazolam (0.05–0.2 mg/kg) or butorphanol (0.1–0.3 mg/kg) are drugs often used in neonates.

10. Can acepromazine or medetomidine be administered in neonates?

Acepromazine can produce significant hypotension and heat loss due to vasodilation, and is best avoided in the immature patient. α_2-Adrenergic agonists can cause significant bradyarrhythmias, as well as dramatic afterload increases. Phenothiazines and α_2-agonists also require extensive hepatic metabolism and renal clearance, resulting in prolonged and exaggerated effects. Both are best avoided in immature animals.

11. What should I use for anesthetic induction of neonates?

Inhalant induction via mask or chamber is probably the most common method of induction. Foals can be induced with inhalant via a nasotracheal tube. Isoflurane or sevoflurane is most commonly used. Maintenance of anesthesia is typically a continuation of either gas anesthesia via a mask or connection to a circuit after endotracheal intubation. Intubation is preferable when possible, as it decreases contamination of room air with inhalants and allows mechanical ventilation.

12. How do I intubate a neonate?

Neonates typically have large tongues and a wide, flat mouth. They tend to be nasal breathers, and the palate may therefore block the glottis from view. A laryngoscope with a small blade is extremely useful. Many puppies and kittens can be intubated with a 2.0 or 2.5 mm ID endotracheal tube. Stylets may be used but should not extend past the tip of the tube. Large intravenous catheters (with the needle removed!) may be used if these tubes are too big. It is important to reduce mechanical dead space as much as possible. Foals are relatively easy to nasotracheally intubate, and can be switched to an orotracheal tube if desired when induced.

13. Can I use the same anesthesia circuit for neonates that I use on adults?

Typically, a non-rebreathing circuit (e.g., Bain circuit, Jackson-Reese circuit) should be used on neonates to reduce the work of breathing. Unfortunately, these circuits are not as good at maintaining body temperature and extra care has to be taken to preserve body heat. Their high flow rates (200–300 ml/kg/min) also put the animal at risk of barotrauma more quickly if the relief valve ("pop-off" valve) is left closed. Foals less than about 110 kg are usually placed on a small animal circle circuit rather than the typical large-animal anesthesia machine.

14. Are injectable anesthetics used in neonates?

Great care must be taken in the neonate due to the extensive metabolism required to excrete these drugs. Redistribution typically results in the termination of anesthetic effects, but prolonged recoveries and/or sedation may result. Propofol has been used with success in foals.

15. How do I achieve venous access in a neonate?

If the animal is large enough, standard over-the-needle catheters may be used at the typical sites (cephalic, saphenous, jugular veins). Intraosseous catheters or needles may be used in animals in which veins are too small or otherwise inaccessible.

16. Should I give fluids during anesthesia?

Some procedures may be short enough that attempting intravenous or intraosseous access may excessively prolong the procedure. However, my rule of thumb is, if I would give fluids to an adult for cardiovascular support for the procedure, I will try to do the same for a neonate. Care must be taken to prevent volume overload; using a syringe pump, buretrol, or at least a microdrip set will help prevent accidental administrations of high volumes of fluid. Typically, 5–10 ml/kg/hr of LRS or 0.9% NaCl with dextrose added (2.5–5.0% final dextrose concentration) are administered via the intravenous or intraosseous routes.

BIBLIOGRAPHY

1. Ettinger SJ, Feldman EC (eds): Textbook of Veterinary Internal Medicine: Diseases of the Dog and Cat, 5th ed. Philadelphia, WB Saunders, 2000.
2. Martinez EA: Anesthetizing neonatal foals. Vet Med, Sept: 879–884, 1995.
3. Menon G, Anand KJ, McIntosh N: Practical approach to analgesia and sedation in the neonatal intensive care unit. Semin Perinatol 22(5):417–424 1998.
4. Miller RD (ed): Anesthesia, 5th ed. Philadelphia, Churchill Livingstone, 2000.
5. Mohan CG, Risucci DA, Casimir M, Gulrajani-LaCorte M: Comparison of analgesics in ameliorating the pain of circumcision. J Perinatol 18(1):13–19 1998.
6. Muir WW, Hubbell JAE, Skarda RT, Bednarski RM (eds): Handbook of Veterinary Anesthesia, 3rd ed. St. Louis, Mosby, 2000.
7. Olson TL, Downey VW: Infant physiological responses to noxious stimuli of circumcision with anesthesia and analgesia. Pediatr Nurs 24(4):385–389 1998.
8. Otto CM, Kaufman GM, Crowe DT: Intraosseous infusion of fluids and therapeutics. Compendium 11(4):421–431, 1989.
9. Stoelting RK (ed): Pharmacology and Physiology in Anesthetic Practice, 3rd ed. Philadelphia, Lippincott-Raven, 1999.
10. Thurmon JC, Tranquilli WJ, Benson GJ (eds): Essentials of Small Animal Anesthesia and Analgesia. Baltimore, Lippincott, Williams & Wilkins, 1999.
11. Thurmon JC, Tranquilli WJ, Benson GJ (eds): Lumb and Jones' Veterinary Anesthesia, 3rd ed. Baltimore, Williams & Wilkins, 1996

37. ANESTHESIA OF GERIATRIC PATIENTS

Jeff C. H. Ko, D.V.M., M.S., D.A.C.V.A.,
and David S. Galloway, D.V.M., M.M.A.S.

1. Define "geriatric" as it relates to small animals.

There is no single definition for the term *geriatric* as it relates to dogs and cats. Great variation in life expectancy and the rate of age-related body changes exists between species, breeds, and individuals. Two methods of geriatric classification have be suggested:

• Some suggest that an animal is "geriatric" when it has reached 75% to 80% of its anticipated life expectancy.

*Life Expectancy of Small Animals**

SIZE OF ANIMAL	BODY WEIGHT	GERIATRIC AGE
Small dogs	Less than 9 kg (20 lbs)	9–13 years
Medium dogs	9.5–22.7 kg (21-50 lbs)	9–11.5 years
Large dogs	23.2–41 kg (51-90 lbs)	7.5–10.5 years
Giant dogs	More than 41 kg (> 90 lbs)	6–9 years
Cats	—	8–10 years

*Modified from Goldston RT: Geriatrics and gerontology. Vet Clin North Small Anim Pract 19:1–202, 1989.

• Others suggest that all animals over the age of 8 years be considered geriatric, regardless of species, breed, or current health.

2. List age-related changes to the cardiovascular system. Discuss their impact on anesthetic management.

Decreased blood volume and blood pressure, reduced cardiac output and baroreceptor activity, increased circulation time, and increased vagal tone have been reported in otherwise healthy geriatric patients. Vascular changes include thickened elastic fibers, increased wall collagen content, and vessel wall calcification. The geriatric patient's ability to autoregulate blood flow is decreased. Each of these changes is considered significant, and collectively they produce a severe reduction in cardiac reserve capacity, which may limit the patient's ability to compensate for cardiovascular changes that occur during anesthesia. Clinically, the anesthetic management of geriatric patients should avoid bradycardia or tachycardia, sudden changes in blood pressures, hypotension, or increased vascular resistance.

Geriatric patients commonly have acquired progressive or degenerative myocardial diseases. Changes of the cardiac conduction system associated with myocardial disease increase the chance for geriatric patients to develop cardiac arrhythmias while under general anesthesia. Second-degree heart block, bundle branch block, ventricular premature contractions, or atrial fibrillation may be common existing arrhythmias in geriatric patients. These arrhythmias can be exaggerated when the geriatric patient is exposed to stress from anesthesia or surgery. Anesthetic agents that have the potential to exaggerate arrhythmias, such as xylazine or medetomidine (bradycardia and second-degree heart blocks), thiopental (ventricular premature contractions or ventricular bigeminy), and ketamine (tachycardia) should be avoided altogether or used conservatively and with extreme caution.

Intravenous access is critical in geriatric patient anesthesia as it allows judicious fluid therapy for vascular volume maintenance and the administration of intravenous drugs. Blood pressure measurement and continuous assessment of electrocardiogram during anesthesia is also critical.

3. List age-related changes to the respiratory system. Discuss their impact on anesthetic management.

Decreased lung elasticity, respiratory rate, tidal volume, minute volume, oxygen consumption, carbon dioxide production, and oxygen diffusion capacity; decreased strength of muscles of respiration, chest wall compliance, and loss of elastic recoil; decreased vital capacity and increased residual volume; and loss of protective airway reflexes all have been reported in otherwise healthy geriatric patients. These changes collectively result in decreased respiratory functional reserve. Such changes are significant when anesthetic agents, such as propofol, thiopental, etomidate, or inhalant anesthetics, induce mild to moderate respiratory depression. Clinically, this frequently results in marked hypoxia and hypercapnia. If heavy sedation has to be used, oxygen supplementation via intubation, facemask, or nasal canula should also be considered. The impact of any pathologic lung lesions, such as pulmonary fibrosis, pulmonary neoplasia, pneumonia, pulmonary cysts, bullae, or blebs, will be greatly exacerbated in the geriatric patient. Anesthetic management should avoid any respiratory depression. Intermittent positive pressure ventilation (IPPV) should also be carefully monitored for appropriate peek positive pressures to prevent lung overinflation and subsequent barotrauma. Preoxygenation before induction will be beneficial to the geriatric patient by increasing the oxygen fraction in the lungs and preventing hypoxia during the period between induction and intubation. Pulse oxymetry, capnography, and blood gas analysis allow ongoing assessment of ventilatory efficiency. Geriatric patients have diminished protective airway reflexes; therefore, airway control, patency, and oxygen supplementation should be maintained whenever possible.

4. List age-related hepatic changes. Discuss their impact on anesthetic management.

It has been reported that in the otherwise healthy geriatric patients, there is reduction in functional liver mass, reduction in hepatic blood flow secondary to reduced cardiac output, decreased microsomal enzyme activity, and generalized reduction of metabolic activity. These hepatic functional changes cause prolonged metabolism and excretion of drugs dependent on hepatic conjugation and predispose the geriatric patient to prolonged recovery. Hence, the selection of anesthetic agents should avoid drugs that have a long duration of action (i.e., acepromazine), drugs that rely heavily on hepatic metabolism, or drugs that cannot be reversed. Reduced hepatic function also may lead to hypoproteinemia, impaired clotting function, and a greater susceptibility to hypothermia and hypoglycemia. When managing anesthetized geriatric patients, these changes should be kept in mind. Preanesthetic hematology and serum chemistry evaluation will help assess hepatic function. Clotting profiles are recommended before ultrasound-guided internal organ biopsy or surgery. Hypotension, which can greatly exacerbate the reduction of hepatic blood flow, should be avoided or properly managed with appropriate plane of anesthesia, fluid administration, and inotropic agents.

5. List age-related renal changes. Discuss their impact on anesthetic management.

Renal changes in the otherwise healthy geriatric patients include reduction in renal blood flow secondary to reduced cardiac output, decreased glomerular filtration rate, decreased functional kidney mass due to loss of functional neurons, and decreased ability to concentrate urine and secrete hydrogen ions. As a result of decreased renal functional reserve, geriatric patients are less tolerant of dehydration or acute hemorrhage during surgery. Additionally, overhydration due to excessive fluid administration during the perioperative period may lead to pulmonary edema and compromise the limited functional reserve of the aged respiratory system. Geriatric patients will be more prone to acidosis. Drugs that rely on renal excretion, such as ketamine in cats, should be used with caution. Hypovolemia, hypotension, hypoxia, and hypercapnia, all of which can greatly exacerbate the reduction of renal blood flow, should be avoided. Monitoring of urine production should also be routinely performed. Normal urine production under general anesthesia should be 1–2 ml/kg/hour. Less urine production or no urine production following anesthesia is a strong indication of renal system damage due to severe hypotension or poor renal perfusion. A proper diagnosis and treatment should be instituted as soon as possible before a nonreversible renal injury occurs. Serum chemistry and electrolyte analysis may offer subtle indictors of renal dysfunction in geriatric patients.

6. List age-related nervous system changes. Discuss their impact on anesthetic management.
Geriatric patients often present with alterations of cognitive, sensory, motor, and autonomic nervous functions. Age-related nervous system changes include decreased cerebral perfusion and oxygen consumption, reduction in brain mass due to neuronal degeneration, myelin sheath degeneration, increased destruction and decreased production of neurotransmitters, alterations of neurotransmitter receptors, decreased thermoregulatory center function, and decreased sympathetic response to stress. These changes enhance the effects of local anesthetics, increase the relative efficacy of anesthetic drugs, make geriatric patients more susceptible to anesthesia-induced cardiopulmonary depression and hypothermia, and decrease the patient's tolerance of stressful activities or situations. Total patient management should be geared around these considerations by lowering the regular premedication, induction, and maintenance dosages and by paying attention to detailed monitoring of the cardiorespiratory system and body temperature regulation.

7. What are characteristics of ideal anesthetic agents for use in geriatric patients?
There is no ideal anesthetic agent for use in geriatric patients. Careful selection, conservative dosing, close attention to detail during anesthesia monitoring, and prompt treatments are the hallmarks of appropriate anesthetic drug use in geriatric patients. An anesthetic agent used in geriatric patients should have one or more of the following characteristics:
- Allow rapid and complete recovery (e.g., propofol, inhalants).
- Be fully reversible (e.g., opioids, benzodiazepines, low doses of α_2-agonist sedatives).
- Make minimal metabolic demand for drug elimination (e.g., propofol, etomidate, modern inhalants—isoflurane, sevoflurane).
- Have minimal intrinsic toxicity (e.g., opioids, benzodiazepines, modern inhalants).
- Have minimal adverse side effects if drug activity persists (e.g., benzodiazepines, opioids).

8. What are specific advantages and disadvantages of routinely using anticholinergic agents as anesthetic premedications in geriatric patients?
Atropine and glycopyrrolate are the two most commonly used anticholinergic agents used to decrease respiratory secretions and counteract sinus bradycardia. There is no specific indication or contraindication for using anticholinergic agents as part of premedication in the geriatric patient. The potential danger of indiscriminately administering atropine or glycopyrrolate is that it may precipitate sinus tachycardia. An abnormally increased heart rate produces increased myocardial oxygen demand, which, when compounded by lack of functional cardiac reserve, may result in myocardial hypoxia and precipitate myocardial arrhythmias and failure.
Anticholinergics are indicated to counteract the bradycardic effects of potent vagotonic drugs such as morphine, oxymorphone, and fentanyl. Such anticholinergic use should be titrated to effect, usually starting at one-half to two-thirds of the normal drug dose to avoid potential tachycardia.

9. What are specific advantages and disadvantages of using acepromazine in geriatric patients?
Tranquilizers may be indicated to reduce the stress associated with hospitalization, anesthesia, and surgery of geriatric patients. Low doses of acepromazine (0.025 to 0.05 mg per kg) may be used in such instances for geriatric patients. Undesirable characteristics and side effects of acepromazine should be anticipated. Acepromazine is not reversible and metabolized by the liver. It may produce prolonged tranquilization and prolonged recovery from anesthesia. Acepromazine also causes peripheral vasodilation via α_1-adrenergic blockade. As a result, hypotension may occur, especially in the dehydrated patient. Although acepromazine has antiarrhythmogenic effects, it may precipitate seizures. Volume expansion and blood pressure monitoring are indicated when acepromazine is administered to geriatric patients. In geriatric patients that demonstrate dehydration, acute hemorrhage, liver dysfunction, or are surgical candidates, the use of acepromazine should be avoided.

10. What are specific advantages and disadvantages of using benzodiazepine tranquilizers in geriatric patients?

Benzodiazepines (diazepam or midazolam) are considered minor tranquilizers with minimal sedative effect on young healthy patients. In fact, when used alone in the young animals, they have been reported to cause excitement rather than sedation. These agents have more profound sedative effects on geriatric patients and are usually a better choice than acepromazine because they have minimal cardiorespiratory side effects. They offer the advantages of reversibility (flumazenil is a specific reversal agent for benzodiazepines), minimal cardiopulmonary effects, and short duration of action. These agents are potent anticonvulsants and are suitable for use in patients with a history of seizures. Prolonged sedation may occur after these sedatives are administrated to geriatric patients, probably due to impaired hepatic metabolism. In selected geriatric cases, these agents may also be appropriate for use in combination with dissociatives (ketamine) or opioids (butorphanol, oxymorphone) as a sedative or anesthetic induction combination.

11. What are specific advantages and disadvantages of using α_2-agonist sedatives in geriatric patients?

α_2-Agonist sedatives (xylazine, medetomidine) should be used in geriatric patients only with extreme caution. Despite reversibility with specific α_2-antagonists (yohimbine, tolazoline, atipamezole), these agents have substantial undesirable cardiac, circulatory, respiratory, and central nervous system effects. It is best to leave these agents out of your geriatric anesthetic armamentarium.

12. What are specific advantages and disadvantages of using opioid narcotics in geriatric patients?

Opioids are classified as μ-agonists (morphine, oxymorphone, hydromorphone, fentanyl, meperidine), κ-agonist-μ-antagonists (butorphanol, nalbuphine), and partial μ-agonists (buprenorphine). These agents offer mild to moderate sedation and profound analgesia with minimal cardiovascular depression. They can be used to decrease the requirement for other anesthetic agents for anesthetic induction and maintenance. Some μ-agonists (morphine, oxymorphone, hydromorphone, and fentanyl) can cause bradycardia, which may be prevented with judicious use of anticholinergics. μ-Agonists produce centrally mediated dose-dependent respiratory depression. Such respiratory depression, although rarely of clinical significance in young patients, can cause unwanted complications in geriatric patients with little functional respiratory reserve. When these opioids are combined with isoflurane or sevoflurane, hypoventilation or apnea may occur. κ-Agonist/μ-antagonists and partial μ-agonists have a "ceiling effect" on respiratory depression, making them a popular choice for use in geriatric patients. However, this ceiling effect is also observed as limited analgesic efficacy, making these agents unsuitable for the control of severe pain.

It is recommended that opioids be dosed conservatively, as part of a balanced anesthetic protocol, and that airway control with 100% oxygen administration be offered. Assisted or controlled ventilation may have to be instituted to counter potential respiratory depression. With butorphanol or nalbuphine use, repeated dosing may have to be performed to maintain adequate analgesia when treating severe pain.

13. What are specific advantages and disadvantages of using ultrashort-acting barbiturates in geriatric patients?

Ultrashort-acting barbiturates (thiopental, thiamylal, and methohexital) have been used to induce anesthesia in "healthy" geriatric patients. The margin of safety for these agents is decreased in the geriatric patient. These agents may cause direct cardiovascular depression, pulmonary depression, and initial apnea and vasodilation. Methohexital may precipitate seizures. Arousal occurs upon drug redistribution to the patient's lean body mass and fat compartments, and ultimate drug elimination is via hepatic conjugation. Decreased plasma protein-binding capability, decreased lean mass and body water, lack of hepatic functional reserve, and increased lipid compartment size in geriatric patients may lead to increased physiologic drug effects and prolonged recoveries from ultrashort-acting barbiturates. When administering these agents to geriatric patients, they should be given slowly and titrated to effect for endotracheal intubation. The ultra-short-acting barbiturates cannot be recommended for repeated boluses or use as a continuous infusion in geriatric patients, since prolonged anesthesia and cardiorespiratory depression will occur.

14. What are specific advantages and disadvantages of using dissociative agents in geriatric patients?

Dissociative anesthetic agents (ketamine, tiletamine) are commonly used in veterinary practice for anesthetic induction and for total parenteral anesthesia; however, these agents should be used with caution in geriatric patients. Tachycardia associated with dissociative use may increase myocardial oxygen consumption and precipitate myocardial hypoxia or failure. Increased secretions resulting from these agents may exacerbate pre-existing pulmonary dysfunction by creating a diffusion barrier or airway obstruction, especially in brachycephalic dog breeds. Airway secretions may also induce laryngeal spasm in cats, if the airway is not protected via endotracheal intubation. Dissociative agents may precipitate seizures in both dogs and cats. Existing renal or hepatic disease, or lack of functional reserve of either system, which is common to geriatric patients, may prolong recovery times. Sedatives or tranquilizers, such as diazepam, may be required to preclude muscle rigidity during the surgery or during the delirium associated with recovery from dissociative anesthetics observed in some patients.

15. What are specific advantages and disadvantages of using propofol or etomidate in geriatric patients?

Propofol and etomidate are both excellent choices for anesthetic induction of geriatric patients, offering consistently rapid anesthetic induction and relatively complete recoveries. However, cardiopulmonary depressant effects of propofol are similar to those of thiobarbiturates, and a rapid bolus injection of propofol can cause rapid hemoglobin desaturation, cyanosis, and apnea. As a result, propofol should be given slowly (over a period of 60–90 seconds) to geriatric patients. Propofol should be used cautiously in geriatric patients with pre-existing cardiopulmonary dysfunction (pneumonia). Propofol is rapidly metabolized, even in geriatric patients with minimal hepatic reserve. Residual drug effects are minimal and propofol can be safely used as a constant-rate infusion or a repeatedly bolused injection. Respiratory depression and apnea are the most profound side effects of propofol. If apnea occurs, endotracheal intubation following by positive pressure ventilation should be immediately instituted.

Etomidate is especially useful for patients with cardiovascular dysfunction because it produces minimal changes to heart rate and blood pressure following anesthetic induction. Anesthesia induction is usually rapid and smooth if the patient is premedicated with diazepam or an opioid. Etomidate, used alone as an anesthetic induction agent, may induce retching and involuntary muscle twitching. Premedication will alleviate these problems. Etomidate will inhibit secretion of adrenal corticosteroids for up to 1 week. As a result, it should not be used in the patient that tends to have adrenal corticosteroid deficiency. The respiratory depression produced by etomidate is just as potent as that of propofol and thiopental. Apnea will occur if a large bolus dose of etomidate is given. The same precautions should be taken for preventing and treating etomidate-induced hypotension and apnea.

16. What are specific advantages and disadvantages of using inhalant anesthetic agents in geriatric patients?

Methoxyflurane and halothane elimination requires that 50% and 25%, respectively, of the inhaled portion be metabolized by the liver and kidney. As a result, these agents are not good choices for use in geriatric patients.

Isoflurane and sevoflurane require minimal hepatic and renal metabolism, thereby alleviating metabolic burden from the liver and kidneys. Sevoflurane offers more rapid induction and recovery from anesthesia, making it a good choice for critically ill and geriatric patients. Both isoflurane and sevoflurane minimally sensitize the myocardium to catecholamines and maintain an overall stable cardiac rhythm. However, both agents can cause dose-dependent respiratory depression, vasodilation, and hypotension. These side effects should be taken into consideration if these inhalant anesthetic agents are to be used, especially during facemask or chamber induction, in which a high percentage of the inhalant agent is used. Carefully monitoring the geriatric patients during these procedures is vital.

17. What are specific advantages and disadvantages of using nonsteroidal anti-inflammatory drugs in geriatric patients?

Many nonsteroidal anti-inflammatory drugs (NSAIDs) are currently available and are commonly used in veterinary practice for decreasing inflammation and providing analgesia. Modern NSAIDs such as carprofen and etodolac offer a higher safety margin. They can be used pre-emptively or postoperatively. They are not controlled substances and have a longer duration of action for treating mild to moderate pain. Geriatric patients may already be on long-term NSAIDs for the treatment of osteoarthritis. The side effects of NSAIDs include gastric ulceration and renal and platelet dysfunction. The use of NSAIDs as analgesic agents should be avoided in geriatric patients with liver dysfunction, renal dysfunction, gastrointestinal system dysfunction, or platelet dysfunction. NSAIDs are eicosinoid synthesis inhibitors. Although eicosinoids (prostaglandins, leukotrienes, and thromboxanes) have undesired effects, including inflammation and pain, many are required for normal cellular maintenance activities. Prostaglandin E plays an important role in visceral vasodilation. With decreased renal functional reserve, the indiscriminate use of NSAIDs in geriatric animals can precipitate kidney failure. Such consequences are even more prevalent during anesthetic events in which proper blood pressure has not been maintained, leading to dangerously low kidney perfusion.

18. Isn't sedation safer than general anesthesia for geriatric patients?

Not necessarily. Quite often, using a balanced, multimodal approach to general anesthesia, including maintenance with inhalant anesthetics, is more controllable and safer than parenteral sedatives or tranquilizers, even for procedures requiring minor restraint, such as hip radiographs. Additional advantages of inhalant anesthesia are airway control, administration of 100% oxygen, and minimizing the requirement for drug metabolism by the liver and kidneys.

19. What is considered appropriate monitoring of the anesthetized geriatric patient?

Pulse oximetry for measurement of hemoglobin saturation with oxygen, capnometry for end-tidal CO_2, noninvasive blood pressure monitoring (oscillometric or Doppler ultrasound) for blood pressure assessment, and electrocardiography are the current trend for monitoring geriatric patients. Furthermore, body temperature and electrolytes should be closely monitored during and after general anesthesia.

Case Study for Questions 20–23.

An 8-year-old, intact, female Chihuahua presents with signs attributable to mammary gland neoplasia. A recent cardiac evaluation demonstrated compensation and adequate medical control of left-sided heart failure.

20. What American Society of Anesthesiologists (ASA) category is this patient?

ASA category III (compensated-controlled systemic disease).

21. What diagnostic tests would you consider pre-anesthesia?

A pre-anesthetic diagnostic battery, other than a detailed physical examination, might include the following:
- Plain chest radiography—to assess heart size, functional lung capacity, and the impact of possible pulmonary metastasis of neoplasia.
- Electrocardiogram—to assess baseline conductivity of cardiac tissues and detection of potential arrhythmias.
- Echocardiogram (if not performed routinely in the past 3–4 months)—to assess current medical control and physiologic compensation for heart failure.

- Hematology and serum chemistry evaluation—to assess major organ function and electrolyte balance.

22. Discuss a possible anesthetic regimen for anesthetizing this patient for ovariohysterectomy and resection of the mass.

One possible anesthetic regimen follows:

- Premedication: diazepam (0.2 mg/kg IM) or midazolam (0.2 mg/kg IM) combined with butorphanol (0.2 mg/kg IM)
- Electrocardiograph connected to the dog prior to anesthetic induction
- Preoxygenation with 100% O_2
- Induction: etomidate (1–2 mg/kg) or propofol (4–6 mg/kg) IV to effect
- Maintenance: sevoflurane or isoflurane
- Dobutamine or dopamine (10 µg/kg/min or titrated to effect) for cardiovascular support
- Normasol-R 10 ml/kg/hr for fluid maintenance

23. What anesthetic agents, if any, are contraindicated in this patient?

None.

Case Study for Questions 24–27.

A 14-year-old, female, retired hunting German shorthaired pointer presents with mild neurologic signs attributable to degenerative myelopathy, lumbosacral disease, or type II thoracolumbar disk disease. She has multiple subcutaneous masses that have been diagnosed as lipomas. She also has a severe acral lick granuloma over the right rear metatarsus. Otherwise, she shows no systemic disease.

24. What ASA category is this patient?

ASA category II (localized disease).

25. What diagnostic tests would you consider pre-anesthesia?

A pre-anesthetic diagnostic battery, other than a detailed physical examination, might include the following:

- Plain chest radiography—to assess heart size, and functional lung capacity.
- Electrocardiography—to assess baseline conductivity of cardiac tissues.
- Hematology and serum chemistry evaluation—to assess major organ function and electrolyte balance.

26. Discuss a possible anesthetic regimen for anesthetizing this patient for radiology, myelography, and possible spinal surgery.

One possible anesthetic regimen follows:

- Premedication: diazepam (0.2 mg/kg IM), oxymorphone (0.1 mg/kg IM) or hydromorphone (0.2 mg/kg IM), and glycopyrrolate (0.01 mg/kg IM)
- Preoxygenation with 100% O_2
- Induction: etomidate (1–2 mg/kg IV) or propofol (4–6 mg/kg IV) to effect for endotracheal intubation
- Maintenance: isoflurane or sevoflurane
- Fentanyl CRI (2–10 µg/kg/hour) to decrease total inhalant dose
- Dobutamine or dopamine infusion (5–10 µg/kg/min) for cardiovascular support
- Balanced electrolyte solution at 10 ml/kg/hr

27. What anesthetic agents, if any, are contraindicated in this patient?

Dissociative anesthetics and phenothiazine tranquilizers are contraindicated in this case, as they may precipitate seizures postmyelography.

Case Study for Questions 28–35.

An 8-year-old, male, miniature poodle presents with severe periodontal disease for routine dental prophylaxis and possible extractions of loosening teeth. The dog has a grade III/VI holosystolic heart murmur with a point of maximal intensity auscultable behind the left elbow. The dog exhibits exercise intolerance and appears to have mitral insufficiency.

28. What ASA category is this patient?
ASA category IV (uncompensated-uncontrolled systemic disease).

29. What diagnostic tests would you consider pre-anesthesia?
This patient is presenting as an ASA-IV patient for an elective procedure. Evaluation of and medical control of presented systemic disease is indicated before anesthesia is considered. This patient should be referred for cardiac evaluation and treatment to control suspected left-sided heart failure. It could return as an ASA-III patient, and a much better anesthetic candidate, in as little as 2–3 weeks.

30. Discuss a possible anesthetic regimen for anesthetizing this patient for dental extraction.
The anesthetic combination given in question 34 can be used for anesthesia.

31. What anesthetic agents, if any, are contraindicated in this patient?
None.

Case Study for Questions 32–35.
A 9-year-old, male, German Shepherd dog presents with a 3-day history of lethargy, hepatomegaly, splenomegaly, and progressively decreasing packed cell volume (last recorded at 30%). Intra-abdominal hemangiosarcoma is suspected.

32. What ASA category is this patient?
ASA category IV (uncompensated-uncontrolled systemic disease)

33. What diagnostic tests would you consider pre-anesthesia?
This patient is presenting as an ASA-IV patient for a nonelective procedure. Evaluation of and medical control of presented systemic disease is not possible before anesthesia is considered. A pre-anesthetic diagnostic battery, other than a detailed physical examination, might include the following:
- Plain chest radiography—to assess heart size, functional lung capacity, and the impact of possible cardiac metastasis of suspected neoplasia.
- Electrocardiography—to assess baseline conductivity of cardiac tissues and detection of cardiac arrhythmias.
- Echocardiogram—to assess the possibility of cardiac metastasis or pericardial effusion.
- Hematology and serum chemistry evaluation—to assess major organ function and electrolyte balance. PCV/TP to assess current oxygen carrying capacity and serum protein, as well as baseline data for transfusion therapy decision-making.
- Major and minor cross-match: To prepare for the possibility of transfusion.

34. Discuss a possible anesthetic regimen for anesthetizing this patient for abdominal exploration, possible splenectomy, and multiple tissue biopsies.
Possible anesthetic regimens as follows:
- Premedication: oxymorphone (0.05–0.1 mg/kg IV) or hydromorphone (0.1 mg/kg IV) through the preplaced intravenous catheter.
- Pre-oxygenation with 100% O_2.
- Induction: propofol (4–6 mg/kg). Alternatively, induce with diazepam (0.4–0.6 mg/kg) and oxymorphone (0.1–0.2 mg/kg) via alternating intravenous injection until endotracheal intubation is possible.
- Maintenance: isoflurane or sevoflurane

- Fentanyl CRI (5–10 µg/kg/hr) to decrease total inhalant dose
- Dobutamine or dopamine CRI (5–10 µg/kg/min) for cardiovascular support
- Intravenous balanced electrolyte solution at 10 ml/kg/hr
- If intraoperative hemorrhage occurs, then whole blood transfusion should be commenced.

35. What anesthetic agents, if any, are contraindicated in this patient.
None.

BIBLIOGRAPHY

1. Bronson RT: Variation in age at death of dogs of different sexes and breeds. Am J Vet Res 43:2057–2059, 1982.
2. Crawford P: Anesthesia in aging pets: Physiological considerations. Vet Tech 21:14–19, 2000.
3. Crawford P: A deep sleep: Anesthetics and care of geriatric patients. Vet Tech 21:97–102, 2000.
4. Dodman NH, Seeler DC, Court MH: Aging changes in the geriatric dog and their impact on anesthesia. Comp Contin Educ 6:1106–1113, 1984.
5. Hartsfield SM: Anesthetic problems of the geriatric dental patient. Probl Vet Med 2:24–45, 1990.
6. Harvey RC, Paddleford RR: Management of geriatric patients. Vet Clin North Am (Small Anim Pract) 29:683–699, 1999.
7. Herrtage ME: Management of the geriatric dog. Vet Ann 30:203–210, 1990.
8. Maher ER, Rush JE: Cardiovascular changes in the geriatric dog. Comp Contin Educ 12:921–928, 1990.
9. Paddleford RR: Anesthetic considerations for the geriatric patient. Vet Clin North Am (Small Anim Pract) 19:13–31, 1989.

38. OBESITY

Kurt A. Grimm, D.V.M., M.S., D.A.C.V.A., D.A.C.V.C.P.

1. How is obesity defined?

Obesity has been defined many different ways. Generally, animals with an excessive accumulation of body fat to the point of being 20% or more over ideal body weight are considered obese. Morbidly obese is defined as a body weight twice the ideal body weight. An alternative functional definition is an excessive accumulation of body fat sufficient to impair body functions and be detrimental to good health and well being. Ideal body weight varies with species, age, breed, and sex.

2. Where did the term *pickwickian syndrome* come from?

A morbidly obese character in the 1836 novel, *Pickwick Papers,* by Charles Dickens.

3. What are the signs of pickwickian syndrome in animals?

In the context of veterinary medicine, the term refers to preoperative hypoxemia caused by obesity. Often the patient is lethargic and somnolent and has intermittent respirations with brief periods of apnea. The condition is usually markedly worsened by anesthetic drug administration in the absence of ventilatory support.

4. How does obesity affect respiration?

Obesity decreases the ventilatory capacity of a patient through decreased thoracic compliance and hypoventilation resulting from impaired diaphragmatic motion due to increased weight of abdominal contents. The respiratory pattern is shallow, with decreased tidal volumes, increased work of breathing, and increased rate. Increased mass of pharyngeal tissues and tongue may lead to upper airway obstruction following premedication with sedatives and tranquilizers and during induction of anesthesia before a secure airway has been established.

5. What should I do differently during anesthesia of an obese patient?

It is prudent to constantly observe obese patients for signs of airway obstruction following premedication. During anesthesia, ventilatory support may be required. At a minimum, endotracheal intubation should be performed and tidal volume monitored. Capnography, pulse oximetry, and blood gas analysis will help warn of the need for ventilatory assistance. Obese animals must regain normal muscle function to maintain an adequate tidal volume and patent airway after extubation.

6. How does obesity affect the circulatory system?

Circulating blood volume, plasma volume, and cardiac output increase proportionally with increasing body weight. Since heart rate usually remains within normal limits, the excess cardiac output is generated from increased stroke work. In the worse case, this increase in cardiac work will result in ventricular failure over time.

7. What other conditions commonly occur with obesity?

Pancreatitis, diabetes mellitus, hepatic lipidosis, hypothyroidism, cardiac, orthopedic, and intervertebral disk disease are a few of the conditions commonly diagnosed in obese animals.

8. How should induction drug dosages be altered in obese animals?

Depending on the drug and route of administration, the dosage may need to be increased, be decreased, or remain unchanged. A highly lipophilic drug that has a large apparent volume of distribution (Vd_{ss}) may require a larger initial dose than in a normal weight animal for an equivalent plasma concentration at steady state. Many injectable anesthetics are highly lipid soluble and have large Vd_{ss}, but these drugs are not usually administered with the goal of attaining steady-state plasma levels. Instead, the effective concentrations necessary for anesthesia are achieved soon after drug administration, before distribution into the adipose tissue can occur. Therefore, increased doses are not usually indicated. In fact, often a smaller dose relative to nonobese animals may be equally effective. When administering intravenous anesthetic agents to obese animals, the safest approach is still to administer the drugs slowly to effect.

9. What exactly does *dosing to effect* mean?

Dosing to effect means administering drugs slowly until the desired effect is achieved. For anesthetic induction agents this, is usually until endotracheal intubation can be performed without causing the patient to gag. Dosing to effect is usually the safest method when individual variation makes calculation of a dose difficult. It usually works best for rapidly acting intravenously administered drugs but can also be applied to inhalant agents, inotropic agents, analgesic agents, and many other classes of drugs.

10. Are obese animals at greater risk of complications during anesthesia?

If anesthesia is managed in a similar fashion to anesthesia for a nonobese patient, it would be expected that the incidence of respiratory depression, airway obstruction, and hypoxemia would be greater. However, these cases can usually be managed by proper drug selection, airway management, and perioperative monitoring, reducing the risk of morbidity or mortality.

11. Why do obese animals appear to require a longer time to recover from inhalant anesthetics?

Most inhalant anesthetics are variably soluble in lipids (see table). In fact, anesthetic potency appears to parallel lipid solubility (Meyer-Overton rule). Because adipose tissue has a relatively low rate of perfusion (2–3 ml/100 g tissue/min), and because in obese animals the size of this tissue compartment is larger, it can be predicted that as the length of anesthesia increases, there is more uptake of anesthetic by the adipose tissue.

During recovery, this process reverses. The length of time required to remove the anesthetic is directly proportional to the amount of anesthetic stored in the adipose tissue and indirectly proportional to the blood flow to the tissue. Using agents with high adipose/gas partition coefficients (e.g., methoxyflurane) should result in slower removal than poorly soluble agents (e.g., nitrous oxide) if all other factors remain equal. In the clinical setting, many factors, such as duration of anesthesia, cardiac output, minute ventilation, and metabolism, can alter the disposition of an anesthetic agent, resulting in varied recovery rates.

Adipose/Gas Partition Coefficients of Some Inhalant Anesthetics at 37°C*

AGENT	ADIPOSE/GAS PARTITION COEFFICIENT
Methoxyflurane	902
Enflurane	83
Halothane	51
Sevoflurane	48
Isoflurane	45
Desflurane	27
Nitrous oxide	1

*Values are based on data from humans. There are minor species differences in the absolute values.

12. Can opioids be administered to obese patients?

Opioids are not contraindicated in obese patients. However, vigilant monitoring of respiratory function is prudent. Much of the concern for opioid-induced respiratory depression is based on human data. People are more sensitive to the respiratory depressant effects of opioid agonists, and careful dose titration is required in the clinical setting. Dogs and cats appear less sensitive to these effects, especially when in pain. Attention to respiratory function is still required in veterinary patients.

13. Can regional anesthesia and analgesia be used in obese patients?

Regional anesthesia and analgesia appears to be a useful technique to reduce the morbidity and mortality associated with general anesthesia. However, increased thickness of the subcutaneous adipose tissue makes palpation of landmarks difficult.

Epidural anesthesia and analgesia is difficult in obese patients and is often abandoned when proper drug placement cannot be ensured. However, with practice, epidural anesthesia and analgesia can be performed on most patients, but doses of epidural drugs are usually reduced in obese patients because of the increased amount of epidural fat.

14. Is regional anesthesia safer than general anesthesia for obese patients?

In some situations, general anesthesia may be preferable because a secure airway can be maintained and high inspired concentrations of oxygen can be delivered. Respiratory depression from cranial migration of epidural local anesthetics or systemic uptake of opioids may lead to decreased minute ventilation and respiratory embarrassment if assisted or controlled ventilation cannot be instituted. With regional techniques, careful patient monitoring is still required.

BIBLIOGRAPHY

1. Lemke KA, Dawson SD: Local and regional anesthesia. Clin North Am Small Anim Prac 30(4):839–857, 2000.
2. Bednarski, RM: Anesthesia and immobilization of specific species: Dogs and cats. In Thurmon JC, Tranquilli WJ, Benson GJ (eds): Lumb and Jones' Veterinary Anesthesia, 3rd ed. Baltimore, Williams & Wilkins, 1996.
3. Clutton RE: The medical implications of canine obesity and their relevance to anaesthesia. Br Vet J 144(1):21–8, 1988.

39. PREGNANCY

Stephen A. Greene, D.V.M., M.S., D.A.C.V.A., and
G. John Benson, D.V.M., M.S., D.A.C.V.A.

1. What factors determine anesthetic transfer across the placenta into fetal circulation?
Maternal blood concentration is determined by the drug dose, location and route of injection, and maternal metabolism and excretion. The time from beginning administration of anesthetic to the time of delivery of the newborn is the most critical factor under control of the veterinarian during a cesarian surgical procedure. Minimizing the time from the beginning of uterine exteriorization until delivery is critical in reducing the period of decreased uterine blood flow. Other factors that determine the rate of placental transfer arise from the concentration gradient as described by the Fick equation [$Q/t = KA (C_m - C_f)/D$ where Q/t is the amount of diffused substance per unit time; K is the diffusion constant of a given substance which takes into account its pKa, molecular weight, lipid solubility, and protein binding; A is the surface area for diffusion; C_m is the concentration in maternal uterine arterial blood; C_f is the concentration in fetal blood; and D is the thickness of the placental membrane]. The veterinarian has little control over these other factors, since nearly all anesthetics are low molecular weight, highly lipid soluble, and highly protein bound drugs.

2. How does pregnancy affect anesthetic requirement (MAC)?
Pregnancy is associated with a 25–40% decrease in anesthetic requirement. It is believed that the decrease is related to circulating levels of progesterone. Newborns will have a decreased anesthetic requirement for the first month after birth, at which time their MAC requirement will be at a maximum for that animal's lifetime. The decrease in MAC during the first month of life is also related to progesterone that has crossed the placenta to the fetal circulation. MAC values tend to decrease gradually from one month of age until death.

3. What physiologic changes altering the response to anesthetics occur during pregnancy?

Heart rate	Increased
Cardiac output	Increased
Blood volume	Increased
Packed cell volume	Decreased
Hemoglobin	Decreased
Plasma protein	Decreased
Oxygen consumption	Increased
Minute ventilation	Increased
Functional residual capacity	Decreased
Gastric emptying time	Increased
Gastric pH	Decreased
Glomerular filtration rate	Increased
Renal blood flow	Increased

4. Discuss the effect of pregnancy on epidural analgesic technique.
Pregnancy is associated with increased blood volume, increased shunting of abdominal blood to epidural tissues, and, during optimal nutrition, increased epidural fat stores. These factors increase the volume of epidural blood vessels and fat, which decreases the potential volume of the epidural space. Thus, the volume of epidural analgesic injected in a pregnant animal at term will migrate more rostrally than the same volume injected in a nonpregnant animal of similar size

and conformation. Epidural injectate volume can typically be decreased by about one-third for patients at term.

5. Describe an anesthetic protocol suitable for canine cesarian deliveries.

One commonly used anesthetic protocol for inducing bitches for cesarian section is diazepam (0.2 mg/kg, IV) combined with either propofol (5–8 mg/kg, IV) or ketamine (3–5 mg/kg, IV). Light anesthesia is induced after she is clipped and prepared for surgery. Ideally, the patient is placed on the surgery table prior to induction of anesthesia. Once induced, the trachea is intubated and isoflurane is administered in low concentrations. After the newborn are delivered, oxymorphone or hydromorphone (0.1 mg/kg) can be administered IV or IM for maternal analgesia. If opioids are used prior to delivery, reversal in the newborn can be achieved by administering 3–4 drops of naloxone sublingually. Intravenous fluid therapy and vigilant monitoring of the anesthetized patient are important in the anesthetic management of cesarian surgeries.

6. Describe an anesthetic protocol suitable for feline cesarian deliveries.

The protocol described above for use in dogs can be applied to cats with minor modifications. The ketamine dose is frequently decreased to 2–4 mg/kg, IV. Lidocaine should be sprayed on the glottis to prevent laryngeal spasm during tracheal intubation. The dose of oxymorphone or hydromorphone for the cat is 0.03 mg/kg. Alternatively, meperidine (3 mg/kg, IV or IM) or butorphanol (0.3 mg/kg, IV or IM) can be used with less likelihood of an excitatory reaction.

7. Describe an anesthetic protocol suitable for equine cesarian delivery.

Induction of anesthesia for cesarian delivery in the mare may be accomplished using a low dose of xylazine (0.3 mg/kg, IV) for premedication followed by IV administration of the technique of your choice. For example, induction can be accomplished using guaifenesin (100–300 ml of 5% solution per 450 kg) and ketamine 1.5 mg/kg, IV. (Body weight used for calculation of doses should be the estimated nonpregnant weight.) Alternatively, xylazine (0.5-1.0 mg/kg, IV) followed by ketamine (2 mg/kg, IV) has been used successfully in mares at term.

8. What precautions should be taken when anesthetizing pregnant mares?

Anesthesia during the first or second trimester of pregnancy is generally uneventful for the mare. However, during the third trimester, the gravid uterus may compress the vena cava, resulting in hypotension when the mare is positioned in dorsal recumbency. Tilting the mare off her back to one side may minimize compression of the vena cava. Attention to monitoring cardiovascular function and maintenance of arterial blood pressure and oxygenation is paramount.

8. Which drugs are susceptible to "ion trapping" in the fetal circulation?

Drugs that are weak bases cross the placenta into fetal circulation as unionized molecules and enter fetal circulation. Because fetal blood is more acidic than maternal blood, the drug ionizes, thus becoming trapped and unable to readily diffuse back across the placenta. The most commonly used weak bases are opioids. Thus, use of sublingual or intravenous injection of naloxone is frequently effective in reversing depression in neonates that have been exposed to maternal administration of opioids.

9. What precautions should pregnant women take when working near anesthetized animals?

Pregnant women should discuss their work environment with their physician. While there are no convincing studies to document health benefits from reduced exposure to inhaled anesthetics during pregnancy, this remains the common practice. Means of reducing environmental exposure to inhaled anesthetics include vigilant use of scavenging equipment, avoidance of areas with high anesthetic use, elimination of mask or chamber induction techniques, recovery of patients connected to their breathing circuit with oxygen administered, and use of properly fitted personal facemasks (for the person) that are equipped with filters effective against hydrocarbons.

BIBLIOGRAPHY

1. American Society of Anesthesiologists: Waste Anesthetic Gases. 2001. Internet website: http://www.sahq. org/ProfInfo/wasteanesgases.html
2. Taylor PM, and Clarke KW: Anesthesia in special situations. In Taylor PM, Clarke KW (eds). Handbook of Equine Anaesthesia. London, WB Saunders, Co., 1999, pp 158-160.
3. Thurmon JC, Tranquilli WJ, and Benson, GJ: Anesthesia for special procedures and patients. In Thurmon JC, Tranquilli WJ, and Benson, GJ (eds). Essentials of Small Animal Anesthesia & Analgesia. Philadelphia, Lippincott Williams and Wilkins, 1999, pp 483-491.

40. CANINE BREED-SPECIFIC PROBLEMS

*Sophie Cuvelliez, D.M.V., M.S., D.A.C.V.A., D.E.C.V.A.,
and Yves Rondenay, D.M.V.*

There are urban legends and there are real facts about the importance of breed on anesthesia management. Breeders will often offer recipes for the best way to anesthetize the dogs they are raising. Every dog breed is particular, just as every dog is particular and every episode of anesthesia unique. Some dogs manifest breed-specific characteristics that will affect the perianesthetic choices available to the veterinarian. Problems may be associated with conformation characteristics (such as malformation of the upper airways in brachycephalic breeds), use and training of the animal (such as aggressiveness in defense dogs), or an important consanguinity (such as von Willebrand disease in Doberman pinschers). Some diseases have increased presentation in certain breeds of dogs, and their occurrences are increased with continued inbreeding.

1. What is a breed?

As defined in Webster's dictionary, "A breed is a particular group of domestic animals related by descent from common ancestors, visibly similar in most characteristics and usually is incapable of maintaining its distinctive characteristics in nature." The dog is the oldest domesticated animal that has been bred extensively, and familial sensitivity to certain drugs may be present. The canine genome has been manipulated by humankind, and the thorough study of its composition will shed light on its specificity.

2. What are the breeds referred to as "sighthounds"?

Classification of a dog breed as a sighthound is purely subjective. It is based on body conformation similarities and breed purpose. These dogs were primarily bred to hunt by sight. Nowadays, in countries where it is allowed, some of these breeds are used as racing dogs. These breeds are part of the Hound group of the American Kennel Club (AKC). They are:

Afghan Hound
Borzoi
Greyhound
Ibizan Hound
Italian Greyhound
Irish Wolfhound
Pharaoh Hound
Saluki
Scottish Deerhound
Whippet

Dogs such as the Rhodesian Ridge Back and the Basenji are sometimes included in this group. The sighthound is considered the oldest breed of dogs. Some non-sighthound breeds of dogs, such as collies, the Belgian tervueren shepherd dog, and the soft-coated Wheaton terrier, may therefore share some common ancestry with the sighthounds.

3. What are the significant characteristics of sighthounds and how will they affect your choice of anesthetic drugs?

They are usually nervous and are more prone to develop stress-related clinical complications such as gastrointestinal upset and hyperthermia. To prevent these complications, sedation and analgesia are important.

Sighthounds tend to have higher packed cell volumes (50%–60%) and lower serum proteins

(6.5 mg/dl). Lower serum albumin concentrations may result in a relatively increased effect of drugs that are highly protein bound (e.g., anesthetics).

Two factors play an important role in the recovery from the effects of drugs in sighthounds:

- Their morphology is characterized by a lack of fat tissue that will affect the redistribution of drugs.
- They have different abilities to metabolize drugs used to induce or maintain anesthesia. Most of the research has been done on greyhounds, but those data have been, truly or falsely, applied to the other sighthounds.

4. Several environmental factors are important to control when anesthetizing any patient (e.g., noise level). What environmental factor is essential to control with a greyhound or a whippet?

The body temperature needs to be maintained as close as possible to physiologic level. Sighthounds are lean animals with a low body fat to muscle ratio. This makes them susceptible to hypothermia, especially when thermoregulatory mechanisms are depressed by general anesthesia. In dogs with a short thin coat, such as greyhounds or whippets, the heat loss is exacerbated. Prevention of hypothermia is essential, as those dogs tend to cool down very rapidly and the problems associated with hypothermia can be significant (e.g., bradycardia unresponsive to anticholinergic drugs). Warming the patient (e.g., circulating warm water blankets) is the treatment to put in place.

5. Is the hepatic metabolism of drugs different in greyhounds compared with mixed breed dogs?

Yes. In fact, the liver metabolism of several drugs is different in this breed of dogs. There is an alteration in the activity of liver enzymes of the cytochrome P450 family. This mostly affects the metabolism of thiobarbiturates, but propofol and methohexital also appear to be cleared more slowly. For thiobarbiturate, the effect is more significant because this class of drug is much more slowly metabolized than propofol or methohexital.

6. What induction drugs should be avoided in greyhounds? Why?

Recovery from thiobarbiturate anesthesia in dogs occurs by redistribution of the drug from brain tissue to muscle and fat with concomitant liver metabolism and elimination of the drug. Thiobarbiturates (thiopental, thiamylal) are known to provoke a delayed recovery in greyhounds. The absence of significant adipose tissue for redistribution of the drug and the alteration of liver metabolism of the drug are the two main reasons to avoid thiobarbiturates in sighthound anesthesia. Greyhounds have a significantly lower hepatic clearance of thiobarbiturates compared with mixed-breed dogs. The rate of elimination is nonlinear, suggesting a saturation of the enzymatic clearance process. When the hepatic enzymes are induced with pentobarbital, the recovery time in the greyhound is reduced and is similar to that of mixed-breed dogs.

7. What are recognized and acceptable methods of performing anesthesia in a sighthound?

A sedative premedication to reduce perioperative stress with a drug such as acepromazine is recommended. Low dosages (< 0.05 mg/kg) should be used because acepromazine can exacerbate hypothermia via α-adrenoceptor blockade. Analgesic drugs, such as opioids, should be given prior to procedures likely to be painful. Therefore, a technique of neuroleptanalgesia is recommended.

Propofol (Rapinovet), a diazepam-ketamine mixture, and methohexital (Brevital) are drugs used for induction of anesthesia in greyhounds. Even though they are metabolized more slowly in greyhounds, they provide an acceptable recovery. Telazol (tiletamine-zolazapam) is not recommended in sighthounds because of the possibility of poor recoveries. Opioid and benzodiazepine combinations for premedication followed by etomidate can also be used, especially in animals with cardiac disease. Inhalation induction is a safe alternative in compromised animals, provided they are sufficiently sedated or obtunded by their disease state to avoid struggling during mask induction. The comfort of the veterinarian with a given technique and the status of the patient will lead to the right choice.

8. What is meant by "boxer sensitivity to acepromazine" or "boxer-ace syndrome"? What could be the factors influencing its occurrence?

The administration of acepromazine to some boxers can induce a profound bradycardia, associated with hypotension and collapse of the animal. This is a dramatic event experienced by a generation of veterinary clinicians, especially in the United Kingdom. Some clinicians report that doses as low as 0.01 mg/kg given subcutaneously have induced collapse in an otherwise healthy animal. It appears to be related to certain strains of the breed. An explanation for this problem such as excessive vagal response or epinephrine reversal has not been documented.

9. Are large-breed dogs more sensitive to the cardiovascular and respiratory depressant effect of drugs used in an anesthesia protocol?

Not per se. Large dogs are more easily overdosed, and the effects and duration of actions of the drugs will be increased. Drug doses for large dogs ideally should be calculated in relation to body surface area rather than by body weight. Body surface area is difficult to calculate in practice, but an acceptable approximation is to dose the drug in relation to the metabolic weight. Metabolic Weight = Body Weight $(kg)^{3/4}$.

10. Newfoundland dogs do not respond well to anesthesia and tend to be overly depressed by the anesthetic drugs. Is this statement true?

Yes and no. Hypothyroidism is frequently present as a subclinical disease in the Newfoundland dog. Already on the quiet side of the behavior scale, these animals tend to be easily depressed. This can be due to the hypothyroid state and the associated depression of physiologic functions. Whenever in doubt, the health status should be assessed preoperatively with assay of thyroxine (T_4) and triiodothyronine (T_3). A thyroid-stimulating hormone (TSH) response test may be required in equivocal cases.

11. Is it true that toy breeds are more sensitive to the effects of isoflurane?

No. Isoflurane is a potent and hypotensive anesthetic. The rate of rise of the alveolar concentration of this agent when using a high oxygen flow rate on a non-rebreathing system (e.g., Bain) is rapid, and the equilibration time for small body sizes and weights is much faster than for larger dogs. Facemask inductions in toy breeds can be much more rapid than in medium or large breeds.

12. What is the brachycephalic syndrome?

The brachycephalic syndrome is an upper airway obstruction process found in certain breeds of dogs characterized by one or more of the following anatomical or functional abnormalities:
- Stenotic nares
- Elongated soft palate
- Laryngeal saccule eversion
- Laryngeal collapse
- Hypoplastic trachea

Clinical signs are typical of upper airway obstructive disease and include snoring, stridor, exercise intolerance, cyanosis, and collapse.

13. What are brachycephalic breeds?

The following breeds are considered brachycephalic:
- Boston terrier
- Chinese shar pei
- English bulldog
- Pug
- French bulldog
- Lhasa apso
- Pekinese
- Shih tzu

Cross-bred dogs from these breeds can also exhibit signs of the brachycephalic syndrome.

14. What are the preanesthetic considerations when performing anesthesia on a brachy-cephalic dog?

When premedicating these dogs, it is preferable to avoid deep sedation. Deep sedation can be associated with excessive relaxation of upper airway muscles and worsened obstruction. Therefore, if a sedative is to be used, we recommend using a low dose.

Analgesic agents should be used for surgical procedures. Opioids are the most frequently used preanesthetic analgesic agents. Although opioids may cause respiratory depression, this is not a contraindication for their use in brachycephalic dogs. Low doses of opioids should be used to avoid this complication. It is essential to closely monitor the patient after the premedication is administered.

Brachycephalic dogs have strong vagal tone. We therefore recommend using anticholinergic agents (atropine or glycopyrrolate) in the premedication. In addition to preventing bradycardia, these agents will clear the airway from excessive salivary secretions.

15. How should brachycephalic dogs be induced?

It is essential to preoxygenate these breeds of dogs before induction of general anesthesia. This will provide an additional reserve of oxygen in case intubation is difficult and an airway obstruction should occur at induction. Preoxygenation for 5 minutes before induction is time well spent!

Any rapid intravenous induction technique is adequate for brachycephalic dogs. This will allow the veterinarian to rapidly control the airway. It is generally not advised to use slow induction techniques such as mask or chamber inductions.

Intubation is mandatory. Several sizes of endotracheal tubes should be ready. You should always plan to have available an assortment of tubes.

16. When is the best time to extubate a brachycephalic dog?

Recovery is a critical anesthetic phase for any patient, but special attention should be taken for brachycephalic dogs. Time of extubation is an important factor in this phase. Some controversy exists concerning this topic.

Some clinicians prefer a rapid extubation, before signs of the animal waking up have been observed. In this situation, the brachycephalic patient is at a greater risk of upper airway obstruction, but this obstruction will be much easier to manage than in a dysphoric animal emerging from anesthesia. Correct head positioning and reintubation will be accomplished smoothly if the patient is still anesthetized.

Other clinicians prefer to wait for the patient to be almost totally awake and react to the presence of the endotracheal tube before removing it. The advantage of this technique is a lower risk of obstruction and a good protection of the airway at the moment of extubation. If obstruction does occur, however, there is a greater risk of panic from the patient (which can be easily transferred to the anesthetist). Therefore, everything should be ready for rapid reinduction of the animal to allow reintubation, if necessary.

17. What are other specific considerations for the recovery of brachycephalic dogs?

It is important to have drugs and equipment set up for rapid induction and intubation during the recovery phase. Supplemental oxygen should be provided as needed, delivered by face mask or nasal insufflation.

Correct positioning of the patient is often crucial for adequate ventilation. The dog should be kept sternal with the head in extension. Pulling the tongue out (considering that the patient is cooperative!) might help to relieve the obstruction.

If inflammation of the larynx or pharynx is suspected (e.g., in laryngeal surgery), it might be helpful to administer a steroidal anti-inflammatory agent prior to the extubation.

Constant monitoring of the patient should obviously be maintained as long as the animal is still not fully recovered.

18. What special consideration should you have in mind during preanesthetic assessment of a Doberman pinscher?

Dobermans are highly susceptible to von Willebrand disease, a genetic disorder affecting platelet function. It is characterized by a lack of synthesis or an abnormal function of the von Wille-brand factor (vWf). The vWf is essential to the activity of factor VIII, required for platelet adhesion. Coagulation should therefore be assessed before anesthesia of these dogs. A simple bleeding time measurement can be accomplished. It is also possible to measure plasma levels of vWf.

19. Is it possible to prevent hemorrhage in a Doberman pinscher with von Willebrand disease undergoing a surgical procedure?

It is possible to supply active vWf to dogs prior to a surgical procedure by transfusion with fresh whole blood, fresh plasma, fresh frozen plasma, or platelet-rich plasma. The use of desmopressin, a synthetic vasopressin analog, has been suggested because it stimulates the secretion of vWf from storage sites in the vascular endothelium. The response to this therapy is extremely variable and can therefore not be recommended as the sole prophylactic agent to be used in these cases. Good surgical hemostasis is essential.

20. Can stored whole blood or packed red cells be used to provide vWf?

No. Packed red cells do not contain vWf. Blood that has been stored for more than 6 hours does not contain therapeutic levels of vWf.

21. What are the drugs that should be avoided in the anesthetic management of a von Willebrand-positive Doberman pinscher?

There is little information in veterinary anesthesia on the effects of drugs on coagulation. It is reported that phenothiazine tranquilizers (e.g., acepromazine) decrease platelet aggregation and should therefore be avoided. Nonsteroidal anti-inflammatory drugs should also be avoided because they increase clotting time.

22. Are Doberman pinschers the only breed of dogs affected with von Willebrand disease?

No. This disease has been reported in more than 60 breeds of dogs. It is more prevalent in the Doberman pinscher but can be seen in many other dogs, such as the Shetland sheepdog, the Pembroke Welsh corgi, the Scottish terrier, the Airedale, and the standard poodle. DNA detection tests are available for all these breeds.

23. Why are small breed dogs more susceptible to hypothermia?

Small dogs (e.g., Yorkshire terrier, Chihuahua) are more susceptible to hypothermia because they have a lower body weight to surface ratio. The surface exposed for heat loss is therefore larger in these breeds. Techniques should be used to prevent heat loss starting immediately after induction. These techniques include circulating heated water and air blankets, heat lamps, and fluid warming devices. Anesthesia time should be reduced to the minimum possible. Hypothermia can lead to several complications, including increased postoperative infection, coagulopathies, and cardiac morbidity.

24. Can carprofen be used in Labrador retrievers?

A recent study reported idiosyncratic hepatotoxicosis in 21 dogs following carprofen use. More than half of the cases reported were Labrador retrievers. A similar case observed by the authors occurred in a Labrador retriever. Whether this really represents a genetic predisposition remains unknown. Therefore, caution should be taken at this stage for this breed.

BIBLIOGRAPHY

1. Ackerman L: The genetic connection: A Guide to Health Problems in Purebred Dogs. AAHA Press, 1999.
2. Brock N: Acepromazine revisited. Can Vet J 35(7):458–459, 1994.
3. Court M: Anesthesia of the greyhound. Clin Techn Small Anim Pract 14(1):38–43, 1999.
4. MacPhail CM, et al: Hepatocellular toxicosis associated with the administration of carprofen in 21 dogs. J Am Vet Med Assoc 212(12):1895–1901, 1998.
5. The New Lexicon Webster's Dictionary of the English Language, 1989.

41. FELINE ANESTHESIA

Yves Rondenay, D.M.V.,
and Sophie Cuvelliez, D.M.V., M.S., D.A.C.V.A., D.E.C.V.A.

Cats may be pets but will never be entirely domesticated. They are always, or at least often, on the wild side, and this can make them difficult to handle. Furthermore, their small size makes their handling like trying to manipulate delicate flowers with boxing gloves. Even if they are supposed to have nine lives, the utmost care must still be taken when anesthetizing them. Tricks of the trade are useful when working with cats, and this is what we will try to give you in this chapter.

1. A cat is a cat, they all weigh about the same, and a visual examination is enough to evaluate their weight. True or false?

Beware of cats with long hair! They appear a lot heavier than they really are. It is IMPORTANT (if not essential) to have an accurate measurement of the weight. Overdosage of anesthetic drugs is perhaps one of the most common reasons for problems encountered when anesthetizing long-haired cats (e.g., respiratory depression, long recovery).

2. A cat in a box is your next patient. It escaped from its home, was captured by the local humane society, and has to be examined for a skin laceration. He is showing signs of intense aggressiveness. How will you handle this situation?

Aggressive cats are often a veterinarian's nightmare. The use of pheromone (Feliway) in the examination area and on the veterinarian's hand can help to settle the animal. But more often than not, chemical restraint of the animal is needed.

Tranquilization of such a patient is like doing wild animal anesthesia. You do not know the exact weight or the physical status of the animal, and your first goal is to be able to touch and examine the beast in a relatively safe situation for both you and the animal.

Oral administration of ketamine is a practical way to handle such cases. For an average cat (3–4 kg), 1 ml of ketamine (100 mg/ml) is drawn into a 3 ml syringe. A urinary catheter is inserted at the end of the syringe. Tickle the cat on its nose with the catheter to encourage him to bite the catheter. Once the catheter is bitten, a rapid push will squirt the ketamine into the cat's mouth. Considerable salivation is expected; recumbency and a characteristic catatonic position are observed. Prudence is still required when manipulating the cat, but the speed of each parry is greatly reduced!

3. Intravenous catheterization is not easy in all cats, and on tomcats the skin is thick and difficult to go through. How would you handle this situation?

First of all, adequate premedication and restraint are mandatory. Inserting a catheter on a moving target is an unnecessary trial. Even if the skin is thick, and the feline-sized catheter (22-gauge) is unable to penetrate the skin, changing to a bigger catheter will not be the answer; the vein may be small and easily traumatized by a larger catheter. An insertion path (knick) through the skin is needed and can be performed with a 20-gauge needle while the skin is pushed to the side of the vein. The catheter is then inserted though the skin tunnel and does not encounter the resistance from the surrounding tissues.

4. Lidocaine should be used with caution in the cat. Is it true?

Local anesthesia has been rarely used in cats. One reason is the cat is more sensitive than the dog to the toxic effects of lidocaine. Lidocaine is used as an antiarrhythmic agent (class Ib). Its use is associated with neurologic signs of toxicity (e.g., seizures, depression) and with pacemaker depression at dosages as low as 0.5 mg/kg IV. The toxic dose of lidocaine in cats is not readily defined, but we need to be aware of the potential of neurotoxicity. It has been reported that a dose in the order of

10 mg/kg of lidocaine given as an infiltration is a maximum before toxic signs (neurologic signs, seizures and cardiovascular collapse) are seen. This is about 1 to 2 ml of 2% lidocaine for a cat.

5. What is the treatment for lidocaine toxicity?

Diazepam (0.25–0.5 mg/kg), given intravenously.
Barbiturates can be used if the animal is refractory to benzodiazepines, but this is rarely the case.

6. What are the potential uses of local anesthetics in cats?

- Laryngeal desensitization
- Local infiltration (ring block) for declawing
- Local infiltration (local midline block) for caesarian section
- Epidural anesthesia for abdominal procedures or procedures on the hind limbs

7. Describe the technique and dosage for laryngeal desensitization.

Surface analgesia of the larynx to allow endotracheal intubation after induction of anesthesia is performed using 0.1 to 0.2 ml of 2% lidocaine in a 1 mL syringe. The needle is removed and the lidocaine is spread on the arythenoids, or it may be sprayed using an indwelling catheter as a nozzle.

8. Describe the technique and dosages for ring block.

We like to use a mixture of lidocaine (1.5 mg/kg) and bupivacaine (1.5 mg/kg) to achieve a fast onset (in 5–10 minutes) and long duration (4–6 hours) of local analgesia. This dose is for each cat and there are three injection sites per paw (see figure). The superficial branches of the radial nerve are on the dorsomedial aspect of the carpus, the medial nerve and palmar branch of the ulnar nerve are medial to the accessory carpal pad, and the dorsal branch of the ulnar nerve is lateral and proximal to the carpal pad. Therefore, the total volume should be divided by the number of infiltration sites. We use sterile water to dilute the local anesthetic when needed, and a volume of 0.2 ml per site is injected. After insertion of the needle in the subcutaneous tissue, aspiration is performed to avoid intravenous injection.

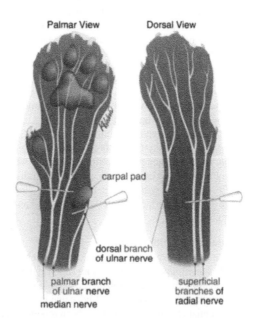

From Tranquilli WJ, Grimm KA, Lamont LA: Pain Management. Jackson WY: Teton New Media, 2000, p. 44, with permission.

9. Describe the technique and dosages for local midline block.

After dilution to a concentration of 1% (10 mg/ml), 1.5 mg/kg of lidocaine can be infiltrated at the site of the incision.

10. Describe the technique and dosages for epidural anesthesia.

As in other species, a sterile preparation of the injection site is mandatory. Local anesthetics are injected at the lumbosacral junction. The spinal cord ends between L7 and S3 in the cat, and the risk of penetrating the subarachnoid space is greater than in the dog.

When in the subarachnoid space, the dose of drugs injected should be reduced to a quarter of the prepared dose. The duration of analgesia provided by lidocaine (45 minutes) is often too short for the surgical procedure and therefore bupivacaine is usually used (4–6 hours' duration).

Dosage is as follows: Lidocaine (2%) or bupivacaine (0.5%), 1 ml/5 kg for a block to L1 and 1 ml/3.5 kg for a block to T4.

11. What are the rationales for using lidocaine to desensitize the arytenoids at the time of intubation? What are the important steps for a successful intubation?

Feline upper airways are fairly reactive. Laryngospasm can be associated with mechanical or chemical stimulation.

• Cats need to be adequately anesthetized prior to intubation. Lack of proper anesthesia can lead to laryngeal spasm, traumatic intubation, or regurgitation of gastric content.

• A laryngoscope will provide a clear view of the larynx. The tip of the laryngoscope should rest on the base of the tongue and **not** touch the epiglottis, as it can cause trauma and edema. Visualization of the larynx is essential.

• A few drops of local anesthetic (0.1–0.2 ml of lidocaine 2% in a 1 mL syringe) squirted directly on the arytenoids will facilitate intubation and minimize the risk of laryngospasm. The spray preparations contain some additives, potentially causing chemical irritation of the larynx. In addition, the rapid flow of air associated with the spray can induce a laryngeal spasm. The content of lidocaine is fairly high in some sprays (about 10 mg of lidocaine per vaporization) and toxic levels are rapidly reached in a small cat. Benzocaine sprays should be avoided for topical laryngeal desensitization, as their use has been associated with development of methemoglobinemia in dogs and cats.

• The use of a stylet may provide some rigidity to a flimsy endotracheal tube. Be careful not to let it protrude from the distal tip (the tip going down the trachea), as tracheal laceration can occur.

12. What should be done if a cat has a laryngeal spasm during tracheal intubation?

If the larynx does not relax within 10 to 20 seconds after the first attempt, it may be necessary to deepen the anesthesia. In any case oxygen should be supplied by mask, so that any mixture of gas that does enter the trachea is oxygen enriched. Local anesthetic could be used if it has not already been applied.

If extra time and deepening anesthesia do not resolve the spasm (which they usually do), neuromuscular blockade is indicated. Neuromuscular blocking agents such as succinylcholine or atracurium can be used.

A male canine polypropylene urinary catheter (6–8Fr) can be manipulated gently between closed arytenoids. Once through the glottis, an endotracheal tube can often be slipped into position over the catheter. It is advisable to preplace the catheter through the endotracheal tube before insertion.

A temporary airway can also be provided with a large needle or catheter placed in the trachea percutaneously.

13. Hyperthyroidism is a pathologic condition typically developed in older cats. Thyroidectomy is the treatment often performed. What are the important problems for anesthesia associated with this multisystemic disease?

• Age
• Temperament, hyperactivity, and aggression
• Weight loss, muscle weakness, and polyphagia

- Polyuria, polydypsia, and altered renal function
- Tachycardia and potential arrhythmias

Cats with hyperthyroidism tend to be older skinny cats with a bad temper (or an attitude). The weight loss will affect their ability to maintain normothermia. Polyuria, polydipsia, and vomiting are frequent. They tend to have an accelerated metabolic rate and a hyperdynamic circulation. They have an elevated heart rate and increased cardiac output and glomerular filtration rate and frequently develop hypertrophic cardiomyopathy. They are prone to arrhythmias and are sensitive to the arrhythmogenic effects of catecholamines. It is hypothesized that the number and the sensitivity of β-receptors on the myocardium are increased during hyperthyroidism. The use of β-blocking drugs (propanolol, esmolol) preoperatively is often part of the stabilization of the animal prior to anesthesia. Drugs that have catecholamine-like effects (e.g., ketamine) should be avoided, as well as arrhythmogenic (e.g., xylazine) drugs and drugs that increase heart rate (e.g., atropine, glycopyrrolate).

14. After stabilization of the patient, what anesthetic protocol could be used in a cat with hyperthyroidism?

The physical status of the animal *must* be assessed prior to any medication and a euthyroid state is obtained with adequate medical treatment. Neuroleptanalgesia, the combination of an opioid and low dose of acepromazine, for example, is a good premedication for these cats.

Induction should be as stress-free as possible, and (after 5 minutes of preoxygenation) a rapid induction technique such as intravenous administration of propofol or thiopental is suggested. The use of thiopental is controversial because even though it has antithyroid effects, it sensitizes the myocardium to the arrhythmogenic effects of catecholamines. After intubation and connection to an anesthesia machine, anesthesia is maintained with isoflurane in oxygen.

Close monitoring of heart and respiratory rate, electrocardiographic activity, arterial blood pressure, and body temperature are essential.

15. What are the potential complications during a thyroidectomy?

Stimulation of the thyroid can induce a "thyroid storm" associated with an acute and persistent tachycardia. A β-blocker (e.g., propranolol 0.01–0.05 mg/kg IV) can be used to treat this problem. Caution should be taken with a cat in congestive heart failure because of the negative inotropic effect of the drug.

Bleeding at the surgery site is another potential intraoperative complication. The anesthetist should guard against compression of the trachea by the surgeon's hands, the instruments, or the gauzes used on the surgery site.

16. What are the potential complications after a thyroidectomy?

Recovery from anesthesia is an important step in the management of such cases. *Hypothermia* is to be controlled and body temperature restored to normal level. The occurrence of *obstruction of the airways* in the recovery period is to be monitored. It can be progressive or acute, associated with the development of seromas or hematomas at the level of the surgery site. An acute occurrence may be associated with trauma to the recurrent laryngeal nerve, larynx paralysis, or airway obstruction at the time of extubation. Emergency anesthesia and intubation or tracheotomy are treatments for this problem.

The parathyroid glands are sometimes accidentally included in the removed thyroid tissue. Subsequent *hypocalcemia* can appear in the 12–24 hours postoperative period (monitoring for 3 days). Muscle tremors, tetany, or convulsions will respond to intravenous treatment with calcium and vitamin D.

17. Hepatic lipidosis often requires the insertion of a gastric tube to provide adequate nutrition. It can be done through an esophagostomy or a gastric tube. Whatever the choice, general anesthesia is required. What are the concerns associated with anesthetizing a cat in hepatic lipidosis?

Cats with hepatic lipidosis are usually fat, have been eating very little or nothing for the past few weeks, and may show signs of muscle wasting. Hepatic lipidosis is associated with liver dysfunction. The extent of the dysfunction can be variable; therefore, evaluation of both clinical signs and serum chemistry prior to anesthesia is essential. The consequences of this condition as they affect anesthetic management are the following:

• Alteration of thermoregulation and modification of body tissue composition: hypothermia is often a problem encountered when body temperature is not aggressively controlled.

• Alteration of drug metabolism: The duration of the effects of drugs metabolized in the liver will be increased.

• Hypoproteinemia: for equal amounts of drug injected in the bloodstream, there will be more free, and therefore active, form of the drug.

• Anemia and coagulopathy: the anemia may be nonregenerative and the coagulopathy, even if unusual, can modify the management of the patient.

• The animal usually is not eating or drinking adequately and the hydration status may be deficient. Dehydration must be corrected prior to anesthesia.

18. What factors will guide your choice of drugs to anesthetize a cat with hepatic lipidosis?

Evaluation of the animal's health status prior to medication is essential. The choice should be based on the following rules:

• Minimal side effects.

• Lack of liver metabolism. Drugs such as acepromazine are contraindicated.

• Short duration of action or reversibility of its effects. Propofol with its short duration of action at a low dose (3–4 mg/kg) is a good induction drug; ketamine is another good choice.

• No effect on coagulation. Drugs such as acepromazine or nonsteroidal anti-inflammatory drugs are contraindicated.

• No or little effect on hepatic blood flow. Drugs with minimal cardiovascular effects are recommended.

19. Should pure μ-agonist opioids be used in cats?

Yes, they should be used. There is a traditional fear that pure opioids (e.g., morphine, oxymorphone, meperidine) may cause paradoxical excitement in the feline patient. Athough this is true in some cases, this excitement is easy to control if the analgesic is combined with a sufficient dose of a sedative agent such as acepromazine. Furthermore, this excitement is seen only with high doses of opioids and will not be seen when appropriate feline doses are used (e.g., 0.1 mg/kg morphine). Pure μ-agonists opioids provide the most reliable analgesia in cats, and we strongly support their use for any painful surgical procedures.

20. Can doses of μ-agonist opioids used in dogs be extrapolated to cats?

No, they should not be. Cats appear to be more sensitive to opioids than dogs, so more conservative dosages should be used. This is because of the paradoxical excitement that can be seen in cats (see question 19) and new evidence that the pharmacokinetics of opioids differs greatly in cats when compared with dogs.

21. Can propofol be used to induce a cat with hepatic lipidosis?

Yes, it is an induction agent of choice for cats with hepatic lipidosis. Although it is primarily metabolized in the liver, alternate routes of extraction exist, with the lung being an important one. It is reported that up to 61% of the propofol is extracted after the first pass through the lungs in cats.

22. Can cats be anesthetized repeatedly or maintained long term on propofol?

Propofol is a phenolic compound. Phenolic compounds are metabolized using glucuronide conjugation. Cats have a limited concentration of enzymes responsible for this pathway. Feline red blood cells can be damaged by oxidative compounds following repeated exposure to propofol. This results in excessive Heinz body formation, delayed recovery and signs of general illness such as anorexia, diarrhea, and malaise.

Propofol is not recommended for repeated or long-term maintenance of anesthesia in cats. This is in contrast to dogs or humans, in whom propofol is the agent of choice in this situation because of lack of accumulation and absence of delayed recoveries.

23. Can propofol cause compulsive behavior in cats?

It is an anecdotal observation that cats recovering from propofol anesthesia frequently exhibit compulsive pawing of the face. From that experience, we prefer to avoid this drug for ophthalmic procedures or any facial surgery in cats. The exact reason for this phenomenon is not known. Compulsive pawing of the face has also been observed in cats during anesthesia that did not include propofol.

24. Should acepromazine be avoided in a cat suffering from hypertrophic cardiomyopathy?

Not necessarily. It is true that high doses of acepromazine will have a peripheral vasodilation effect (α_1-antagonist) and will cause severe hypotension and decreased cardiac filling. However, low doses (0.03–0.05 mg/kg) can be beneficial because they will decrease afterload, myocardial oxygen consumption and the incidence of catecholamine-induced arrhythmias. It is obvious that if the condition is an end-stage disease process and the cat is in heart failure, acepromazine will be contraindicated; otherwise, its use at the lower end of the dosage can be beneficial.

25. What drugs are contraindicated for the induction of a cat suffering from hypertrophic cardiomyopathy?

Dissociative anesthetic agents (tiletamine, ketamine) should be avoided. This class of drugs increases sympathetic activity and by consequence increases heart rate and myocardial oxygen consumption; it also decreases diastolic filling time. The use of dissociatives could cause rapid decompensation and fatal arrhythmias in these cats.

Barbiturates can induce transient tachycardia, and they sensitize the myocardium to catecholamine-induced arrhythmias. They should therefore be avoided for the induction of cardiomyopathic cats.

26. What fluid rate should be used in cats suffering from hypertrophic cardiomyopathy?

It is essential to avoid fluid overload and subsequent pulmonary edema in these patients. Fluid administration should be carefully monitored and be adjusted according to the central venous pressure, blood pressure, and fluid losses. Fluid rate should be approximately 5 to 10 ml/kg/hr.

27. I do not like injectable anesthetics in cats. Can I anesthetize all my patients using an induction chamber or by mask induction?

This approach is not recommend for several reasons:

• Induction with volatile agents is more stressful than with injectables.
• Stress can cause severe cardiac arrhythmias and increase morbidity and mortality.
• If no premedication is used, this protocol would not provide any postanesthetic analgesia.
• Monitoring is difficult in an induction chamber.
• Environmental contamination when opening the chamber or from leaks from the induction mask is greater with this technique.

BIBLIOGRAPHY

1. Andres, JL, Day TK, Day DG: The effect of consecutive day propofol anesthesia on feline red blood cells Veterinary Surgery 24(3) 277-288, 1995.
2. Bedford PGC:, Small Animal Anaesthesia. London, Baillière Tindall, 1991.
3. Hall and Taylor. Anaesthesia of the Cat. London, Baillière Tindall,1994.
4. Tranquilli WJ, Grimm KA, Lamont LA: Pain management for the small animal practitioner. Teton New Media, 2000.

42. EQUINE ANESTHESIA

Stephen A. Greene, D.V.M., M.S., D.A.C.V.A.,
and Robert D. Keegan, D.V.M., D.A.C.V.A.

1. What are the effects of anesthetics on the equine alimentary system?

Many drugs used in the perianesthetic period can have effects on the gastrointestinal system of horses. **Opioids** may decrease intestinal motility, but this effect is usually of minor importance. **Xylazine** prolongs gastrointestinal transit time in a variety of species. In the horse, xylazine (0.55 mg/kg IV) decreases the motility index of circular and longitudinal muscle layers for 30 minutes. In ponies, xylazine (1.1 mg/kg IV) increases vascular resistance, motility, and oxygen consumption. In a study of cecal and right ventral colon myoelectric activity in ponies, xylazine (0.5 mg/kg IV) and/or **butorphanol** (0.04 mg/kg IV) resulted in decreased coordinated spike bursts for 20 minutes or longer. Clinically, these effects are rarely a disadvantage to using xylazine for preanesthetic medication in horses.

Succinylcholine is a depolarizing neuromuscular blocking agent that initially causes contraction of skeletal muscle. Distention of the stomach, abdomen, or bladder predisposes to rupture of these organs if succinylcholine is administered prior to relief of the excess pressure.

Halothane has been associated with a 62% decrease in intestinal blood flow in ponies anesthetized at 1 minimal alveolar concentration (MAC). Halothane anesthesia in ponies is associated with decreased bile acid excretion and increased conjugated bilirubin excretion. In ponies anesthetized with isoflurane, only biliary bilirubin excretion was increased.

Isoflurane increases hepatic artery blood flow at both 1 and 2 MAC in humans, whereas halothane preserves hepatic arterial flow at 1 MAC but decreases it at 2 MAC. The use of halothane in horses with hepatic disease is not contraindicated unless previous exposure to halothane resulted in unexplained hepatitis. The presence of hepatic disease does not necessarily result in increased hepatotoxicity when the patient is subsequently exposed to an unpredictable hepatotoxin such as halothane. Effects of **sevoflurane** on equine hepatic or intestinal blood flow have not been determined.

2. What are the effects of anticholinergic agents on equine gastrointestinal motility?

Anticholinergic agents are occasionally used in horses for treatment of vagal-induced bradycardia. When used in high doses (e.g., 0.04 mg/kg), the anticholinergics decrease gastrointestinal motility for up to 12 hours in horses. Recently fed horses that are anesthetized have developed colic. However, recently fed horses treated with anticholinergics are more likely to develop colic or cardiopulmonary distress. Horses withheld from feed for 4–6 hours before administration of anticholinergics are less likely to develop gastrointestinal distress. Horses that are fasted and given low doses of atropine (e.g., 2–5 mg total dose for a 450-kg horse) for treatment of bradycardia during anesthesia are not particularly likely to develop significant gastrointestinal stasis.

3. Describe the anesthetic management of horses with acute abdominal distress.

Horses with acute abdominal distress often present with pain as a primary problem. It is difficult to perform diagnostic procedures or a physical examination on a horse in pain. Pain may elicit various responses, including release of catecholamines and corticosteroids. The stress response and the sympathetic nervous system stimulation that result from pain are detrimental to the animal's well-being. Judicious use of analgesics in the painful horse with acute abdominal distress is advised.

The **alpha-2 agonists** such as xylazine and detomidine (Domosedan, Farmos Laboratories) are often the first analgesics administered because they are sedatives as well as potent analgesics. It is important to know how much xylazine or detomidine has been administered as an analgesic in the preoperative period to evaluate anesthetic depth accurately during surgery because, even though the sedative and analgesic effects of these drugs may be diminished, the anesthetic requirement for other drugs is still decreased. The induction dose of xylazine may be decreased or avoided to prevent deleterious cardiovascular effects. A decreased dose of xylazine should be given followed by **diazepam** (0.02–0.04 mg/kg) or guiafenesin (55–80 mg/kg) IV. Induction is accomplished with **ketamine** (0.35–0.45 mg/kg) or thiopental (4–5 mg/kg) IV. The horse is maintained with **halothane**, isoflurane, or sevoflurane in oxygen.

Opioid agonists such as oxymorphone (Numorphan, DuPont), morphine, butorphanol, and meperidine can be safely used in horses experiencing pain. These agents frequently induce undesirable excitement in horses that are not painful unless preceded with a suitable sedative or tranquilizer.

In addition to pain control, **support of the respiratory and cardiovascular systems** is paramount in managing anesthesia for colic surgery. Evaluation of acid–base status aids in determining adequacy of ventilation. Extreme respiratory acidosis (pH < 7.2) should be avoided by use of controlled ventilation. Aggressive fluid therapy with lactated Ringer's solution aids in correcting mild-to-moderate metabolic acidosis if normovolemia is re-established. It is common for a horse to require 30 or more liters of intravenous fluids during the course of colic surgery.

Monitoring of arterial blood pressure is recommended to prevent decreased tissue perfusion which has been implicated in the occurrence of post-anesthetic myositis. Mean blood pressure may be maintained above 60 mm Hg by fluid administration, adjustment of anesthetic depth, and careful infusion of a catecholamine such as dobutamine (3–5 ug/kg/min). Cardiac output improves when intravenous fluids are administered to the hemoconcentrated patient. A packed cell volume of less than 55% helps reduce blood viscosity and improves cardiac output.

Compromised intestine may release toxins into the systemic circulation and can lead to cardiovascular dysfunction and decreased tissue perfusion. Administration of flunixin meglumine (1 mg/kg) may counteract deleterious effects of toxins released during abdominal surgery.

4. What are the effects of anesthetics on the equine respiratory system?

In general, anesthetics and anesthetic adjuncts cause dose-dependent respiratory depression. Anesthetics increase the threshold of carbon dioxide tension necessary to stimulate the respiratory center. Thus, hypercapnia is a frequent finding in anesthetized horses.

In standing, awake horses, the matching of pulmonary perfusion with alveolar ventilation is optimized. In anesthetized horses, however, dramatic imbalances in ventilation and perfusion may be observed. This is often referred to as ventilation/perfusion mismatch or V/Q mismatch. When V/Q mismatch occurs, arterial oxygen tension may decrease, producing hypoxemia. In large animals, the lowest portions of the lung are at greatest risk for atelectasis and decreased alveolar ventilation. Positioning of the anesthetized horse can affect the degree of V/Q mismatch. Dorsal recumbency impairs V/Q matching the most and usually causes low arterial oxygen tension. Laterally recumbent horses tend to mismatch less than horses in dorsal recumbency. Because the left lung is smaller than the right, better V/Q matching is expected with horses in left lateral recumbency compared with right lateral recumbency.

5. How can we support the equine respiratory system during general anesthesia?

Controlled ventilation using a mechanical ventilator is an effective way to decrease arterial carbon dioxide tension and may improve the arterial oxygen tension in anesthetized, hypercapnic, healthy horses. However, controlled ventilation does not necessarily increase arterial oxygen tension in compromised patients. Positive pressure ventilation has the potential to decrease venous return to the heart and thus decreases cardiac output. Decreased perfusion of the lung and peripheral tissues may result. In addition, when atelectasis has occurred, positive pressure ventilation may produce overexpansion of the uncollapsed alveoli while opening only a few atelectic alveoli. This can further impair lung perfusion and decrease arterial oxygen tension. The decision to mechanically ventilate the anesthetized horse should be based on some measure of respiratory efficiency such as P_aCO_2. Positive pressure ventilation in horses may be most effective when begun immediately after induction. Delay in instituting positive pressure ventilation may allow atelectasis to progress to such an extent that reversal with conventional ventilators is not possible without producing detrimental effects on cardiovascular function.

During anesthesia, the hemodynamic responses to either hypocapnia or hypercapnia differ from those observed in conscious subjects because the sympathetically mediated component of the circulatory response to changes in P_aCO_2 can be obtunded by some anesthetic agents or enhanced by others. Carbon dioxide is a direct dilator of systemic vascular beds. In addition, increased P_aCO_2 is a potent stimulus for medullary vasomoter centers and results in increased sympathetic nervous system activity and increased secretion of catecholamines. Hypercapnia has been associated with acidosis and with dysrhythmias. The net effect of carbon dioxide on cardiovascular performance is a product of the relative balance between its direct and indirect effects. The relationship between cardiac output and P_aCO_2 is greatly dependent on the anesthetic agent used. Mild-to-moderate hypercapnia (P_aCO_2 between 45–80 mmHg) was associated with positive inotropic effects on the heart in halothane-anesthetized horses. However, further study of hypercapnia in anesthetized horses is required to determine whether myocardial performance is improved enough to outweigh the effects of respiratory acidosis or potential dysrhythmias associated with varying degrees of increased P_aCO_2.

Antagonism of V/Q mismatch has been achieved using special equipment for selective endo-bronchial intubation of the caudal lung lobes. Apparently, much of the pulmonary perfusion in anesthetized horses is directed to the caudodorsal lung regions, regardless of body orientation with respect to gravity. Thus, V/Q matching improved when ventilation was selectively directed to the better-perfused lung lobes. In addition, arterial oxygen tension in hypoxemic, anesthetized horses has improved following IV administration of the beta agonist, clenbuterol.

6. What special anesthetic considerations are recommended for equine laryngeal surgery?

Laryngeal surgery predisposes the equine patient to postoperative airway obstruction. Blood and secretions in the larynx may stimulate laryngospasm. Laryngeal paralysis or laryngospasm may occur after extubation of the horse, resulting in airway obstruction. Horses extubated late (i.e., when awake) may be more likely to develop laryngospasm than those extubated early (i.e., at the first sign of swallowing). Acute airway obstruction is a life-threatening situation. Acute, fulminant pulmonary edema may occur following laryngeal obstruction. If laryngeal obstruction occurs, emergency tracheostomy or immediate orotracheal intubation (usually under general anesthesia) is required.

Before induction of anesthesia for laryngeal surgery, a tracheostomy may be performed and the horse intubated through the stoma. This technique avoids problems associated with edema or altered laryngeal function in the recovery period.

When orotracheal intubation is used, the endotracheal tube is periodically removed during some surgeries. Usually, the trachea is easily reintubated with digital guidance by the surgeon and/or manipulation of the patient's head and neck. For difficult reintubation, a sterile stomach tube or canine endotracheal tube (9–10 mm) can be passed retrograde through the glottis by the surgeon to guide the endotracheal tube into the trachea.

If laryngostomy or tracheostomy is not performed, astute observation of the horse during recovery is necessary, especially at the time of tracheal extubation. Nasal congestion is a frequent occurrence in horses anesthetized for a long period. Laryngeal obstruction can be differentiated from nasal congestion, which presents as flaring of the nostrils with stridorous passage of air through the nasal passages and into the lungs. True laryngospasm is silent with no flow of air through the larynx. Laryngeal paralysis allows only small amounts of air to pass the larynx. Nasal congestion can be relieved by spraying the nasal mucosa at inspiration with aerosolized 0.5% or 1.0% phenylephrine. Phenylephrine has little or no effect in horses that develop laryngospasm or laryngeal paralysis.

7. Describe the cardiovascular effects of anesthetics in horses.

Most drugs used during anesthesia, including barbiturates, halothane, isoflurane, sevoflurane, xylazine, detomidine, ketamine, Telazol, acepromazine, guaifenisen, anticholinergics, and opioids, exert some significant effect on cardiovascular function. Alpha-2 agonists and opioids may decrease heart rate and, therefore, cardiac output. Other drugs, including isoflurane, halothane, sevoflurane, guaifenesin, and acepromazine may decrease arterial blood pressure. These cardiovascular effects are usually dose-related. Sevoflurane and isoflurane produce less reduction of cardiac output than halothane at equipotent levels of anesthesia.

Combinations of injectable anesthetic agents may produce variable cardiovascular effects. The combination of guaifenesin, xylazine, and ketamine for IV infusion maintains adequate blood pressure in horses and ponies.

8. How can we support the cardiovascular system in anesthetized horses?

Cardiovascular support during equine anesthesia is usually best managed by attention to anesthetic depth and IV fluid administration. Inhaled anesthetics are potent vasodilators and decrease cardiac output in a dose-dependent manner. Judicious use of lactated Ringer's solution or other balanced electrolyte solutions can promote improved arterial blood pressure by increasing cardiac preload and subsequently increasing cardiac output. In some instances, a catecholamine such as dobutamine (3–5 ug/kg/min) may be infused to improve cardiac output. Monitoring of blood pressure and the electrocardiogram or pulse for increased heart rate and dysrhythmias is recommended when infusing catecholamine solutions.

Bradycardia is treated by intravenous infusion of the beta agonist, isoproterenol (0.01–0.2 µg/kg/min), administration of atropine (0.005–0.01 mg/kg), or glycopyrrolate (0.01 mg/kg). If atropine is used prior to catecholamine infusion, severe tachycardia or conduction disturbances may occur.

9. How are intraoperative dysrhythmias managed in horses?

When possible, routine evaluation of the electrocardiogram should be part of the preanesthetic evaluation. Auscultation of the heart and palpation of the pulse may alert the clinician to the presence of conduction disturbances. Significant dysrhythmias (e.g., atrial fibrillation) should be corrected prior to anesthesia when possible. Many unmedicated athletic horses and most horses given xylazine IV demonstrate bradycardia and/or first- or second-degree heart block. Athletic horses usually develop a normal heart rate and rhythm when exercised. The presence of a first- or second-degree heart block should prompt close monitoring of the cardiac rate and rhythm following preanesthetic medication. It is preferable to avoid the use of xylazine in debilitated horses or horses exhibiting severe bradycardia and heart block. Diazepam (0.03 mg/kg IV) or acepromazine (0.044 mg/kg IV) can be used effectively before a barbiturate/guaifenesin induction.

Premature ventricular contractions (PVC's) during anesthesia are encountered infrequently, but they require immediate attention. Hypoxia, hypercapnia, electrolyte abnormalities, improper anesthetic depth, catecholamine infusion, and pain can be associated with development of PVCs. The cause of the PVCs should be determined and corrected. Lidocaine (1 mg/kg IV) is often effective for treatment of PVC's during anesthesia.

10. What are common causes of postanesthetic lameness in horses?

Postanesthetic lameness may occur after anesthesia of poorly positioned or inadequately padded horses. Particularly susceptible to damage are the facial, radial, and peroneal nerves. The head, shoulder, and extremeties should be properly padded to prevent these neuropathies. Limbs that hang over the edge of a table are at risk for neurologic damage and should be well supported and adequately padded. The nondependent rear limb should be elevated to relieve the dependent limb of the excess weight. Although many neuropathies will resolve in 24–72 hours, the lameness that occurs may prevent a horse from standing after anesthesia. Unfortunately, this scenario occasionally results in agitation, frenzied behavior, self-inflicted trauma, and, possibly, euthanasia.

11. Describe the technique for local anesthesia of the eye in horses.

To facilitate examination of the eye, blockade of the motor nerve supplying the eyelids is desirable. The auriculopalpebral nerve is blocked at the dorsal point of the zygomatic arch with 5 ml of 2% lidocaine via a 22-gauge needle. The auriculopalpebral nerve is a branch of the facial division of the trigeminal nerve and carries only motor fibers to the orbicularis oculi muscles. Additional motor fibers come from the palpebral branch of the supraorbital nerve. Blockade of the supraorbital nerve with 2 ml of 2% lidocaine at the supraorbital foramen prevents perception of sensations from the middle portion of the upper eyelid. Note that blocking the auriculopalpebral and supraorbital nerves does not provide complete analgesia of the orbit. For minor eye surgery topical analgesia can be combined with sedation from xylazine, tranquilization by acepromazine, or other methods of chemical restraint. However, surgery of the equine eye is best facilitated through the use of general anesthesia.

12. What are the major considerations for eye surgery under general anesthesia in horses?

Significant amounts of topical medications such as anticholinergics, local analgesics, or epinephrine applied to the eye or conjunctiva may be absorbed and produce systemic effects. Gentamicin and other aminoglycoside antibiotics can potentiate neuromuscular relaxation produced by general anesthetics, potentially affecting the quality of ventilation or rate of recovery from anesthesia. Phenylbutazone can displace highly protein-bound drugs such as barbiturates and may prolong recovery when administered during anesthesia.

Manipulation of the eye during surgery may elicit the oculocardiac reflex and cause bradycardia. Premedication with atropine may prevent this reflex. If the cornea is to be incised, an oil-based ophthalmic ointment should not be used because it may result in uveitis.

For intraocular surgery, the horse should be maintained at an adequate anesthetic depth to prevent nystagmus or rotation of the globe. Usually, surgical conditions are adequate with routine general anesthesia, but nondepolarizing neuromuscular blocking agents may provide appropriate muscle relaxation to stabilize the eyeball. Pancuronium (0.08 mg/kg IV), and atracurium (0.07 mg/kg IV) have been used successfully for this purpose. These agents can be antagonised using edrophonium. Avoid the use of depolarizing neuromuscular blocking agents such as succinylcholine during ophthalmic procedures. The muscle fasciculations produced by depolarizing agents may eviscerate a weakened or opened eye by increasing intraocular pressure when the extraocular muscles contract.

13. What are effects of sedatives/tranquilizers on penile relaxation in horses?

For examination of the penis, sufficient penile relaxation can be achieved with xylazine or detomidine. Occasionally, "high-flanking" retained testicles descend into the scrotum after administration of an alpha-2 agonist. Prolonged prolapse of the penis has not been associated with use of alpha-2 agonists in horses. However, paralysis of the retractor penis muscle and persistent penile prolapse have been associated with the use of phenothiazine tranquilizers including promazine, chlorpromazine, propriopromazine, and acepromazine.

14. What special concerns should be kept in mind during anesthesia for ovariectomy in mares?

Ovarian tumor removal or ovariectomy may be performed using routine anesthetic protocols. Hemorrhage may be excessive in difficult cases, and placement of one or two-large bore intravenous catheters permits aggressive fluid administration. Significant hypotension may occur at the time of ligation of the ovarian stump. Standing ovariectomy has been performed through a flank incision using sedative and analgesic combinations such as xylazine (1.0 mg/kg IV) and butorphanol (0.01 mg/kg IV), with additional doses of butorphanol administered as needed. In addition, the incision site may be blocked with a local anesthetic using an inverted "L" technique. Ovariectomy performed via laparoscopy may necessitate tilting the horse in a "head-down" position to facilitate visualization. A severe angle of tilt may dramatically impede respiratory function. Mechanical ventilation should be instituted before tilting the table. Ventilator settings that would normally induce hyperventilation may be required to prevent atelectasis and severe ventilation/perfusion mismatch during this positioning.

15. How can analgesia for perineal procedures be provided to standing horses?

Sedation and perineal analgesia for horses may be accomplished using various combinations. Xylazine or detomidine may be given with an opioid and then combined with epidural analgesia for many procedures such as repair of rectovaginal fistula. Avoid use of acepromazine when performing epidural administration of local anesthetics to minimize the potential for systemic hypotension.

16. Describe the technique for epidural analgesia in horses.

Epidural analgesia may be accomplished by using local anesthetics such as 2% lidocaine, dilute solutions of xylazine, or combinations of xylazine and local anesthetics. The epidural space can be entered at the sacrococcygeal interspace or at the first and second coccygeal interspace. Epidural injection of 8–10 ml of 2% lidocaine provides about 90 minutes of analgesia. Horses may lose motor coordination of the hind limbs if larger doses of local anesthetic are administered. Xylazine has been injected into the epidural space of ponies and horses. Advantages of using xylazine instead of local anesthetics in the epidural space include less loss of motor nerve function and longer duration of analgesia. Xylazine (0.15 mg/kg diluted to 10 ml with isotonic saline) injected in the sacrococcygeal interspace provides up to 3 hours of analgesia. Epidural injection of the combination of xylazine (0.15 mg/kg) and lidocaine has the advantage of providing a rapid onset of analgesia (seen with administration of lidocaine) as well as a long duration of analgesia that is characteristic of xylazine administration.

17. What are the effects of alpha-2 adrenoceptor agonists on urinary output in the horse?

Xylazine and detomidine can dramatically increase urinary output and reduce urinary osmolality. To prevent possible rupture of the urinary bladder, alpha-2 agonists should not be used in animals with urethral obstruction.

18. Describe anesthetic management of ruptured urinary bladder in foals.

Rupture of the urinary bladder is an emergency situation in foals. Animals may become hyperkalemic, hyponatremic, hypochloremic, and acidotic after rupture of the urinary bladder. Intravenous fluids, such as isotonic saline, should be given to aid in correcting electrolyte imbalances. An electrocardiogram should be performed before induction to determine if cardiac dysrhythmias are present. Anesthesia may be induced using an inhalant. In larger foals, xylazine (1.1 mg/kg IV) and ketamine (2.2 mg/kg IV) can be used for induction; anesthesia is maintained with sevoflurane or isoflurane. Foals that are depressed may be induced with greatly decreased doses of injectable induction agents. Large foals that are greatly depressed may also be induced with inhalation agents. Isoflurane or sevoflurane is preferred over halothane because of minimal myocardial depression and relative lack of cardiac dysrhythmia potentiation.

19. Which horses are at greater risk for development of postanesthetic myopathy?

Heavily muscled horses and horses with a history of muscle cramping, apprehensiveness, or recent hard exercise are at a higher risk for developing myopathy during anesthesia. Adequate padding should be used, and mean arterial blood pressure should be maintained above 60 mm Hg since hypotension is a probable causative factor for postanesthetic myopathy. Extreme flexion or overextension of limbs should be avoided. In one clinical study, flexion of the hind limbs in halothane-anesthetized horses positioned in dorsal recumbency coupled with a period of hypotension (mean arterial blood pressure < 70 mmHg for more than 45 minutes), was associated with ischemic necrosis of the adductor muscles. Serum biochemical profiles from affected horses usually demonstrate increased creatine kinase.

20. How is postanesthetic myopathy treated?

Treatment is directed at relief of pain and swelling of affected muscles. Stall rest, intravenous fluid administration (e.g., lactated Ringer's solution), nonsteroidal anti-inflammatory agents (e.g., flunixin meglumine, 10 mg/kg IV), prednisolone (0.25 mg/kg IV), and dantrolene have been recommended for treatment of postanesthetic myopathy. Skeletal muscle relaxants such as methocarbamol and opioids for analgesia have also been advocated. Severe cases may require euthanasia.

21. What is "tying up" syndrome?

"Tying up" syndrome, postanesthetic myopathy, and malignant hyperthermia (MH) may be various manifestations of a common metabolic disturbance. MH is a generalized condition that appears as progressive hyperthermia, hypercapnia, and acute myopathy. It is occasionally seen in horses and represents an abnormality in excitation-contraction coupling of the sarcoplasmic reticulum with a disturbance in intracellular calcium transport. Inhalation anesthetics, succinylcholine, and local anesthetics with an amide structure have been implicated as triggering agents that may induce MH. Horses with familial history of MH-like reactions should not be anesthetized with these agents. If signs of MH occur during anesthesia, the anesthetic agents should be changed to drugs not associated with this syndrome (e.g., guaifenesin and thiopental). Anesthesia should be stopped as soon as possible. Cardiac and respiratory function should be supported as necessary; body temperature should be reduced with cool IV fluids and an ice water or alcohol bath. Dantrolene sodium (2–3.5 mg/kg IV) is effective for treatment of MH. Dantrolene decreases calcium release from the sarcoplasmic reticulum while calcium uptake continues. MH-susceptible horses can be premedicated with dantrolene, 10 mg/kg, via nasogastric tube.

22. How is susceptibility to malignant hyperthermia determined?

Muscle biopsy for preanesthetic identification of MH-susceptible horses has been described. Muscle samples are tested in-vitro using sensitivity to halothane- and/or caffeine-induced contracture as a reliable measure of susceptibility. Biopsy sample preparation and shipping requirements for halothane-caffeine contracture testing vary among laboratories. A familial history of MH is a good reason to avoid inhaled anesthetics.

23. What are common induction techniques for foals?

Foals weighing less than 120 kg are readily anesthetized by face-mask administration of halothane, isoflurane, or sevoflurane. An alternative is nasotracheal intubation followed by inhalation anesthetic induction. The technique involves insertion of a 9 or 10 mm (id) silicone endotracheal tube lubricated with 10% lidocaine gel into a nostril. The tube is gently advanced to the pharynx. The neck is extended, and the tube is advanced through the glottis during inspiration. The awake foal tolerates this procedure well. Xylazine can be used (0.5 mg/kg IM) to facilitate intubation in larger or less cooperative foals. The tube is secured to the muzzle and connected to the anesthetic circuit. Following preoxygenation, the cuff is inflated as needed, and the seal is checked by applying positive pressure. An adequate seal prevents the foal from smelling the inhalation agent and decreases airway irritation during induction. Inductions are usually smooth and rapid using 5% isoflurane or 8% sevoflurane delivered in oxygen (5 L/min).

24. How does anesthesia differ in ponies compared with horses?

Adult ponies can be anesthetized in a manner similar to horses. Ponies generally are less responsive (on a mg/kg basis) to the sedative effects of xylazine or detomidine, and the dose is frequently increased by about 20% to obtain the desired effect, especially when used before ketamine induction.

25. How does the sedative effect of xylazine differ in donkeys and mules compared with horses?

Donkeys and mules are typically less sensitive to the sedative effects of xylazine than horses. The xylazine dose for donkeys or mules is 1.3–1.5 mg/kg IV or 2.6–3.0 mg/kg IM.

BIBLIOGRAPHY

1. Hubbell JAE: Anesthesia and immobilization of specific species: horses. In Thurmon JC, Tranquilli WJ, Benson GJ (eds): Lumb and Jones' Veterinary Anesthesia. Philadelphia, Lippincott, Williams & Wilkins, 1996, pp 599–609.
2. Muir WW, Hubbell JAE: Equine Anesthesia: Monitoring and Emergency Therapy. St. Louis, Mosby, 1991.
3. Taylor PM, Clarke KW: Handbook of Equine Anaesthesia. Philadelphia, W.B. Saunders, 1999.

43. RUMINANT ANESTHESIA

Thomas Riebold, D.V.M., D.A.C.V.A.

1. What general considerations are necessary for general anesthesia in ruminants?

Consideration should be given to acquisition of the necessary supplies, drugs, expendable goods, etc., prior to inducing the first case. These items can be gathered and stored in a large tackle box (approximately 50 cm × 23 cm × 25 cm). Consideration should be given to methods used to handle awake cattle including provision of the necessary head gates, chutes, alleyways, stalls, etc. when building or remodeling an existing facility.

2. What type of equipment do I need for anesthetizing ruminants?

Anesthesia Supplies Included in a Tackle Box for Use during Anesthesia

1	50 ml acepromazine	3	3 ml syringes
1	50 ml xylazine (100 mg/ml)	3	6 ml syringes
1	50 ml butorphanol (10 mg/ml)	2	12 ml syringes
2	10 ml ketamine (100 mg/ml)	2	20 ml syringes
1	125 ml guaifenesin (5–10%)	2	60 ml syringes
2	lactated Ringers (liters)	4 ea	18, 20, 25 gauge needles
2	250 ml saline	2 ea	14, 20, 22 gauge catheters
1	250 ml heparinized saline		alcohol cotton balls
1	100 ml atropine (0.5 **or** 15 mg/ml)	1	bottle alcohol (4 oz)
1	20 ml glycopyrrolate	1	cuff syringe (60 ml)
1	500 ml 23% calcium borogluconate	1	1" tape
1	250 mg vial dobutamine	1	2" roll gauze
2	ampules ephedrine (25 mg/ml)	1	2" Elastikon
1	20 ml doxapram	1	ophthalmic ointment
1	10 ml heparin (1,000 units/ml)	1	demand valve
2	500 ml sodium bicarbonate (5–8.4%)	1	oxygen flowmeter
1	50 ml lidocaine w/o epinephrine (2%)	1	equine nasogastric tube
2	ampules isoproterenol (0.2 mg/ml)	1	oxygen tubing
1	30 ml epinephrine (1:1000)		peripheral nerve stimulator
2	vented IV sets	1	bandage scissors
1	14 gauge × 5.5" needle	1	hand towel

Little specialized equipment is needed when intravenous anesthesia is used. If desired, use of infusion pumps will make administration of drugs given as infusions more precise and convenient. When inhalation anesthesia is used, an anesthesia machine is required. The most commonly used system is a circle system. Veterinary anesthesia machines are available for both large animal and small animal patients. Human anesthesia machines are also available. The size of the patient will determine which machine is used. Large animal machines have 50 mm tubing diameter and are used when patients weigh greater than 200 kg. Small animal machines have 22 mm tubing diameter and usually a single soda lime canister. They are used when patients weigh less than 45 kg. Human machines have 22 mm tubing diameter with dual soda lime canisters and are used when patients weigh between 45 and 150 kg.

Other necessary equipment includes appropriate surgical table padding (vinyl covered foam pads, water beds, or dunnage bags), endotracheal tubes of various sizes (6–26 mm internal diameter), and a suitable area (approximately 12' × 12', non-slip surface, smooth walls, etc.) for recovery from anesthesia.

3. What type of preanesthetic preparation is necessary for the patient?

The animal should be fasted and deprived of water prior to induction of anesthesia to decrease the fluid content and overall volume of fermentable ingesta in the rumen. Doing so will decrease the incidence of ruminal tympany and regurgitation in anesthetized ruminants. Even with these precautions, as high as 25% of anesthetized ruminants will regurgitate. Regurgitation is more common in animals placed in dorsal recumbency, particularly during abdominal surgery. Calves and small ruminants should be fasted for 12 hours and deprived of water for 8–12 hours. Adult cattle should be fasted for 12–24 hours and deprived of water for 12–24 hours. Large mature bulls should be fasted for 24–36 hours and deprived of water for 24–36 hours. Fasting neonates is not advisable because hypoglycemia may result. While fasting and water deprivation decreases the incidence of tympany and regurgitation, it will also produce bradycardia in cattle. Additionally, pulmonary functional residual capacity may be better preserved in the fasted anesthetized ruminant.

4. Do ruminants need to be sedated or treated with an anticholinergic prior to induction of anesthesia?

Animals are sedated prior to induction of anesthesia to make the animal easier to handle during induction, decrease the amount of anesthetic agent needed for induction, and to make the recovery period smoother with fewer premature attempts to arise. This allows more of the general anesthetic agents to be either expelled or metabolized before the animal makes its attempt(s) to rise. Ruminants have a different temperament than horses and seldom make premature attempts to rise and tend to remain in sternal recumbency until able to stand. Thus, sedation is often not used assuming that the animal is tractable enough to be handled or suitable equipment is available to allow handling of the animal.

Ruminants salivate copiously while under anesthesia. Use of either atropine or glycopyrrolate may decrease the volume of secretions while increasing their viscosity, making it more difficult for tracheal cilia to clear the secretions should they be aspirated. Additionally, ruminants have high levels of atropinase, requiring higher and more frequent doses of atropine to maintain an effect. Usually anticholinergics are not used.

5. What sedatives are available for use in ruminants?

Acepromazine is a phenothiazine-derivative tranquilizer that can be used in ruminants to provide standing sedation. It provides mild sedation and is given at 0.03 mg/kg IV. It is recommended that the injection not be given in the coccygeal vein because of the risk of inadvertent injection in the coccygeal artery and subsequent sloughing of the tail distal to the injection site. Prolapse of the penis does occur following administration of acepromazine with risk of trauma to that organ in mature bulls. Contraindications to its use in ruminants, for example, in debilitated or hypovolemic patients, are similar to its use in other species.

The alpha-2 agonists, xylazine, detomidine, medetomidine, and romifidine, are the most commonly used sedatives in ruminants. Xylazine is often used to provide sedation or, in higher doses, restraint (recumbency and light planes of general anesthesia) in cattle. There appears to be some variation in response to xylazine within a species. Hereford cattle have been shown to be more sensitive to xylazine than Holstein cattle, and anecdotal evidence indicates that Brahmans are the most sensitive of the breeds. High environmental ambient temperature will cause a pronounced and prolonged response to xylazine in cattle. Xylazine also will cause hyperglycemia and hypoinsulinemia in cattle and sheep. Additionally, it will cause hypoxemia and hypercarbia in cattle and can cause pulmonary edema. Finally, xylazine has an oxytocin-like effect on the uterus of pregnant cattle and sheep. The degree of sedation or restraint produced by xylazine depends on the amount given and the animal's temperament. Low doses (0.015–0.025 mg/kg IV or IM) will provide sedation without recumbency in cattle. Higher doses of xylazine (0.1 mg/kg IV or 0.2 mg/kg IM) will provide recumbency and light planes of general anesthesia in cattle for approximately one hour. Higher doses can be expected to induce longer periods of recumbency.

Detomidine has been used to a lesser extent in the United States but is also effective for providing sedation and/or analgesia in cattle. Detomidine is given at 2.5–10.0 µg/kg IV in cattle to provide standing sedation of approximately 30–60 minutes duration. Detomidine at 40 µg/kg IV will produce profound sedation and recumbency. Higher doses of detomidine (100 µg/kg) administered by dart have been used to immobilize free ranging cattle. Approximately 15 minutes was required for onset of action. Detomidine does not appear to have the same effect on the gravid uterus as xylazine in cattle and would appear to be the drug of choice for sedation in pregnant cattle.

Medetomidine and romifidine are less commonly used in the United States. Medetomidine has been given at 30.0 µg/kg IM to produce recumbency in calves lasting 60–75 minutes or at 10 µg/kg IV to produce recumbency in sheep. Romifidine has been used at 50 µg/kg IV to produce recumbency in sheep.

Historically, pentobarbital has been used as a general anesthetic. It can also be used in cattle for standing sedation and tranquilization and is given at 2 mg/kg IV. Caution must be exercised to avoid administering pentobarbital in a large enough amount to cause excitement. Pentobarbital provides moderate sedation for 30 minutes and mild sedation for an additional 60 minutes.

Finally, combinations of xylazine and butorphanol have been used in cattle to provide neuroleptanalgesia. Doses are 0.01–0.02 mg/kg IV of each drug given separately in cattle. Duration of action is approximately 1 hour. Combinations of detomidine (70 µg/kg) and butorphanol (0.04 mg/kg) have also been used to immobilize free-ranging cattle.

6. What are the drugs available for injectable induction techniques?

Drugs that are available are thiopental, ketamine, tiletamine-zolazepam, and propofol. Pentobarbital is also available but its use has been largely replaced by contemporary techniques.

7. What are the advantages and disadvantages of thiopental?

Thiopental is a thiobarbiturate that has enjoyed widespread use in veterinary anesthesia. Changes in acid-base status and physical status of the patient affect the action of this drug. Acidemia increases the nonionized fraction (the active portion) of the drug, increasing its activity, thus decreasing the dose required. In addition, the heart, brain, and other vital organs receive a larger portion of cardiac output when patients are in shock. Because patients in shock are often acidemic, altered kinetics and altered hemodynamics can result in relative overdose. Recovery from induction doses of thiobarbiturates is based upon redistribution of the drug from the brain to other tissues in the body. Metabolism of the agent continues for some time following recovery until final elimination occurs. Maintenance of anesthesia with thiobarbiturates is not recommended because saturation of tissue depots with thiobarbiturate causes recovery to be dependent on metabolism and recovery will be prolonged. Concurrent use of nonsteroidal antiinflammatory drugs is contraindicated because they will displace the thiobarbiturates from protein and delay recovery.

Thiopental is given at 6–10 mg/kg IV in unsedated animals and will provide approximately 10–15 minutes of anesthesia and offers the advantage of small injection volume. Thiopental (2 gm) can also be combined with guaifenesin (50 gm). This combination is administered rapidly to effect with the calculated dose being 110 mg/kg (guaifenesin)–4 mg/kg (thiopental). If the ruminant has not been sedated prior to induction, one can expect that induction will require an amount that approaches the calculated dose. While this technique allows one the opportunity to administer the drugs to effect, it also carries the disadvantage of a large injection volume.

8. What are the advantages and disadvantages of ketamine?

Ketamine is a very versatile anesthetic agent and has been used in many species. It provides mild cardiovascular stimulation and is safer than thiobarbiturates when used in sick animals. Although ketamine does not eliminate the swallowing reflex, tracheal intubation can be accomplished. Given intravenously, it quickly induces anesthesia. It also offers the advantage of being effective following intramuscular injection. Although ketamine will induce immobilization and incomplete analgesia when given alone, addition of a sedative or tranquilizer will improve muscle relaxation and quality of anesthesia. Commonly, diazepam or an alpha-2 sedative is recommended. Diazepam (0.1 mg/kg IV) followed immediately by ketamine (4.5 mg/kg IV) can be used in cattle. Muscle relaxation is usually adequate for tracheal intubation, although the swallowing reflex may not be completely obtunded. Anesthesia usually is of 10–15 minutes duration following diazepam-ketamine with recumbency of up to 30 minutes.

Xylazine is the most commonly used alpha-2 sedative prior to ketamine administration. It is given at 0.1–0.2 mg/kg IM followed by ketamine (10–15 mg/kg IM) in calves. Anesthesia usually lasts about 45 minutes and can be prolonged by injection of 3–5 mg/kg IM of ketamine or 1–2 mg/kg IV. The longer duration of action of xylazine obviates the need for readministration of xylazine in most cases. Alternatively, xylazine (0.03–0.05 mg/kg IV) followed by ketamine (3–5 mg/kg IV) can be used to provide anesthesia of 15–20 minutes duration. Adult cattle can be anesthetized with xylazine (0.1–0.2 mg/kg IV) followed by ketamine (2.0 mg/kg IV). The lower dose of xylazine is used when cattle weigh greater than 600 kg. Duration of anesthesia is approximately 30 minutes; anesthesia can be prolonged for 15 minutes with additional ketamine (0.75-1.25 mg/kg IV). Medetomidine has been combined with ketamine to provide anesthesia in calves. Because medetomidine (20 µg/kg IV) is much more potent than xylazine, very low doses of ketamine (0.5 mg/kg IV) can be used. However, use of a local anesthetic at the surgical site may be required when ketamine is used at this dose.

9. What are the advantages and disadvantages of tiletamine-zolazepam?

Tiletamine-zolazepam is a proprietary mixture of tiletamine, a dissociative anesthetic agent, and zolazepam, a benzodiazepine tranquilizer. Although there are differences in potency, it could be considered to be similar to a mixture of diazepam and ketamine. In contrast to the horse, tiletamine-zolazepam can be used either singly or in combination with xylazine and can be given either intravenously or intramuscularly. When used alone in unsedated ruminants, it is given at 2.0 mg/kg IV and provides anesthesia of approximately 25 minutes duration with recumbency of up to 45 minutes. When given at 4.0 mg/kg IV to unsedated calves, it causes minimal cardiovascular effects and provides anesthesia of 45–60 minutes duration.

Xylazine (0.1 mg/kg IM) followed immediately by tiletamine-zolazepam (4.0 mg/kg IM) produced onset of anesthesia within 3 minutes and duration of anesthesia of approximately 1 hour with the calves being able to stand approximately 130 minutes following injection. Increasing xylazine to 0.2 mg/kg IM increased duration of anesthesia and recumbency and the incidence of apnea. Apnea was short-lived but still required intubation and manual or mechanical ventilation. If desired, the drugs can be administered intravenously. Xylazine can be given at 0.05 mg/kg IV followed by tiletamine-zolazepam at 1.0 mg/kg IV.

10. What are the advantages and disadvantages of propofol?

Propofol is a nonbarbiturate, nonsteroidal hypnotic agent that will provide brief periods (5–10 minutes) of anesthesia. The dose for induction in unsedated sheep and goats is 4.0–6.0 mg/kg IV. A similar dose could be used in cattle. Sedation of the animal prior to induction with propofol will decrease the amount of propofol required. Constant infusion can be used to maintain a light plane of anesthesia. Induction and recovery are smooth. If injected rapidly, apnea may occur, although slow administration will usually prevent that complication. Except during special circumstances (for example, during MR imaging), economic considerations will dictate its use in ruminants.

11. What are the drugs available for inhalation induction techniques?

Induction of anesthesia can be performed with inhalation agents in certain instances. When one wishes to avoid administration of intravenous anesthetic agents—for example, in neonates or compromised animals weighing less than 125 kg—induction with inhalation agents can be very useful as recovery tends to be much quicker because it is based upon elimination of the agent by the respiratory tract rather than metabolism of the agents. Halothane, isoflurane, and less commonly sevoflurane and desflurane are available. Halothane has enjoyed widespread use with isoflurane finding less widespread use mainly because of economic implications. Halothane does not provide the speed of induction and recovery that isoflurane provides but is still a very useful agent. Sevoflurane and desflurane impart very quick induction of anesthesia and recovery from anesthesia. Currently, sevoflurane is an expensive agent to use. Desflurane is less expensive, but the vaporizer used to administer the agent is very expensive. Economic considerations will dictate both drugs' entry into ruminant anesthesia. Typically, a face mask is applied to the muzzle of the calf. Depending on the calf's size, commercial canine masks can be used or a mask can be fabricated from a plastic gallon jug or other suitable sized container. The mask is connected to the Y-piece of the rebreathing tubes. One must be certain that the mask does not occlude the nares of the calf. Typical flow rates of oxygen are 3–6 liters/minute with a vaporizer setting of 3–5% halothane or isoflurane. If desired nitrous oxide can be given in addition to oxygen at 3–6 liters/minute. Induction will be accomplished within five minutes. Typical flow rates of oxygen are 3–6 liters/minute with a vaporizer setting of 5–7% sevoflurane. If desired, nitrous oxide can be given in addition to oxygen at 3–6 liters/minute. Induction will be accomplished quickly. Typical flow rates of oxygen are 3–6 liters/minute with a vaporizer setting of 10–15% desflurane. If desired nitrous oxide can be given in addition to oxygen at 3–6 liters/minute. Induction will be accomplished quickly. Flow rate and vaporizer settings should be decreased following intubation to appropriate levels.

12. What are the injectable anesthetic drugs available for maintenance of anesthesia?

Agents used for induction of anesthesia, thiopental, ketamine, tiletamine-zolazepam, propofol, and guaifenesin can also be used for maintenance. Following induction with the agents, supplemental injections of 25–50% of the original dose can be administered intermittently as needed to maintain anesthesia. A mixture of 0.1% ketamine (1.0 mg/ml) – 0.005% xylazine (0.05 mg/ml) –5% guaifenesin (50 mg/ml) can be infused at 2.0 ml/kg/hour. Recovery usually occurs within 30 minutes of discontinuing the infusion. Propofol can be infused in unsedated ruminants at 0.3–0.5 mg/kg/min IV. The infusion rate should be decreased in sedated ruminants. Ruminants maintained under intravenous anesthesia should be intubated, as regurgitation remains a possibility.

13. Can intravenous infusion pumps be used?

Infusion pumps can be used as a very convenient method for administering intravenous fluids or anesthetic agents in a controlled and precise manner. An infusion pump with a maximum administration rate of 999 ml/hr should be selected as it offers more flexibility when dealing with the variety of patient size (10 kg to > 1000 kg) than pumps limited to 499 ml/hr. For example, if one were administering 0.01% xylazine (0.1 mg/ml)–0.2% ketamine (2.0 mg/ml)– 10% guaifenesin (100 mg/ml) solution at 1.0 ml/kg/min for maintenance of anesthesia the pump would be suitable for use on an animal weighing up to 900 kg. These pumps can also be used for administering infusions of dobutamine or calcium gluconate. Syringe pumps are also available for use. Their maximum infusion rate is not as large thus their use for administration of fluids or anesthetic agents is limited to smaller patients. They can also be used for administration of cardiovascular support drugs to any size patient.

14. How difficult is tracheal intubation?

Intubation can be difficult in ruminants because visibility of the larynx is limited. The animal's mouth will not open very widely, and considerable distance may exist between the animal's incisors and larynx. In addition, the larynx of sheep and goats reacts vigorously to tactile stimulation. In those species, use of topical lidocaine to desensitize the larynx is helpful. One can use a syringe with a 12-cm catheter attached to it or plant misters to spray the larynx.

Some cattle can be intubated blindly. Following hyperextension of the neck, the endotracheal tube is placed in the buccal cavity and manipulated into the trachea. When this technique is not successful, a laryngoscope is used to visualize the larynx or the animal is intubated by digital palpation if its mouth is big enough to accommodate the person's hand and arm. One would insert their hand with the endotracheal tube under it into the animal's mouth. After locating and depressing the epiglottis, the arytenoid cartilages are identified. The endotracheal tube is guided through the larynx and into the trachea. While the operator's hand is in the animal's mouth, the animal will have its airway obstructed. It is recommended that intubation be accomplished in an expedient manner. If intubation is not possible in a timely fashion, the hand should be removed from the animal's mouth for a short period of time to allow it to ventilate before intubation is reattempted.

Intubation is accomplished with the aid of laryngoscopy in sheep, goats, and calves that cannot be intubated blindly. It is also helpful to use an extended stylet during intubation. When the appropriate size endotracheal tube is used it will hinder visualization of the larynx as it is advanced towards the larynx and one will have difficulty seeing the endotracheal tube enter the larynx. Use of a stylet that extends 10 cm beyond the bevel of the tube will aid intubation. The stylet and tube are advanced together and the stylet is placed in the larynx and trachea during inspiration as maximum adduction of the arytenoid cartilages will occur then. The endotracheal tube is then advanced into the trachea and the stylet removed. Choice of stylet depends on the size of the animal. Feeding tubes, male canine urinary catheters, or colt urinary catheters or similar devices can be used.

Following intubation, correct placement of the endotracheal tube can be confirmed by detecting passage of air from the endotracheal tube during breathing, noticing steaming and clearing of transparent endotracheal tubes during breathing, absence of stertorous breathing sounds, synchrony of movement of the chest and rebreathing bag on the anesthesia machine, and, if a capnograph or capnometer is available, CO_2 will be detected. Compressing the rebreathing bag to help confirm correct placement of the endotracheal tube is best avoided because ruminal distention will occur following esophageal placement of the tube and can increase the likelihood of regurgitation.

15. What are the inhalation anesthetic drugs available for maintenance of anesthesia?

Halothane, isoflurane, and, less commonly, sevoflurane and desflurane are available for maintenance of general anesthesia in ruminants. Halothane has enjoyed widespread use, with isoflurane finding less widespread use mainly because of economic implications. Halothane does not provide the speed of induction and recovery that isoflurane provides but is still a very useful agent. Sevoflurane and desflurane impart very quick induction of anesthesia and recovery from anesthesia. Currently, sevoflurane is an expensive agent to use. While desflurane is less expensive than sevoflurane, larger volumes of the agent are used because it is less potent and the vaporizer used to administer the agent can be very expensive. Economic considerations will dictate both drugs' entry into ruminant anesthesia.

16. What types of anesthesia machines are available for use in ruminants?

Conventional large animal anesthesia machines with airway diameters of 50 mm are used for ruminants weighing greater than 200 kg. Anesthesia machines manufactured by Mallard Medical, Matrx, and SurgiVet/Anesco are available. When ruminants weighing less than 150 kg are anesthetized, conventional human anesthesia machines can be used. These machines are identical to veterinary machines in that they have airway diameters of 22 mm but they have dual absorber canisters and thus offer more absorptive capacity for animals that exceed 45 kg. There are many machines available. Manufacturers of veterinary machines among others include AM Bickford, Lawson Enterprises Inc., Matrx, SurgiVet/Anesco, and Vasco. Manufacturers of human anesthesia machines include North American Dräger and Ohmeda.

17. What are the advantages and disadvantages of halothane?

Halothane is a drug that has long been used for induction and maintenance of anesthesia in ruminants. It is relatively insoluble and provides quick induction of, and recovery from, anesthesia. It is relatively potent, with a MAC (minimal alveolar concentration) of 0.8%. Typically, anesthesia is induced with vaporizer settings of 4–5% in adult cattle and 3–4% in small ruminants, with vaporizer settings of 2–3% used for maintenance in spontaneously ventilating ruminants. It can cause dose-related bradycardia, and hypotension and has been associated with postoperative liver dysfunction in goats.

18. What are the advantages and disadvantages of isoflurane?

Isoflurane is a drug that has been more recently used for induction and maintenance of anesthesia in ruminants. It is more insoluble than halothane and provides quicker induction of, and recovery from, anesthesia. It is relatively potent, with MAC being 1.3%. It can cause dose-related bradycardia and hypotension. The agent is less prone to cause arrhythmias than halothane. Very little of the drug is metabolized (<1%).

19. What are the advantages and disadvantages of sevoflurane?

Sevoflurane is a drug that has been recently used for induction and maintenance of anesthesia in ruminants. It is much more insoluble than halothane, and isoflurane provides very rapid induction of and recovery from anesthesia. It is not as potent as halothane or isoflurane with MAC being 3.3% in ruminants. It can cause dose-related bradycardia and hypotension.

20. What are the advantages and disadvantages of desflurane?

Desflurane is a very insoluble anesthetic and is characterized by rapid onset of and recovery from anesthesia. It is not as potent as other inhalation agents and thus higher concentrations are needed to maintain anesthesia. The vaporizer used to deliver the agent is very expensive and may limit usefulness of desflurane. It is the least potent of the modern inhalation anesthetic agents, with MAC being 8.4–11.1% in ruminants. It can cause dose-related bradycardia and hypotension.

21. What about field use of inhalation anesthesia?

If desired, portable inhalation anesthesia equipment can be obtained to allow one to perform inhalation anesthesia in the field. Patient size is limited to about 175 kg. Use of aluminum gas cylinders adds to convenience when oxygen must be transported. Some manufacturers of anesthesia devices—for example, Matrx—have portable units for use in nontraditional locations.

22. What is needed for supportive care?

Supportive therapy consists of proper padding and positioning of the patient, techniques to help maintain normal body temperature, administration of intravenous fluids and cardiovascular support drugs, good monitoring techniques, and mechanical ventilation. Anesthetized ruminants should be placed on a flat, padded surface. Padding can be vinyl covered foam pads, water beds, or dunnage bags. Padding of 4" thickness is sufficient for adult cattle. Padding of 1–2" thickness is sufficient for calves, sheep, and goats. Hypothermia in young calves, sheep, and goats can be a problem, and they will benefit from placement of circulating warm water blankets. Hypothermia is less of an issue in adult cattle because of their surface area to mass ratio.

23. What type of fluids should be administered during anesthesia?

Usually a polyionic isotonic fluid with an alkalinizing effect is chosen for fluid administration/replacement during anesthesia. Choices are lactated Ringers or Normosol-R. Fluid is usually given at 10 ml/kg/hour. When the patient is hypochloremic, sodium chloride is indicated. Sodium bicarbonate is indicated when metabolic acidosis is present and is replaced according to the formula: mEq $HCO3^-$ = body weight (kg) $\times$ base deficit $\times$ 0.3.

Usually 50% of that amount is given over 30–60 minutes and then the need for additional sodium bicarbonate is reassessed.

24. What type of monitoring techniques should be used during anesthesia?

Monitoring is similar to that performed during equine cases. Heart rate, pulse strength, muscle relaxation, respiratory rate, capillary refill time, blood pressure, color of mucous membranes, and ocular rotation to monitor depth of anesthesia. Normal values are listed in the table. Heart rate will usually decrease as depth of anesthesia increases and usually remains above 80 beats/minute. Animals who have received an alpha–2 agonist will have slower heart rates, as will cattle weighing more than 600 kg.

The common digital arteries are easily palpated just dorsal to the dewclaws. The caudal auricular artery is also easily palpated and the saphenous artery can be palpated. The facial artery is palpable at the ramus of the mandible in calves; however, as the animal matures, the sternomandibularis muscle increases in size, making the facial artery less easily palpable.

Normal Values for Anesthetized Ruminants

VARIABLE	VALUE
Respiratory rate	
Adult cattle	20–40 breaths/minute
Calves, sheep, goats	30–40 breaths/minute
Tidal volume	7.0–8.0 ml/kg (3.1–3.6 ml/lb)
Heart rate	
Adult cattle	70–100 beats/minute
Calves, sheep, goats	80–120 beats/minute
Gingival perfusion time	1-2 seconds
Arterial pressure (systolic/diastolic)	
Cattle	120–150/75–100 mm Hg
Sheep, goats	100–130/65–80 mm Hg
Arterial pressure (mean)	
Cattle	90–120 mm Hg
Sheep, goats	75–100 mm Hg
Central venous pressure	5–10 cm H_2O
End tidal CO_2 (controlled ventilation)	30–40 torr
End tidal anesthetic agent (controlled ventilation)	
Halothane (with premedication)	0.8–0.9%
Halothane (without premedication)	1.0–1.2%
Isoflurane (with premedication)	1.3–1.4%
Isoflurane (without premedication)	1.6–1.9%
Sevoflurane (with premedication)	2.3–2.6%
Sevoflurane (without premedication)	2.9–3.5%
Desflurane (with premedication)	8.0–10%
Desflurane (without premedication)	10–12 %

Movement of the animal's eye is useful for assessing depth of anesthesia in cattle. When the patient is in surgical anesthesia, the iris and pupil are centered between the two lids; during minimal depth of surgical anesthesia, the globe is rotated ventrally so that the iris and pupil are obscured by the lower lid. Depth of anesthesia may not be sufficient for invasive procedures when the eye is rotated ventrally. When mask induction of a calf is performed, slight dorsal rotation of the globe would be noted before ventral rotation occurs.

Following the administration of the intravenous anesthetic agent, the eye is usually rotated ventrally. The vaporizer setting is initially 4–5% for halothane or isoflurane and decreased to 3% as the globe begins its upward rotation. After the globe is centered, the concentration of halothane is decreased until downward rotation of the globe begins, finding the point where the anesthetic plane begins to become inadequate. Increasing the concentration of halothane slightly will center the globe again. Ocular rotation does not occur in goats or sheep. Other ocular reflexes, other than rotation of the globe in cattle are not very reliable in assessing the depth of anesthesia. The palpebral reflex disappears with minimal depth of anesthesia. Nystagmus is of little value.

Because cattle have a relatively small tidal volume during spontaneous ventilation compared to horses or swine, expired gas sampled by end tidal CO_2 and anesthetic agent monitors may not contain sufficient alveolar gas and results may be inaccurate. These analyzers are accurate when cattle are mechanically ventilated. Additionally, some anesthetic agent analyzers will detect methane present in the expired gas of herbivores and report it as anesthetic agent. Values obtained from blood gas analysis are similar to normal values of other species.

25. What type of ventilation should be employed during anesthesia?

Spontaneous ventilation is usually sufficient when ruminants are anesthetized. When the procedure is expected to be lengthy (> 90 minutes), consideration can be given to instituting mechanical ventilation. Controlled ventilation must be used during thoracotomy or when muscle relaxants are used. Common ventilator settings are a respiratory rate of 6–10 breaths/minute with a tidal volume of 15 ml/kg. Final ventilator settings are dependent on results of blood gas analysis. Unexplained bradycardia in the absence of blood gas analysis is often due to hypocarbia, and minute volume should be decreased.

26. What types of mechanical ventilators are available for use in ruminants?

Both pneumatic and electronic ventilators are available. Examples of ventilators for adult cattle are the JD Medical LAV 2000®, Mallard Medical Model 2800®, and SurgiVet/Anesco DHV 1000®. These ventilators have a bellows capacity of approximately 20 liters. Most calves, sheep, and goats are small enough that ventilators designed for human use are applicable for use. Specific ventilators designed for veterinary use are also available. Examples of ventilators available for calves, sheep and goats are the Hallowell 2000®, JD Medical SAV-75®, Mallard Medical 2400®, Matrx 3000®, North American Dräger AVE®, and Ohmeda 7000® and 7400®. These ventilators have a bellows capacity of 1.4 to 3.0 liters. Final choice of ventilator is determined by patient size, cost, and availability.

27. What type of cardiovascular support is required during anesthesia?

When hypotension is present and cannot be corrected by administering intravenous fluids and adjusting anesthetic depth without the animal moving, several different drugs are available for use. They include calcium borogluconate, ephedrine, dobutamine, and dopamine. When hypotension without bradycardia occurs, inotropes are used to increase stroke volume and cardiac output. Calcium borogluconate (23% solution) increases myocardial contractility and is given as a slow infusion (0.5–1.0 ml/kg/hr) to effect. Often, calcium administration can be discontinued after mean arterial pressure returns to normal values. Ephedrine, a mixed alpha- and beta-sympathomimetic drug, can be used at 0.02–0.06 mg/kg IV to increase mean arterial pressure through an increase in cardiac contractility and vasomotor tone. Dobutamine and dopamine, synthetic beta-catecholamines, can be used to improve cardiac output. At low doses they increase myocardial contractility and at higher doses can increase heart rate. Overdosage causes tachycardia and arrhythmias. Dobutamine is recommended over dopamine because improvement in hemodynamics occurs with smaller increases in heart rate and because its effect is more predictable. Each is administered at 1.0–2.0 µg/kg/minute IV to effect. Following correction of hypotension, rate of administration can usually be decreased to maintenance levels. Use of an infusion pump is recommended for convenience and accuracy of administration.

28. What arrangements must be made for recovery?

The preferred location for recovering ruminants from anesthesia would be a stall with solid walls and a nonslip floor under moderate ambient temperature. If less than ideal facilities are available, the ruminant should at least be allowed to recover in an area where no other animals can injure it. If recovery is expected to be lengthy, greater than 30 minutes, then adult cattle should be placed on a vinyl-covered foam pad with an automobile inner tube under the down elbow. Padding will help to prevent myopathy/neuropathy while use of the inner tube helps prevent injury to the radial nerve. The animal should remain intubated until it is able to swallow, chew, cough, and is actively trying to expel the tube. If possible, the tube could be left in place until the ruminant is able to assume sternal recumbency. An assistant should remain nearby to offer assistance if it is needed, particularly if the stall walls are not solid and it is possible for the animal to get a leg or its head through the fence. For the most part, ruminants tend to remain in sternal recumbency until they are able to stand and then do so. After the ruminant is no longer ataxic, it can be moved to its stall.

29. Is sedation necessary for recovery?

A very high number, if not all, ruminants recover very well from anesthesia without experiencing emergence delirium. This characteristic is more a reflection of their personality, as ruminants do not feel the urgency to arise that horses experience and respond more favorably to restraint. If a ruminant should experience emergence delirium, minute doses of xylazine could be given intravenously.

30. What agents are available for reversal of alpha-2 agonists?

Sedation following use of alpha-2 agonists can be reversed by alpha-2 adrenoceptor antagonists, yohimbine, tolazoline, atipamezole, and idazoxan. Yohimbine is given at 0.12 mg/kg IV although there is some variability in response to its administration in cattle. Tolazoline is given at 0.5–2.0 mg/kg IV. Tolazoline given at 2.0 mg/kg IV will cause hyperesthesia in unsedated cattle. Idazoxan is given at 0.05 mg/kg IV to calves. Atipamezole is given at 20–60 μg/kg IV. Doxapram, an analeptic, can be used to augment the response of yohimbine or tolazoline to alpha-2 agonist sedated cattle. Doxapram (1.0 mg/kg IV) given alone has been shown to be effective in cattle. None of these agents are cleared for use in ruminants by the FDA.

31. Any precautions for use of alpha-2 antagonists?

There are anecdotal reports of death associated with tolazoline administration in cattle, usually following higher doses of the drug given to animals with compromised physical status. Tolazoline has both alpha-1 and alpha-2 activity and thus will cause vasodilatation. Animals that are dehydrated or in shock try to maintain their blood pressure in spite of falling cardiac output by vasoconstriction. Administration of tolazoline, acepromazine, and other compounds that cause alpha-1 blockade eliminate this protective response and can cause severely affected animals to decompensate. If an alpha-2 agonist has been used to provide sedation in this instance and antagonism of sedation is desired, an agent with high specificity for alpha-2 receptors is indicated. If tolazoline is the only available agent it should be given at 0.5–1.0 mg/kg IV. If sufficient arousal does not occur, additional tolazoline could be given.

BIBLIOGRAPHY

1. Carroll, GL, SM Hartsfield: General anesthetic techniques in ruminants. Vet Clin North Am—Food An Pract 12:627-661, 1996.
2. Daunt DA: Supportive therapy in the anesthetized horse. Vet Clin North Am—Eq Pract 6:557-574, 1990.
3. Hall LW, Clarke KW, Trim CM: In Veterinary Anaesthesia. 10th ed. Philadelphia, WB Saunders, 2001, pp. 275-289.
4. Heath RB: General anesthesia in ruminants. In Jennings PB (ed): The Practice of Large Animal Surgery. PB Jennings, ed. Philadephia, WB Saunders, 1984, pp. 202-204.
5. Riebold TW. Anesthetic techniques in ruminants. In Thurmon JC, Tranquilli WJ, and Benson GJ (eds): Lumb and Jones' Veterinary Anesthesia, 3rd ed. Philadelphia, Lea and Febiger, 1996, pp. 610-626.
6. Short CE: Preanesthetic medications in ruminants and swine. Vet Clin North Am—Food An Pract 2, 553-566, 1986.
7. Swanson CR, ed. Anesthesia update. Vet Clin North Am—Food An Pract 12: 1996.
8. Tranquilli WJ: Techniques of inhalation anesthesia in ruminants and swine. Vet Clin North Am—Food Anim Pract 2: 593-619, 1986.
9. Tranquilli WJ, Greene SA: Cardiovascular medications and the autonomic nervous system. In Short CE (ed): Principles and Practice of Veterinary Anesthesia. Baltimore, Williams and Wilkins, 1987, pp. 426-454.
10. Trim CM: Special anesthesia considerations in the ruminant. In Short CE (ed): Principles and Practice of Veterinary Anesthesia. Baltimore, Williams and Wilkins, 1987, pp. 285-300.
11. Thurmon JC, Benson GJ: Anesthesia in ruminants and swine. In Howard JC (ed): Current Veterinary Therapy, Food Animal Practice 3rd ed., Philadelphia, WB Saunders, 1993, pp 58-76.

44. ANESTHESIA IN SOUTH AMERICAN CAMELIDS

Thomas Riebold D.V.M., D.A.C.V.A.

1. What are the perianesthetic considerations for general anesthesia in camelids?

Anesthesia of llamas and alpacas is very similar to anesthesia of ruminants. As in other species, consideration should be given to acquisition of the necessary supplies, drugs, expendable goods, etc., prior to anesthetizing the first case. Consideration could also be given to purchase of a chute specifically designed for llamas, which can facilitate catheter placement and performance of other clinical procedures.

Body weight of the camelid must be determined either by weighing the animal or estimating its weight so that accurate drug administration is possible. It is easy to overestimate body weight because camelids are fairly tall and have a long haircoat that obscures their body type. Adult male llamas usually weigh from 125–160 kg, although some males can exceed 180 kg. Adult female llamas usually weigh from 100–150 kg, but some will also exceed 180 kg. Adult male alpacas usually weigh 55–80 kg, and adult female alpacas usually weigh 45–70 kg. Body weight of crias and small juveniles may be estimated by lifting the camelid, or a bathroom scale can be used to weigh the individual holding the camelid and again without it.

2. What type of equipment do I need for anesthetizing camelids?

Little specialized equipment is needed when intravenous anesthesia is used. If desired, use of infusion pumps will make administration of drugs given as infusions more precise and convenient. When inhalation anesthesia is used, an anesthesia machine is required. The most commonly used system is a circle system. Small animal machines have 22-mm tubing diameter and usually a single soda lime canister, while human anesthesia machines have dual soda lime canisters. Small animal machines can be used when patients weigh less than 45 kg, which would include many alpacas and juvenile llamas. Human anesthesia machines are preferred when anesthetizing larger alpacas and most llamas. Anesthesia ventilators that have 1.4–2.2 liter bellows capacity are sufficient for ventilating llamas.

Other necessary equipment includes appropriate surgical table padding, endotracheal tubes of various sizes (6–16 mm internal diameter), a laryngoscope with a 300 mm blade, and a suitable area (approximately 12' × 12', non-slip surface, smooth walls, etc.) for recovery from anesthesia.

3. What type of preanesthetic preparation is necessary for the patient?

The animal should be fasted and deprived of water prior to induction of anesthesia to decrease the fluid content and overall volume of fermentable ingesta in the first compartment. Although camelids seldom bloat during anesthesia, fasting will decrease the incidence of regurgitation. Even with these precautions, as many as 25% of anesthetized camelids will regurgitate. Regurgitation is more common in animals placed in dorsal recumbency, particularly during abdominal surgery. Crias older than six weeks of age should be fasted for 12 hours and deprived of water for 8–12 hours but still allowed to nurse. Adult camelids should be fasted for 12–18 hours and deprived of water for 8–12 hours. Fasting neonates is not advisable because hypoglycemia may result.

4. What technique is used for venous catheterization?

Jugular venous catheterization is recommended prior to induction of anesthesia. Sixteen-gauge catheters are appropriate for adult camelids and 18–20 gauge catheters for smaller camelids. Camelids can have 4–5 jugular venous valves that prevent flow of venous blood into the head when the head is lowered during grazing. Contact with jugular venous valves may prevent successful catheterization; a site caudal to the point where the valve was contacted should be used.

The jugular vein is formed rostrally by the union of the linguofacial vein ventrally and maxillary vein dorsally; in this regard it is comparable to the external jugular vein of domestic ruminants. However, rather than taking a superficial course in the neck, the vein is directed deeply in its caudal course for most of its length and is contained in the carotid sheath with the common carotid artery and vagosympathetic nerve trunk in a relationship similar to the internal jugular vein of domestic animals. Most of the jugular vein lies deep to the sternomandibularis and brachiocephalicus muscles, ventral to cervical vertebral transverse processes. Beginning at a point about 15 cm caudal to the ramus of the mandible, the rostral course of the jugular vein is separated from the carotid artery by the omohyoideus muscle. The origin of the jugular vein is located at the intersection of a line drawn caudally along the ventral aspect of the body of the mandible and another line connecting the base of the ear and the lateral aspect of the cervical transverse processes. Venipuncture or catheterization can be performed at the origin of the jugular vein or at any point caudal to it. Because of the close proximity of the carotid artery to the jugular vein, one must ascertain that the vein has been catheterized, and not the artery, before injecting any medication.

Camelids have a round neck without a distinct jugular groove. The location of the jugular vein can be approximated by placing the four fingers of one's hand at the dorsal midline of the neck and compressing the thumb against the cervical vertebrae. After occlusion of the vessel, one will usually be unable to see the jugular vein distend; however, the vein can be palpated or ballotted particularly rostrally, and more easily in females and altered males because their skin is thinner. On occasion, one will be able to see the jugular vein distend on crias and juvenile camelids. Camelid skin is quite thick and passage of an over-the-needle catheter through the unbroken skin will damage the catheter. After location of the site where the catheter will be placed, the skin should either be pierced with a 14-gauge needle or a #11 scalpel blade. The catheter is place through the skin defect. Local anesthesia at the catheterization site is recommended.

5. Do camelids need to be sedated or treated with an anticholinergic prior to induction of anesthesia?

Camelids have a different temperament than horses and seldom make premature attempts to rise during recovery, and tend to remain in sternal recumbency until able to stand. Thus, sedation is often not used, assuming that the animal is tractable enough to tolerate procedures such as clipping of the surgical site, venous catheterization, etc. Camelids are prone to vagal arrhythmias during intubation, and use of either atropine or glycopyrrolate is recommended. Anticholinergics will eliminate salivation during anesthesia. Atropine can be given at 0.02 mg/kg IV or 0.04 mg/kg IM. Glycopyrrolate can be given at 2–5 µg/kg IV or 5–10 µg/kg IM.

6. What agents are available to provide sedation or restraint in camelids?

Acepromazine is a phenothiazine derivative tranquilizer that has been used in camelids to provide standing sedation. It provides mild sedation and is given at 0.03 mg/kg IV. Contraindications to its use in camelids—for example, in debilitated or hypovolemic patients—are similar to its use in other species.

Xylazine, an alpha-2 agonist, is the most commonly used agent for sedation or, in higher doses, restraint (recumbency and light planes of general anesthesia) in camelids. Other alpha-2 agonists include detomidine, medetomidine, and romifidine. In general, xylazine could be expected to have similar effects as occur in other species, hyperglycemia and hypoinsulinemia, hypoxemia, and hypercarbia. Alpacas are less sensitive to xylazine than llamas. The degree of sedation or restraint produced by xylazine depends on the amount given and the animal's temperament. Low doses (0.1 mg/kg IV or 0.2 mg/kg IM) will provide sedation without recumbency in llamas. Higher doses of xylazine (0.2–0.3 mg/kg IV or 0.2–0.4 mg/kg IM) will provide recumbency and light planes of general anesthesia in llamas for approximately one hour. Higher doses can be expected to induce longer periods of recumbency and usually are not needed.

In a limited number of llamas, detomidine in doses as high as 40 µg/kg IV provided mild sedation but would not provide restraint in llamas. The animals would lie down following detomidine administration at 20–40 µg/kg IV but would arise as soon as a handler approached.

Medetomidine has recently been evaluated for use as a sedative/restraint agent in llamas. Doses as low as 10 µg/kg IM give brief periods of standing sedation (approximately 35 minutes). Onset of sedation is approximately 10–15 minutes. Llamas will not always assume sternal recumbency and, if they do so, duration is brief (5–10 minutes). Analgesia is not present. When medetomidine is given at 20 µg/kg IM, sedation is more profound and lasts approximately 60 minutes. Onset of sedation is approximately 10–15 minutes. Llamas will assume either sternal or lateral recumbency. Analgesia is present about 30 minutes following injection and lasts approximately 30 minutes. When medetomidine is given at 30 µg/kg IM, sedation is more profound and duration of recumbency approaches two hours. Onset of sedation is within 7 minutes. Llamas will assume either sternal or lateral recumbency. Analgesia is present about 15 minutes following injection and lasts approximately 60 minutes.

Butorphanol (0.07–0.1 mg/kg IM) can also be used to provide sedation and analgesia in camelids. While butorphanol does provide sedation, it also causes some degree of dysphoria in camelids, yielding sedation that is qualitatively somewhat less than that usually obtained with tranquilizers and sedatives. The animals usually remain standing but may show slight agitation. Poorly trained animals or berserk males tend to be less responsive and ill or debilitated camelids are more responsive to sedative doses of butorphanol and xylazine.

Neuroleptanalgesia (combinations of analgesic agents and tranquilizers or sedatives) has been used in llamas. Xylazine, 0.2 mg/kg IV, and butorphanol, 0.02 mg/kg IV, have been combined to provide recumbency and profound sedation. They are given simultaneously in separate syringes. Duration of action is approximately 20 minutes.

Xylazine, 0.25 mg/kg IV or 0.35 mg/kg IM, and ketamine, 3.0–5.0 mg/kg IV or 5.0–8.0 mg/kg IM 15 minutes later, usually provide 30–60 minutes of restraint. Xylazine, 0.4 mg/kg IM, and ketamine, 4.0 mg/kg IM, given simultaneously usually provide 15–20 minutes of restraint. When restraint of 15–20 minutes duration is desired, xylazine, 0.2 mg/kg IM, given simultaneously with ketamine, 2.2 mg/kg IM, will provide recumbency within 10 minutes.

Xylazine (0.03 mg/kg), butorphanol (0.3 mg/kg), and ketamine (3.0 mg/kg) have been given simultaneously intramuscularly to llamas to provide restraint for completion of diagnostic procedures. Slightly higher doses, xylazine (0.04 mg/kg), butorphanol (0.4 mg/kg), and ketamine (4.0 mg/kg) are used in alpacas. Recumbency occurs within 7 minutes. Llamas resume sternal recumbency within 45 minutes and stand within 65 minutes. Alpacas resume sternal recumbency within 19 minutes and stand within 22 minutes.

Medetomidine can also be combined with ketamine to provide anesthesia. Medetomidine is given at 40 µg/kg IM with ketamine at 4 mg/kg IM. Induction is rapid, within 5 minutes, and anesthesia is present for about an hour with total time of recumbency being approximately 75 minutes. Cardiovascular variables were well preserved but hypoxemia and hypercarbia were present early during recumbency. Consideration could be given to decreasing the amount of medetomidine in an effort to improve ventilation and oxygenation.

Tiletamine-zolazepam, 4.0 mg/kg IM, can provide up to two hours of restraint. Laryngeal reflexes were present but diminished following tiletamine-zolazepam, affording some airway protection. Tiletamine-zolazepam used in this manner provides quite long duration of recumbency and probably other techniques that provide better airway management are better choices for restraint if up to two hours duration of effect is needed.

Quality of restraint varies because of variable absorption following intramuscular administration, with the amount of agents given, and varies with the camelid's temperament but is usually sufficient for minor procedures such as suturing lacerations, draining abscesses, or cast application. When these combinations provide insufficient anesthetic depth, supplemental local anesthesia may be needed to allow completion of surgery. Muscle relaxation may not be adequate to allow tracheal intubation. However, these combinations do immobilize the animal, facilitating venipuncture and administration of additional anesthetic agent or application of a face mask to increase depth of anesthesia and thus allow one to manage a fractious animal.

7. What are the drugs available for injectable induction techniques?

Thiopental, ketamine, guaifenesin, tiletamine-zolazepam, and propofol.

8. What are the advantages and disadvantages of thiopental?

Use of thiopental in camelids is similar to its use in ruminants. Thiopental is given at 6–10 mg/kg IV in unsedated animals and will provide approximately 10–15 minutes of anesthesia and offers the advantage of small injection volume. Muscle relaxation is usually adequate for tracheal intubation. Intracarotid administration of thiopental must be avoided by confirming correct placement of the venous catheter. Thiopental (2 mg/ml) can also be combined with guaifenesin (50 mg/ml). This combination is administered to effect with the calculated dose being 2.2 ml/kg. If the camelid has not been sedated prior to induction, one can expect that induction will require approximately 65–75% of the calculated dose. This technique allows one the opportunity to administer the drugs to effect. The drugs can be administered via large syringe (60 ml or 140 ml) to provide more precise control over the amount administered. While the combination carries the disadvantage of large injection volume, it is less of an issue in camelids when compared to horses. Camelids tend to cush during induction when they begin to feel the effects of the drugs eliminating the requirement for rapid administration of the agents.

9. What are the advantages and disadvantages of ketamine?

Ketamine is commonly used in camelids. It provides mild cardiovascular stimulation and is safer than thiobarbiturates when used in sick animals. It can be used singly in sedated animals or in combination (1 mg/ml) with guaifenesin (50 mg/ml) given to effect with the calculated dose being 1.5–2.0 ml/kg. Most animals can be intubated following administration of 65–75% of the calculated dose. For convenience, guaifenesin-ketamine may be injected with large (60 ml or 140 ml) syringes rather than administered by infusion.

Xylazine, 0.25 mg/kg IV, and ketamine, 2.5–3.0 mg/kg IV, may be administered 5 minutes apart to obtain a more uniform response and sufficient depth of anesthesia for intubation when compared to intramuscular administration of xylazine-ketamine. If desired, xylazine, 0.5 mg/kg IM, followed by ketamine, 2.2 mg/kg IV, can be used. Duration of anesthesia is 15–20 minutes. Diazepam can be used in place of xylazine in debilitated animals and is given at 0.1 mg/kg IV and followed immediately by ketamine at 2.2–4.4 mg/kg IV. If desired, both drugs may be given mixed in the same syringe. Duration of anesthesia is brief, 5–10 minutes, and muscle relaxation may not be sufficient to allow orotracheal intubation. Transient apnea can occur with all the techniques.

10. What are the advantages and disadvantages of tiletamine-zolazepam?

Tiletamine-zolazepam is a proprietary mixture of tiletamine, a dissociative anesthetic agent, and zolazepam, a benzodiazepine tranquilizer. In a limited number of cases, tiletamine-zolazepam, (2.0 mg/kg IV) provided 15–20 minutes of restraint and 25–35 minutes of recumbency. Depth of anesthesia was adequate to intubate the animals nasally, but muscle relaxation was poor and oral intubation would have been difficult.

11. What are the advantages and disadvantages of propofol?

Propofol is a nonbarbiturate, nonsteroidal hypnotic agent that will provide brief periods (5–10 minutes) of anesthesia in other species. Sedation of the animal prior to induction will decrease the amount of propofol required. Induction and recovery are smooth. If injected rapidly, apnea may occur. Slow administration will usually prevent that complication. Anesthesia was induced with propofol given at 2 mg/kg IV to unsedated llamas. A light plane of anesthesia can be maintained with a constant infusion of propofol at 0.4 mg/kg/min with minimal cardiovascular effects. Mean time from discontinuation of infusion to sternal recumbency was 13 minutes and to standing was 22 minutes. Except during special circumstances (for example, during MR imaging), economic considerations will dictate its use in camelids.

12. What are the drugs available for inhalation induction techniques?

Induction of anesthesia can be performed with inhalation agents in certain instances. When one wishes to avoid administration of intravenous anesthetic agents, for example in crias or compromised animals weighing less than 45 kg, induction with inhalation agents can be very useful as recovery tends to be much quicker because it is based upon elimination of the agent by the respiratory tract rather than metabolism of the agents. Older or less tractable camelids may resent application of the face mask and respond by "spitting." Often, regurgitated ingesta remains in the oral pharynx and hinders intubation or can cause airway obstruction. Halothane, isoflurane, and less commonly sevoflurane and desflurane are available. Halothane and isoflurane have enjoyed widespread use. Halothane does not provide the speed of induction and recovery that isoflurane provides but can still be a useful agent. Sevoflurane and desflurane impart very quick induction of anesthesia and recovery from anesthesia. Currently, sevoflurane is a relatively expensive agent. Desflurane is less expensive, but the vaporizer used to administer the agent is very expensive. Economic considerations will dictate both drugs' entry into camelid anesthesia.

Typically, a face mask is applied to the muzzle of the cria. Depending on the cria's size, commercial canine masks can be used or a mask can be fabricated from a plastic gallon jug, beverage bottle, or other suitable-sized container. The mask is connected to the Y-piece of the rebreathing tubes. One must be certain that the mask does not occlude the nares of the cria. Typical flow rates of oxygen are 3–6 liters/minute with a vaporizer setting of 3–5% isoflurane, 3–5% halothane, 5–8% sevoflurane, or 10–15% desflurane. Recumbency will be accomplished within five minutes with halothane or isoflurane and more rapidly with sevoflurane and desflurane. Flow rate and vaporizer settings with any agent should be decreased to appropriate levels following intubation. If desired, nitrous oxide can be given in addition to oxygen at 3–6 liters/minute with any of the above techniques and will increase the speed of induction.

13. What are the injectable anesthetic drugs available for maintenance of anesthesia?

Agents used for induction of anesthesia, thiopental, ketamine, tiletamine-zolazepam, propofol, and guaifenesin can also be used for maintenance. Following induction with the agents, supplemental injections of 25–50% of the original dose can be administered intermittently as needed to maintain anesthesia for short surgical or diagnostic procedures. A mixture of 0.2% ketamine (2.0 mg/ml), 0.02% xylazine (0.2 mg/ml), 5% guaifenesin (50 mg/ml) can be infused at 1.2–2.4 ml/kg/hr. Final administration rate will vary with patient temperament and the invasiveness of the surgical or diagnostic procedure. Recovery usually occurs within 30 minutes of discontinuing the infusion. Propofol can be infused in unsedated camelids at 0.4 mg/kg/min IV. The infusion rate should be decreased in sedated camelids. It is recommended that camelids maintained under intravenous anesthesia be intubated, as regurgitation remains a possibility. If desired, infusion pumps can be used as a convenient method for administering anesthetic agents in a controlled and precise manner.

12. How difficult is tracheal intubation?

Techniques that combine guaifenesin with a thiobarbiturate or ketamine provide better muscle relaxation during intubation. While xylazine can be given in a high enough dose to allow intubation, muscle relaxation is poor and intubation can be difficult. Techniques that use ketamine or tiletamine-zolazepam as the primary induction agent may also provide difficult conditions for intubation. Intubation can be difficult in camelids because visibility of the larynx is limited. The animal's mouth will not open very widely, and considerable distance may exist between the animal's incisors and larynx. Attempting intubation when anesthetic depth is insufficient will often provoke active regurgitation when the laryngoscope blade contacts the epiglottis or when the endotracheal tube contacts the larynx. With adequate depth of anesthesia, this reflex is eliminated. Desensitization of the larynx with topical lidocaine as is performed in sheep, goats, and swine is usually not necessary in camelids.

Llamas are obligate nasal breathers and are prone to airway obstruction following removal of an oral endotracheal tube. Obstruction is most likely due to dorsal displacement of the soft palate and can be severe and life-threatening, necessitating tracheotomy. Use of agents that promote fast recovery and rapid restoration of airway control by the camelid, sevoflurane, and desflurane, can be advantageous.

Oral intubation (cuffed, 6–14 mm i.d., 50 cm tubes) is performed in a manner similar to that for domestic ruminants. Oral, blind intubation is usually unsuccessful, and laryngoscopy with a 250–350 mm laryngoscope is recommended. Visibility of the larynx is improved by hyperextending the head and neck to make the orotracheal axis approach or exceed 180° and using gauze on a sponge forceps to swab the pharynx if secretions hinder visibility of the larynx. If desired, a guide tube—e.g. a male canine urinary catheter or a feeding tube—could be inserted through the endotracheal tube. The guide tube should extend 6–10 cm beyond the bevel of the endotracheal tube and be passed into the larynx. The endotracheal tube is then threaded off of the guide tube into the trachea.

Nasotracheal intubation is also possible, although it requires an endotracheal tube one size smaller than would be used orally. Blind nasal intubation is technically easier than oral intubation but nasal intubation under laryngoscopic control is technically more difficult than orotracheal intubation. Even though nasotracheal intubation under direct laryngoscopy can be more difficult when blind intubation is not possible, it offers the option of recovering the animal with the endotracheal tube in place as a method of preventing airway obstruction during recovery. The animal can be extubated after it stands when it has full control of its airway.

Camelids are prone to epistaxis, and use of lubricating compounds that contain phenylephrine is recommended. The endotracheal tube is advanced through the external nares into the ventral meatus with slow, gentle pressure. If an obstruction is encountered at approximately 6–10 cm in adult llamas, it is usually due to placement of the tube in the middle meatus. If an obstruction is encountered more caudally, approximately 25 cm in adult llamas, the tube is likely in the pharyngeal diverticulum. In either case, the tube should be withdrawn and redirected. If the endotracheal tube cannot be redirected and manipulated to avoid the pharyngeal diverticulum, placement of a prebent stylet (e.g., a piece of the smallest aluminum diameter rod available for Thomas splints) into the tube to direct the endotracheal tube tip ventrally is usually effective. The pharyngeal diverticulum is not as prominent in alpacas.

After the endotracheal tube has been advanced into the nasopharynx, the camelid's head and neck should be hyperextended and the tube manipulated into the larynx. If the tube will not enter the larynx, placing a slightly bent stylet in the endotracheal tube to direct the tube tip ventrally into the larynx instead of the esophagus is helpful. Although visibility of the larynx is somewhat limited, oral laryngoscopy will aid intubation and confirm correct and incorrect placement of the tube during intubation. Following intubation, correct placement of nasal and oral endotracheal tube can be confirmed by standard techniques.

15. What are the advantages and disadvantages of halothane for maintenance of anesthesia?

Halothane is a drug that has been used for induction and maintenance of anesthesia in camelids. It is relatively insoluble and provides quick induction of, and recovery from, anesthesia. It is relatively potent with a MAC (minimal alveolar concentration) of 0.8%. Typically, anesthesia is induced with vaporizer settings of 4% in adult camelids and 3% in crias, with vaporizer settings of 1.5–2.5% used for maintenance. It can cause dose-related bradycardia and hypotension and has been associated with postoperative liver dysfunction and death in one alpaca.

16. What are the advantages and disadvantages of isoflurane for maintenance of anesthesia?

Isoflurane is a drug that is widely used for induction and maintenance of anesthesia in camelids. It is more insoluble than halothane and provides quicker induction of, and recovery from, anesthesia. It is relatively potent, with MAC being 1.3%. It can cause dose-related bradycardia and hypotension. The agent is less prone to cause arrhythmias than halothane. Very little of the drug is metabolized (<1%).

17. What are the advantages and disadvantages of sevoflurane and desflurane for maintenance of anesthesia?

Sevoflurane is a drug that has recently become available for induction and maintenance of anesthesia in camelids. It is much more insoluble than halothane or isoflurane and provides very rapid induction of and recovery from anesthesia. It is not as potent as halothane or isoflurane, with MAC predicted to be between 2.3% and 2.6% in camelids after extrapolation from other species. It can cause dose-related bradycardia and hypotension.

Desflurane is a very insoluble anesthetic and is characterized by rapid onset of, and recovery from, anesthesia. The vaporizer used to deliver the agent is very expensive and may limit usefulness of desflurane. It is the least potent of the modern inhalation anesthetic agents with MAC expected to be between 7.0% and 8.0% in camelids after extrapolation from other species. It can cause dose-related bradycardia and hypotension. Both drugs' ability to impart rapid recovery from anesthesia should provide rapid restoration of airway control by the camelid and help decrease the incidence of post-extubation airway obstruction.

18. What is needed for supportive care?

Supportive therapy consists of proper padding and positioning of the patient, techniques to help maintain normal body temperature, particularly in crias. Administration of intravenous fluids and cardiovascular support drugs, good monitoring techniques, and mechanical ventilation, and should be managed in a manner similar to domestic ruminants.

19. What type of monitoring techniques should be used during anesthesia?

Monitoring is similar to that performed during equine and ruminant anesthesia. Heart rate, pulse strength, muscle relaxation, respiratory rate, capillary refill time, blood pressure, color of mucous membranes, and palpebral reflexes are used to monitor depth of anesthesia. Normal values are listed in the table. Heart rate is usually above resting values in response to atropine administration. It often decreases as the effects of the chronotrope dissipate and depth of anesthesia increases and usually remains above 60 beats/minute. Animals who have received an alpha-2 agonist will have slower heart rates.

The saphenous artery can be easily palpated. The caudal auricular artery is also easily palpated. The common digital arteries just dorsal to the dewclaws can be palpated. The facial artery is usually not palpable.

Normal Values for Anesthetized Camelids

VARIABLE	VALUE
Respiratory rate	
Adults	10–30 breaths/minute
Juveniles	20–40 breaths/minute
Tidal volume	5.0–10.0 ml/kg
Heart rate	
Adults (following atropine)	60–90 beats/minute
Adults (following xylazine)	28–40 beats/minute
Juveniles (following atropine)	100–125 beats/minute
Gingival perfusion time	12 seconds
Arterial pressure	
Systolic/diastolic	100–130/6580 mmHg
Mean	75–100 mmHg
Central venous pressure	5–10 cm H_2O
End tidal CO_2	30–40 torr
End tidal anesthetic agent	
Halothane (with premedication)	0.8–0.9%
Halothane (without premedication)	1.0–1.2%
Isoflurane (with premedication)	1.3–1.4%
Isoflurane (without premedication)	1.6–1.9%
Sevoflurane (with premedication)	2.3–2.6%*
Sevoflurane (without premedication)	2.9–3.6%*
Desflurane (with premedication)	7.0–8.0%*
Desflurane (without premedication)	9.5–11.5%*

*Predicted from other species

Ocular reflexes are beneficial in assessing anesthetic depth. Usually the palpebral reflex of the dorsal eyelid remains during surgical anesthesia. However, if the animal can move its ventral eyelid without tactile stimulation, anesthetic depth is decreasing and eventually movement is likely. Nystagmus usually does not occur. The corneal reflex should be present, but often is not assessed because of the reliability of the other reflexes and the risk of injury to the eye. Ocular rotation as occurs in cattle in response to changes in depth of anesthesia does not occur in camelids.

Some anesthetic agent analyzers will detect methane present in the expired gas of herbivores and report it as anesthetic agent. Values obtained from blood gas analysis are similar to normal values of other species.

20. What type of ventilation should be employed during anesthesia?

Anesthetized camelids tend to ventilate very well, especially if sedatives were not administered prior to induction, and allowing the camelid to remain on spontaneous ventilation is usually sufficient. When the procedure is expected to be lengthy (> 90 minutes), consideration can be given to instituting mechanical ventilation. Controlled ventilation must be used during thoracotomy or when muscle relaxants are used. Common ventilator settings are a respiratory rate of 6–10 breaths/minute with a tidal volume of 15 ml/kg. Final ventilator settings are dependent on results of blood gas analysis. Ventilators adequate for foals, calves, or other animals of similar size are recommended for llamas.

21. What type of cardiovascular support is required during anesthesia?

When hypotension is present and cannot be corrected by administering intravenous fluids and adjusting anesthetic depth without the animal moving, several different drugs are available for use. They include calcium borogluconate, ephedrine, dobutamine, and dopamine. When hypotension without bradycardia occurs, inotropes are used to increase stroke volume and cardiac output. Calcium borogluconate (23% solution) increases myocardial contractility and is given as a slow infusion (0.5–1.0 ml/kg/hr) to effect. Often, calcium administration can be discontinued after mean arterial pressure returns to normal values. Ephedrine, a mixed alpha and beta sympathomimetic drug, can be used at 0.02–0.06 mg/kg IV to increase mean arterial pressure through an increase in cardiac contractility and vasomotor tone. Dobutamine does not seem to be as effective in camelids as in other species, often causing tachycardia without increasing blood pressure. Dobutamine is administered at 1.0–2.0 µg/kg/minute IV to effect. Following correction of hypotension, rate of administration can usually be decreased to maintenance levels. Use of an infusion pump is recommended for convenience and accuracy of administration.

22. What arrangements must be made for recovery?

The preferred location for recovering camelids from anesthesia would be similar to that used for ruminants. Placing the camelid in sternal recumbency is preferred. If intubated orally, the animal should remain intubated until it is able to swallow, chew, cough, and is actively trying to expel the endotracheal tube. Following removal of the oral tube, confirmation of air exchange during breathing must be performed. Animals with a nasal endotracheal tube can be extubated after they stand. An assistant should remain nearby to offer assistance. For the most part, camelids tend to remain in sternal recumbency until they are able to stand and then do so.

23. Is sedation necessary for recovery?

A very high number, if not all, camelids recover very well from anesthesia without experiencing emergence delirium. This characteristic is a reflection of their personality, as camelids do not feel the urgency to arise that horses experience and they respond more favorably to restraint.

24. What agents are available for reversal of alpha-2 agonists?

Sedation following use of alpha-2 agonists can be reversed by alpha-2 adrenoceptor antagonists, yohimbine, tolazoline, and atipamezole. Although doxapram, an analeptic, will reverse xylazine sedation in cattle, it will not reverse xylazine sedation in camelids even when given in doses as high as 2.0 mg/kg IV. None of the alpha-2 antagonists are cleared for use in camelids by the FDA.

The amount of antagonist required to reverse an alpha-2 sedative will depend on the amount of alpha-2 agonist used and the interval between its administration and administration of the antagonist. If the interval between administration of the two drugs is relatively long, then extensive metabolism of the alpha-2 sedative should have occurred and less antagonist will be needed. Giving the full dose of antagonist after extensive metabolism of the sedative has occurred could cause mild to moderate excitement in the animal.

Yohimbine (Yobine®, 2 mg/ml, Lloyd Laboratories; Antagonil®, 5 mg/ml, Wildlife Laboratories) is given at 0.12 mg/kg IV. Atipamezole is a highly selective alpha-2 antagonist, approximately 200 times greater than yohimbine. Side effects associated with its use in unsedated dogs are increased heart rate, increased motor activity, irritability, panting, sweating, and vomiting. Experience with atipamezole is somewhat limited in llamas. One could expect on occasion to see somewhat similar signs when reversing alpha-2 sedation in llamas if large doses of atipamezole are given relatively long after the alpha-2 sedative was administered. Atipamezole (Antisedan®, 5 mg/ml) has been used in llamas at 125 µg/kg IV following medetomidine. Reversal of sedation occurred in approximately 6 minutes.

Tolazoline (Tolazine®, 100 mg/ml, Lloyd Laboratories), has both alpha-1 and alpha-2 activity and can cause vasodilatation because of its alpha-1 effect. Caution should be exercised when tolazoline is given to animals with compromised cardiovascular status to avoid precipitating shock. Our method of administering tolazoline to llamas and domestic ruminants has been to give 50% of the calculated dose (1.0– 2.0 mg/kg) initially and the remainder if adequate reversal does not occur. In most instances, the initial amount (1.0 mg/kg IV) of tolazoline is adequate to provide sufficient arousal of the animal for it to be able to stand. Following tolazoline at 2.0 mg/kg IV opisthotonus can occur in some llamas, usually those where the interval between alpha-2 agonist and antagonist administration was longer and thus more metabolism of the agonist had occurred. After that period of excitement subsides, recovery is uneventful.

25. Are there precautions for use of alpha-2 antagonists in camelids?

There are anecdotal reports of death associated with tolazoline administration in cattle, usually following higher doses of the drug given to animals with compromised physical status. There have also been anecdotal reports of death associated with tolazoline administration in apparently healthy llamas, usually following higher doses of the drug. The cause of death is undetermined. It may be related to tolazoline's alpha-1 activity. Tolazoline has both alpha-1 and alpha-2 activity and thus will cause vasodilatation. Animals that are dehydrated or in shock try to maintain their blood pressure by vasoconstriction in the face of falling cardiac output. Administration of tolazoline, acepromazine, and other compounds that cause alpha-1 blockade eliminate this protective response and can cause severely affected animals to decompensate. If an alpha-2 agonist has been used to provide sedation in this instance and antagonism of sedation is desired, an agent with high specificity for alpha-2 receptors is indicated. If tolazoline is the only available agent. it should be given at 0.5–1.0 mg/kg IV. If sufficient arousal does not occur, additional tolazoline could be given.

26. What techniques are available for local or regional anesthesia?

Local anesthetic techniques are performed much as they are in domestic ruminants of comparable size. Infiltration, peripheral nerve blocks, and intravenous local anesthesia can be used in camelids to provide regional anesthesia. Because their body weight is lower, one must be cognizant of the amount of local anesthetic agent used to avoid toxicity. In other species, 13 mg/kg is recognized as the maximum amount that can be safely injected at one time for peripheral nerve blocks or infiltrated for regional anesthesia. Techniques for blockade of peripheral nerves could be extrapolated from the equivalent block in horses or domestic ruminants. Techniques for intravenous local anesthesia would be similar to that performed in domestic ruminants of similar size. After application of a tourniquet either distal or proximal to the carpus or tarsus, 5–10 ml of 2% lidocaine is injected into a peripheral vein distal to the tourniquet. Anesthesia will occur rapidly. Following completion of the procedure the tourniquet should be released gradually to avoid toxicity from the local anesthetic agent.

Caudal epidural anesthesia can be performed when indicated. The technique is similar to that used in calves. Usually the injection is made at the sacro-caudal junction with an 18–20 gauge 2.5 cm needle. That space is larger than it is in cattle or horses and the needle usually does not have to be inserted as deeply, approximately 1 cm, before it enters the epidural space. Following placement of the needle, fluid placed in the needle hub will be aspirated into the epidural space or a test injection of air could be used to help confirm correct needle placement. Lidocaine can be injected at 0.22 mg/kg or, if desired, appropriate amounts of bupivacaine, mepivacaine, or procaine could be used. Onset of anesthesia following lidocaine is within 5 minutes and duration of anesthesia is 60–90 minutes. Addition of epinephrine will prolong anesthesia.

Epidural xylazine has been used extensively in cattle and horses to provide anesthesia in the perineal area. This technique provides anesthesia of longer duration than that obtained with traditional local anesthetic agents. When used alone in llamas, 10% xylazine (0.17 mg/kg), diluted in saline or water for injection to a final volume of no greater than 2.0 ml/150 kg provides onset of anesthesia in approximately 20 minutes and duration of anesthesia of approximately 180 minutes. Some llamas will become sedated for about 20–30 minutes beginning 20 minutes after injection but usually remain standing. Onset of anesthesia can be hastened and duration can be lengthened in cattle and horses by combining xylazine with lidocaine. When used in llamas, the combination of xylazine (0.17 mg/kg) and lidocaine (0.22 mg/kg) provides onset of anesthesia within 5 minutes and duration of approximately 325 minutes. When combining the two agents, it is recommended that 10% xylazine be used to minimize injection volume and subsequent ataxia from cranial migration of the agents. Total volume should not exceed 2 ml/150 kg to prevent excessive rostral migration of blockade and subsequent recumbency of the animal.

BIBLIOGRAPHY

1. Amsel SI, and LW Johnson: Choosing the best site to perform venipuncture in a llama. Vet Med 82:535-536, 1987.
2. Barrington GM, TF Meyer, and SM Parish: Standing castration of the llama using butorphanol tartrate and local anesthesia. Eq Pract 15:35-39, 1993.
3. Fowler ME: Medicine and Surgery of the South American Camelid. Ames, Iowa State University Press, 1998, pp 89-107.
4. Fowler ME: The jugular vein of the llama (Lama glama): A clinical note. J Zoo An Med 14:77-78, 1983.
5. Groom S, S Checkley, and B Crawford: Hepatic necrosis associated with halothane anesthesia in an alpaca. Can Vet J 36:39-41, 1995.
6. Grubb TL, TW Riebold, and MJ Huber: Comparison of lidocaine, xylazine, and lidocaine/xylazine for caudal epidural anesthesia in the horse. J Am Vet Med Assoc 201:1187-1190, 1992.
7. Heath RB: Llama anesthetic programs. Vet Clin North Am–Food An Pract 5:71-80, 1989.
8. Klein L, M Tomasic, and K Olson: Evaluation of Telazol in llamas. Vet Surg 19:316-317, 1990.
9. Mama, KR, AE Wagner, DA Parker, PW Hellyer, JS Gaynor: Determination of the minimum alveolar concentration of isoflurane in llamas. Vet Surg 28:121-125, 1999.
10. Mama KR, ML Aubin, LW Johnson: Experiences with xylazine, butorphanol and ketamine for short-term anesthesia in llamas and alpacas. Proceedings 7th World Congress of Veterinary Anaesthesia. [abstract] Berne, 104, 2000.
11. Riebold TW, AJ Kaneps, and WB Schmotzer: Reversal of xylazine-induced sedation in llamas, using doxapram or 4-aminopyridine and yohimbine. J Am Vet Med Assoc 189:1059-1061, 1986.
12. Riebold TW, Kaneps AJ, and WB Schmotzer: Anesthesia in the llama. Vet Surg 18:400-404, 1989.
13. Riebold TW, HN Engel, TL Grubb, JG Adams, MJ Huber, and WB Schmotzer: Orotracheal and nasotracheal intubation in llamas. J Am Vet Med Assoc 204:779-783, 1994.
14. Waldridge BM, HC Lin, FJ DeGraves, and DG Pugh: Sedative effects of medetomidine and its reversal by atipamezole in llamas. J Am Vet Med Assoc 211:1562-1565, 1997.

45. PORCINE ANESTHESIA

Stephen A. Greene, D.V.M., M.S., D.A.C.V.A., and
G. John Benson, D.V.M., M.S., D.A.C.V.A.

1. What are the anatomic features relevant to porcine anesthesia?

Intramuscular injection in swine should be deep into the tissue in order to avoid the thick layer of fat below the skin. A 1.5 inch (3.75 cm) hypodermic needle should be used for intramuscular injections. The lack of readily accessible superficial veins is another complicating feature. The best location for intravenous injection or catheter placement is the marginal ear vein. Intramuscularly administered sedatives or tranquilizers will facilitate procedures for gaining intravenous access. The laryngeal anatomy is somewhat unusual in swine compared to other mammals. The larynx is situated in a sigmoid curve of the airway. Endotracheal intubation is complicated by this feature and frequently results in difficulty passing the tube through the glottis.

2. Why are pigs difficult to anesthetize?

In addition to the anatomic features described above, pigs strongly dislike being restrained. A restraint stanchion or sling can facilitate injections and catheter placement in awake or sedated pigs.

3. Which anesthetics and adjuncts are approved by the Center for Veterinary Medicine (CVM) of the Food and Drug Administration (FDA) for use in food animals?

Atropine, azaperone, chloral hydrate, epinephrine, furosemide, lidocaine, methoxyflurane, and pentobarbital are approved by the FDA for use in food animals. Most of these drugs have no withdrawal time specified and have no established residue tolerance for the pig. Obviously, administration of unapproved agents will be necessary to provide anesthesia and analgesia for pigs. The veterinarian is advised to ensure that at least 10 half-lives of the agent be allowed prior to slaughter as a rule of thumb to eliminate 99.9% of drug residues in pigs intended for food. For most anesthetic agents, this will require a minimum of 48 to 96 hours after administration.

4. Which tranquilizers/sedatives are most useful in pigs?

The group of tranquilizers that is most effective in pigs is the butyrophenone class. Azaperone is a member of this group that is specifically approved for use in pigs by the CVM of the FDA. Phenothiazine tranquilizers are less effective but are also commonly used when butyrophenone tranquilizers are not available. Alpha-2 agonist sedatives are useful, especially in combination with other agents, but relatively high doses must be used (e.g., xylazine, 2.2 mg/kg).

5. How is venous access obtained in a pig?

Pigs can be sedated with xylazine (2.2 mg/kg) and ketamine (2.2 mg/kg) given intramuscularly. The auricular vein is raised by placing a rubber band around the base of the ear. The vein is catheterized and then secured using a roll of gauze or tape that is placed inside the pinna to provide a tube for securing the catheter.

6. Describe tracheal intubation of the pig.

Intubation can be accomplished by use of guide tube technique, or by starting advancement of the tube under direct visualization and then rotating the tube 180 degrees when resistance to further advancement is encountered. The rotation technique is most effective when using endotracheal tubes with a natural curvature versus a straight tube. Swine are predisposed to develop laryngospasm when the airway is physically manipulated. Use of topical lidocaine for laryngeal desensitization is recommended prior to attempting endotracheal intubation.

7. Discuss an anesthetic protocol suitable for a Vietnamese pot-bellied pig.

The combination of Telazol with xylazine and ketamine is useful for providing immobization and anesthesia in Vietnamese pot-bellied pigs. Telazol is reconstituted with 250 mg of xylazine and 250 mg of ketamine. This yields 5 ml of the combination with the following concentrations: xylazine, 50 mg/ml; ketamine 50 mg/ml; tiletamine 50 mg/ml; and zolazepam 50 mg/ml. The combination (referred to as TKX) is dosed using 1 ml/50 kg for deep intramuscular injection. It can also be administered IV at the dose of 1 ml/75 kg. Surgical anesthesia achieved with TKX will last about 30 minutes. Recovery from Telazol combinations may take 1–2 hours.

8. Describe the epidural technique for a cesarian operation in a sow.

Lumbosacral (L6-S1) epidural anesthesia is commonly performed to facilitate the cesarean operation in sows. A crate or stanchion is helpful for restraint. Ideally, sedatives that may cause hypotension or ataxia are not administered. As in the dog, the site for lumbosacral needle placement is on the midline and just caudal to the transverse line connecting the most cranial aspect of the iliac crests. If the ilium cannot be palpated, the vertical line through the patella of a standing sow will be about 2.5 cm cranial to the lumbosacral junction. Lidocaine (2%) has been used for local anesthesia at a dose of 10 ml for 100 kg of body weight, 15 ml for 200 kg, up to a 20 ml maximum dose in larger pigs. Alternatively, 1 ml of lidocaine is injected for the first 40 cm of distance from the base of the tail to the occipital protuberance plus 1.5 ml for each additional 10 cm of back length. Lidocaine will provide about 90 minutes of analgesia with complete recovery in 2 hours.

9. Describe the triggers, symptoms, and treatment of malignant hyperthermia in swine.

Malignant hyperthermia is a rapidly progressing condition characterized by increased metabolism and CO_2 production, muscle rigidity, and increased body temperature. It has been triggered by inhaled halogenated anesthetics, succinycholine, and stress in susceptible individuals. While any animal may develop malignant hyperthermia, white swine appear to be more likely than others. Red, splotchy patterns develop on the ventral skin surface in white swine early in the progression of the syndrome. Anesthetized swine become overheated and temperatures may exceed 105° F. Frequently the soda-lime in the anesthetic circuit becomes quickly depleted and changes to the characteristic blue color in the presence of exhaled CO_2. Hyperpnea may be observed. Lactate production, muscular contraction, sympathetic nervous system activation, and cardiac dysrhythmias occur. Myoglobinuria may be observed in animals that survive long enough.

Dantrolene (2–5 mg/kg, IV) is the treatment of choice for malignant hyperthermia. The inhaled anesthetic should be terminated and oxygen should be delivered from a new anesthesia machine (that has not been used that day). Symptomatic treatment consists of procaine (1–2 mg/kg, iv), corticosteroids, bicarbonate, and body cooling using ice water–alcohol mixtures applied topically. Intravenous or rectal administration of cold saline solutions may also be effective. Orally administered dantrolene, while less expensive than the injectable formulation, is unlikely to be effective when treating an acute episode. Oral dantrolene (10 mg/kg) has been administered as a prophylactic measure in individuals with a familial or individual history of susceptibility when undergoing anesthesia. Acepromazine for premedication of swine may inhibit development of malignant hyperthermia.

BIBLIOGRAPHY

1. Papich MG: Drug residue considerations for anesthetics and adjunctive drugs in food-producing animals. Vet Clin North Am (Food Animal) 12:693-706, 1996.
2. Riebold TW, Goble DO, and Geiser DR: Clinical techniques for food animal anesthesia. In: Large Animal Anesthesia—Principles and Techniques. Ames, IA, Iowa State University Press, 1982, pp 75-87.
3. Skarda RT: Local and regional anesthesia in ruminants and swine. Vet Clin North Am (Food Animal) 12:579-626, 1996.
4. Thurmon JC: Injectable anesthetic agents and techniques in ruminants and swine. Vet Clin North Am (Food Animal) 2:567-592, 1986.
5. Thurmon JC, Benson GJ: Anesthesia in ruminants and swine. In: Howard JC (ed)., Current Veterinary Therapy, Food Animal Practice, 3rd ed., Philadelphia, WB Saunders, 1993, pp 58-76.
6. Thurmon JC, Tranquilli WJ, and Benson GJ: Swine. In: Thurmon JC, Tranquilli WJ, Benson GJ (eds): Lumb and Jones' Veterinary Anesthesia, 3rd ed. Philadelphia, Williams and Wilkins, 1996, pp 627-644.

46. AVIAN ANESTHESIA

Luisito S. Pablo, D.V.M., M.S., D.A.C.V.A.

1. Enumerate the anatomic and physiologic peculiarities in the avian respiratory system that will have an impact on anesthesia.
- The air sacs serve as bellows to ventilate the lung.
- There is no diaphragm to separate the thoracic cavity from the abdominal cavity. The avian thoracic cavity is at atmospheric pressure.
- The total volume of the respiratory system in birds is larger than that in mammals of comparable size. However, birds have smaller functional residual volume.
- Birds have a much higher surface to volume ratio and a thinner blood–air barrier, resulting in more efficient gas exchange.
- Both inspiration and expiration are active processes requiring the contraction of respiratory muscles
- The tracheal volume is about 4.5 times larger in birds, resulting in more dead space.
- The trachea is composed of complete cartilaginous rings.

2. How do you prepare birds for anesthesia?
Anesthetic preparation should include a complete history taking. Birds that will require general anesthesia should have a thorough physical examination. Some birds may not tolerate restraint and should be observed from a distance, with emphasis on the bird's disposition, awareness of the surrounding, feather condition, body form, and posture. This same approach should be used in some debilitated birds to minimize stress and struggling. Focus must be put on preoperative evaluation of the cardiovascular and respiratory functions. The patient should be observed for abnormal breathing patterns, tachypnea, and tail bobbing. The nares should be examined for secretions and possible obstruction. Exercise tolerance can be gauged by the ability of the bird to return to normal respiration following physical restraint. The heart should be auscultated and any abnormalities in rate and rhythm and the presence of murmurs should be noted. Some abnormalities may require more diagnostic testing, such as an electrocardiograph. The hydration status of the bird should be assessed. Skin turgor can be determined by rolling the skin between fingers. The mouth should be examined for dryness, and the peripheral vein can be palpated for turgidity. During the preanesthetic examination, baseline vital signs and accurate body weight (grams in small birds; kilograms in bigger birds) should be recorded.

3. Is fasting before anesthesia necessary in birds?
Fasting is highly recommended in birds because they can regurgitate during anesthesia. Large birds, greater than 500 g, should fast for at least 12 hours. In smaller birds, fasting can be shortened depending on their body weights and it can be as short as 2 to 3 hours before anesthesia. The main concern with fasting in smaller birds is their high metabolic rate and poor hepatic glycogen storage. Water can be offered until 2 to 3 hours before anesthesia.

4. What are the minimum laboratory data needed for birds before anesthesia?
The following laboratory data should be obtained as a minimum requirement:
- Packed cell volume (35–55%)
- Plasma total protein (3.5–5.5 g/dl)
- Blood glucose (200 mg/dl)

Some birds may require more hematologic, and clinical chemistry tests, depending on the presenting problems and findings from physical examination.

5. How do you manage anemic birds before anesthesia?

Blood transfusion is indicated in patients with a packed cell volume (PCV) less than 20%. Blood should also be collected and be ready for transfusion in patients with PCV less than 35% who will undergo a surgical procedure that is commonly associated with hemorrhage. Homologous donors are preferred, although single heterologous transfusions have been successfully administered. About 10% of the donor's blood is collected into a heparinized syringe. The collected blood is immediately transfused to the recipient. The normal blood volume of birds ranges from 5 to 10% of body weight. The volume for transfusion should be 10 to 20% of the recipient's calculated blood volume. If possible, two donors should be available.

6. Is preanesthetic medication necessary in avian anesthesia?

Preanesthetic medication is not routinely employed in birds because:
- Sedatives or tranquilizers will prolong recovery and may lead to rough recovery.
- Anticholinergic (atropine or glycopyrrolate) will make the respiratory secretions more viscous.

There are situations in which preanesthetic medication is necessary:
- Diving birds when mask induction with inhalant agent is contemplated (to minimize diving response).
- Ratites or bigger birds that require chemical sedation before anesthetic induction.
- Birds in pain.

7. If preanesthetic medication is necessary, what are the most commonly used drugs?

For smaller birds (<15 kg), midazolam or diazepam can be given at 0.5–1.0 mg/kg IM. Xylazine should be used with caution in sick birds because of its depressant effect on the cardiovascular and pulmonary systems. In healthy birds, xylazine can be given at 1.0–6.0 mg/kg IM for sedation.

For the bigger birds (ratites), xylazine can be given at 0.2–0.4 mg/kg IM for sedation. As an alternative, tiletamine-zolazepam (Telazol) at 2.0–5.0 mg/kg IM can be used.

8. What is a dive response?

Dive response is considered a stress response manifested by diving birds when trigeminal receptors in the beak and nares are stimulated. The response can be elicited by simply putting a facemask snugly over the beak and face of the bird. The presence of the inhalant anesthetic in the inspired gas is not required for the response. The signs of the dive response include apnea and bradycardia and can last for 3 to 5 minutes. Administration of premedicants, such as diazepam or midazolam, before mask induction appears to blunt this response.

9. What is a renal portal system and does it have any significance in relation to the administration of injectable agents given intramuscularly?

Birds have a renal portal circulation. Venous blood from the legs and the lower intestine, which is in the process of returning to the heart, enters the kidneys first through the renal portal system. It is estimated that 50 to 70% of the total renal blood flow is contributed by the renal portal vein. There is a prevailing concern that injection of drugs into the leg muscles will result in drug loss through the kidneys. This is partly supported by a study showing a difference in the bioavailability of a drug between the pectoral and leg muscles. In practice, the renal portal circulation will have more of an impact in drugs that require constant blood level as in antibiotics. The impact of the renal portal system in intramuscular injectable agents is minimal considering that these drugs are given to effect. If the desired effect is not observed, incremental doses can be given as needed. In general, the pectoral muscles are used for intramuscular administration of drugs in walking birds, whereas in the flying birds, the leg muscles are preferred.

10. What is the most common and effective anesthetic induction technique used in birds that are amenable to physical restraint?

By far the most common anesthetic induction technique in birds that can be restrained physically is the use of inhalant agent, mainly isoflurane, administered using a facemask. A review of our avian cases revealed the use of isoflurane as an induction agent in all the birds anesthetized in 1999. Sevoflurane, which produces quicker induction and recovery than isoflurane, may be a better alternative in birds. The minimum anesthetic concentration (MAC) of sevoflurane in chickens is 2.21%. It can be used in other birds with the assumption that its MAC will be within the range of minimum alveolar concentration in mammals.

11. Describe the technique of mask induction in birds.

A mask that is appropriate to the size and shape of the head of the bird is used. For medium-sized birds, commercially available facemasks for dogs and cats can be used. Smaller birds may require a facemask made of syringe cases. Birds with long bills need an elongated mask made from 60 ml syringe case or plastic soda bottles with the bottom cut and the sharp edges covered with some bandaging material.

The bird is restrained properly with careful attention paid to the adequacy of ventilation. Some birds can be wrapped in a towel during this process. Place the mask over the beak, making sure that the nares are included. A high concentration of oxygen is then administered. The vaporizer setting is turned on to about 0.5% after about 3–5 minutes of oxygen administration. The vaporizer setting is increased by 0.5% every five breaths until 3.0% is reached. This is done to prevent breath-holding. Sevoflurane can be administered to as high as 5.0%. If the bird starts to struggle, increase the concentration immediately. Anytime the bird relaxes, the vaporizer setting should be turned down to maintenance setting (1.25–1.5 MAC). If the bird appears to be in a deep plane of anesthesia, further reduction in the vaporizer setting is warranted.

12. In large birds weighing more than 15 kg, mainly the ratites, what are the most commonly used induction techniques?

Mask induction in ratites, except in young or moribund ones, is very dangerous and can take a long time. Induction in most cases is accomplished with the use of injectable agents either given intramuscularly or intravenously. The table lists the different anesthetic combinations that can be used.

Drugs	Dose and Route	Comments
Xylazine (premed)	1.0–2.0 mg/kg IM	Wait for 15 minutes before giving ketamine.
Ketamine (induction)	4.0 mg/kg IV given to effect	
Xylazine (premed)	0.25 mg/kg IV	Wait for sedation and wing drooping (3–5 minutes)
Ketamine (induction)	2.2 mg/kg IV	
Zolazepam-tiletamine	4–12 mg/kg IM	If unable to intubate, can complete induction using isoflurane via face mask
Zolazepam-tiletamine	2.0–8.0 mg/kg IV	Rapid and smooth induction, but recovery may be stormy and prolonged
Midazolam (premedicant)	0.2 mg/kg IM	Wait for about 35 minutes before giving
Butorphanol (premedicant)	0.4 mg/kg IM	ketamine IV
Ketamine	9 mg/kg IV to effect	
Diazepam	0.2–0.3 mg/kg IV	Given after premedication with xylazine
Ketamine	2.2 mg/kg IV	Can be mixed in a single syringe

13. What is the best anesthetic protocol for maintaining anesthesia in birds?

The best anesthetic protocol for maintenance in birds is the use of an inhalant agent. At present, isoflurane is the agent most commonly used. Its use results in rapid induction and recovery, less depression of cardiac output compared with halothane, and better perfusion of the liver. Sevoflurane, a newer inhalant agent, has much lower blood–gas partition coefficient than isoflurane. It should produce quicker induction and recovery in birds. In a study in psittacines, recovery times for isoflurane and sevoflurane were not significantly different. However, the birds that had sevoflurane were less ataxic.

Precision vaporizer for isoflurane and sevoflurane should be used. For birds smaller than 10 kg, anesthesia is maintained using a non-rebreathing circuit. The oxygen flow rate should be three times the minute ventilation. However, for accurate anesthetic output of the vaporizer, a higher oxygen flow rate should be used. A circle breathing system is used in birds weighing more than 10 kg.

14. Describe tracheal intubation in birds.

Birds are intubated in a sternal position with the head above the body to minimize regurgitation. The mouth of the bird is opened. In some cases, a piece of gauze can be placed around the upper and lower beak to facilitate visualization. The glottis is identified at the base of the tongue. A cotton-tipped applicator or gauze can be used to pull the tongue forward. If the bird is breathing, there is a rhythmic opening of the glottis and the insertion of the endotracheal tube can be timed during inspiration. Since the glottis is slit-like, the tube bevel should be turned sideways during insertion. The glottis of some birds, such as the parakeets, is located at the base of the humped and fleshy tongue, which makes visualization more difficult. If visualization of the glottis is extremely difficult, as in the flamingo, the tube can be passed blindly aided by external palpation of the trachea and placing of the head and neck in extension. In general, tracheal intubation in most birds is easy and should be considered every time. The endotracheal tube is usually secured to the lower beak.

15. What is the size limit for tracheal intubation in birds?

Birds that are larger than 100 g can be intubated.

16. What are the hazards associated with tracheal intubation in birds?

Rupture of the tracheal mucosa and rings can occur as a result of overly inflated cuff. Other possibility is a fibrotic narrowing of the trachea following tracheal intubation. These problems are more likely to happen in birds because their trachea is composed of complete rings of cartilage. To prevent these complications, the use of uncuffed tubes in birds is recommended. The cuffed tubes can be used, but they should not be inflated. In case of excessive leak around the cuff, inflation of the cuff should be undertaken with extreme care.

In small birds, dried mucus can partially or completely obstruct the endotracheal tube. The signs of airway obstruction include airway noises, prolonged expiratory phase, and slow emptying of the air sacs during the expiratory phase following an artificial sigh. If an obstructed tube is diagnosed, the tube should be replaced by a clean and patent tube.

17. How do I monitor the depth of anesthesia in birds?

The principles behind monitoring of the depth of anesthesia in birds are similar to the principles in mammals. All parameters have to be weighed and correlated before a reasonable judgment on the anesthetic depth can be made. Movement as a result of painful stimulus is an obvious manifestation of very light plane of anesthesia. In addition, there will be tachycardia, tachypnea, coughing, and the presence of brisk eye reflexes. The tricky aspect of monitoring the depth of anesthesia is the distinction between deep and medium planes of surgical anesthesia. The depth of anesthesia should correspond to the degree of pain involved with the procedure. Birds in a good plane of anesthesia will have a corneal reflex, regular respiratory pattern, and constricted pupil. The muscle relaxation, as assessed using the jaw tone, is present. The palpebral reflex may be absent. A deep plane of anesthesia is usually characterized by severe hypotension, bradypnea, irregular respiratory pattern and depth, and the absence of response to monitored reflexes. Sudden piloerection and mydriasis are usually followed by cardiac arrest.

18. How would you monitor the cardiovascular function of a bird during anesthesia?

Depending on the availability of equipment and the size of the patient, a bird can be monitored with a combination of the following:
- Clinical skills: Emphasis is placed on observing the mucous membrane color and color of the cere, beak, or bill. The capillary refill time and pulse quality should also be noted.
- Auscultation: A stethoscope is used to obtain heart rate and rhythm. The heart sound is best heard below the sternum and at the thoracic inlet. Changes of 20% above or below the predicted heart rate are abnormal. The esophageal stethoscope can be used in some species. The presence of the crop makes the positioning of the esophageal stethoscope difficult in some birds. A stethoscope can be a useful tool in detecting and confirming cardiac arrest. It is not very sensitive in detecting developing circulatory collapse.

- Electrocardiography: The electrocardiograph will detect dysrhythmias during anesthesia. Depending upon the dysrhythmias, appropriate action can be taken. It is important that the ECG machine be capable of monitoring high heart rates and have a freeze feature for rapid electrocardiogram interpretation. The ECG clips can be attached to hypodermic needles or stainless steel wires inserted through the skin in each prepatagial area and in the medial thigh region. Lead contact is improved by using electrode gel. Either lead I or II can be used.
- Doppler flow apparatus: The Doppler flow probe is very useful in detecting blood flow and changes in pulse rate and rhythm. The sites for probe placement include the ulnar artery, metatarsal artery, under the tongue, or against the carotid artery in the neck. A pediatric probe works well in smaller birds. The Doppler flow can also be used in determining blood pressure indirectly with the aid of a sphygmomanometer. The cuff is placed proximal to the site of probe placement, which in this case is on the metatarsal area. This technique works well if an appropriately sized cuff can be used.
- Indirect blood pressure monitor: Blood pressure can be monitored indirectly using Doppler or oscillometric technology. The oscillometric technique requires that pulsations be detectable by the machine to produce results. It has been used in bigger birds such as ostrich and emu. The cuff is placed over the tibial artery, located above the tarsus.
- Direct blood pressure monitor: Direct blood pressure gives second-to-second changes in the systemic blood pressure. It is very useful in critical cases. However, its application is limited by the size of the artery that can be catheterized. Birds larger than 4 kg should have arteries that are suitable for catheterization. The arteries that can be used are the ulnar and metatarsal arteries. The catheter is connected to a heparizined-saline-filled pressure tubing attached to a pressure transducer. Arterial pressures in most birds are considered higher than in mammals. Significant reduction in arterial pressures should be managed by decreasing the inspired anesthetic concentration and administration of fluid boluses.

19. How would you monitor the respiratory function of the bird under anesthesia?

- Clinical skills: The adequacy of ventilation can be judged subjectively by observing the frequency and degree of motion of the sternum and the movement of the breathing bag of the breathing circuit. The respiratory rate can also be taken by watching the rhythmic condensation in a clear endotracheal tube. The color of the mucous membrane, cere, beak, or bill should also be noted.
- Blood gas analysis: Blood gas analysis is the definitive indicator of ventilatory adequacy and optimal gas exchange. As long as adequate arterial blood can be collected, blood gas analysis can be performed. The requirement for a certain volume of blood by the blood gas machine will lead to hypovolemia in small birds. $PaCO_2$ should be maintained in the 30 to 40 mm Hg range. In birds breathing a high concentration of oxygen, PaO_2 is expected to be in 300 to 500 mm Hg range. The use of blood gas analysis is also limited by the cost.
- Capnography: Capnography determines the CO_2 tension in the expired and inspired gases of the patient. It mainly detects hypoventilation, hyperventilation, airway obstruction, and disconnection from the breathing circuit. Its use in birds is limited by the size of the bird. Both mainstream and sidestream capnographs will pose erroneous results in very small patients because of additional dead space in the mainstream capnograph and the relatively high aspiration rate in the sidestream capnograph. The author has success using the capnograph in ostriches and emus. The expired CO_2 is also kept in the 30 to 40 mm Hg range.

20. How applicable is pulse oximetry in birds?

Pulse oximetry, which measures oxygen saturation of hemoglobin, is not very reliable in avian anesthesia. The existing pulse oximeters are beset by failure to continually display values, readings affected by motion, and inability to foretell critical incidents.

21. How do you monitor body temperature in birds during anesthesia?

Body temperature in birds can be monitored with an electronic thermometer or a thermistor probe. The thermistor probe can be inserted into the esophagus to the level of the heart. Placement of the thermistor probe in the esophagus is preferred over cloacal placement. The sphincter muscle of the cloaca will relax over time, resulting in lower body temperature reading. However, placement of the esophageal probe is hindered by the crop in some birds.

22. Is fluid administration necessary during avian anesthesia?

For short-term procedures (less than 30 minutes) in healthy birds, administration of fluids is not essential. Fluid administration during anesthesia is important in dehydrated animals, during prolonged procedures, especially if the body cavities are open, and during very invasive procedures with associated bleeding.

23. What are the fluids that can be given to birds? What should be the rate of administration during anesthesia?

Balanced electrolyte solutions (lactated Ringer's, Plasmalyte, Normosol) are the fluids that can be administered during anesthesia at a rate of 5.0 to 10.0 ml/kg/hour. The small volume needed necessitates the use of commercial syringe infusion pump for accurate dosing. The fluid rate used to replace the sensible and insensible loss in birds is an extrapolation from the rate used in mammals. Hypoglycemic birds require the use of crystalloid solution that contains dextrose. Half-strength LRS and 2.5% dextrose is an example. In very small birds that will be under anesthesia for longer than 30 minutes, the author supplements the fluid with dextrose. This is brought about by the difficulty of obtaining a blood sample during anesthesia to check for glucose level. Slight hyperglycemia is less of a concern than hypoglycemia during anesthesia.

24. What veins could I use for fluid administration? In case of small birds, are there any alternate routes for fluid administration?

The veins that can be used in birds are:
* Jugular vein (recommended for patients with long neck)
* Basilic vein (useful in birds weighing at least 300–400 g)
* Medial metatarsal vein (useful in long-legged birds)

In very small birds, the intraosseous route can be used. The sites used are the distal ulna and the proximal tibiotarsus.

25. What are the signs of pain in birds postoperatively?

Clinically, determining pain in birds is difficult. The signs of pain shown in birds will differ among species and individuals. The clinician should be aware of the normal behavior of a given species of bird and, if possible, the particular patient at hand. Information about the normal behavior of the patient can be gathered from the client.

There are specific signs that can be attributed to pain in birds. A bird will try to escape or avoid a painful stimulus. The bird may show signs of restlessness and anxiety. Some will also vocalize and may become aggressive. Some will be immobile when under extreme pain. Pain can also be shown as guarding behavior manifested as less social interaction and decreased interest in the surroundings after surgery. Inappetence, lack of grooming, or overgrooming of the surgical site may be associated with pain. The variability of the signs associated with pain in birds makes it difficult to assess pain accurately. The author believes that if there is any doubt about the presence of pain, analgesic should be administered.

26. What are the analgesic options available for birds that will have or had a painful procedure?

Preemptive analgesia should be administered in birds. Before the surgical procedure, the patient should be treated with an opioid, a nonsteroidal agent, and, if possible, a local anesthetic.

Butorphanol, an agonist-antagonist opioid has been used preoperatively, intraoperatively and postoperatively in birds at a dose of 1.0–3.0 mg/kg. Birds have more κ opioid receptors than μ opioid receptors. This explains the efficacy of butorphanol in birds. It appears that the duration of action of butorphanol is less than 4 hours. Hence, its administration should be repeated postoperatively.

Ketoprofen and carprofen are the two nonsteroidal anti-inflammatory drugs (NSAIDs) more commonly used in birds. They are used in surgical patients to reduce the tissue inflammation that contributes to pain. Ketoprofen can be administered intramuscularly or subcutaneously at 2.0 mg/kg once a day. Because the injectable preparation is not available in the United States, carprofen is given orally at 2.0–4.0 mg/kg two to three times a day. For a preemptive effect, the author prefers ketoprofen because it can be given systemically, resulting in predictable bioavailability. The use of NSAID in birds should be approached with caution. The bird should be well hydrated to minimize nephropathy. The administration of an NSAIDs should be stopped immediately if blood is seen in the feces. It is also prudent to limit the duration of NSAID administration to 2 to 3 days postoperatively.

Lidocaine can be used as part of preemptive treatment by infiltrating the incision line. The total dose should be below 4.0 mg/kg. In very small birds, the lidocaine should be diluted at least 1:10 with saline.

Postoperatively, providing a quiet and warm environment will help a bird in pain by reducing apprehension. The cage should be set so as to allow easy access to food and water. The perches should be lowered, and there should be plenty room for the bird to move around.

27. What are the important points to remember when recovering birds from anesthesia?

The birds should be kept intubated during the recovery phase. This is to prevent aspiration if the bird regurgitates. Birds tend to struggle and flop around during recovery. To prevent struggling and injuries, birds should be lightly wrapped with a towel. The wrapping should not be too tight as to impede sternal movement and breathing. Body temperature should be monitored in recovery. Either hyperthermia or hypothermia can occur and appropriate steps need to be taken if there is extreme change in body temperature.

If the recovery is prolonged, the patient should be monitored and supported continuously. Blood glucose level should always be checked in case of prolonged recovery.

28. For surgery involving the airway, specifically the trachea, how can you control ventilation?

Ventilation and gas exchange can be maintained in birds by cannulating the air sac. It has been shown that normal and acceptable PaO_2 and $PaCO_2$ can be maintained by this technique. Increased minute ventilation was associated with the normal PaO_2 and $PaCO_2$.

28. Is there a need for assisting or controlling ventilation in birds during anesthesia?

There is a need to assist or control the ventilation of birds during anesthesia. General anesthesia causes muscle relaxation of the inspiratory and expiratory muscles in birds. The activity of these muscles is essential for ventilation. Depression of the muscle activity will result in hypoventilation. In addition, anesthetics may have an effect on the responsiveness of the peripheral control mechanisms that affect ventilation. Positioning of the bird during anesthesia also can affect ventilation, especially in dorsal and sternal recumbency. In the dorsal position, the weight of the abdominal viscera compresses the air sacs limiting the effective volume for ventilation. In the sternal position, the movement of the keel will be impaired by the weight of the body.

29. What are some of the variables used when controlling ventilation in birds?

The frequency ranges from 8 to 25 breaths per minute. For smaller species, the rate can increase to 30 to 40 breaths per minute. The peak inspiratory pressure should not exceed 20 cm of water. Some birds can be effectively ventilated even with a peak inspiratory pressure of 10 cm of water. It is important to observe the movement of the abdominal wall and keel during the inspiratory phase. Effective ventilation should produce detectable excursion of the keel.

BIBLIOGRAPHY

1. Abou-Madi N: Avian anesthesia. Vet Clin North Am Exotic Animal Pract 4:147–167, 2001.
2. Bailey JE, Heard D, Schumacher J, et al: Midazolam/butorphanol/ketamine and the clinically effective dose of isoflurane anesthesia of ostriches (Struthio camelus). Proceedings of the Annual Meeting of American College of Veterinary Anesthesiologists, San Francisco, 2000, p 37.

3. Heard DJ: Anesthesia and analgesia. In Altman RB, Clubb SL, Dorrestain GM, et al (eds): Avian Medicine and Surgery. Philadelphia, WB Saunders Co, 1997, pp 807–827.
4. Ludders JW, Matthews N: Birds. In Thurmon JC, Tranquilli WJ, Benson GJ (eds): Lumb & Jones' Veterinary Anesthesia, 3rd ed. Baltimore, Williams & Wilkins, 1996, pp 645–669.
5. Muir WW, Hubbell JAE, Skarda, RT, et al: Handbook of Veterinary Anesthesia, 3rd ed. St. Louis, Mosby, 2000, pp 373–387.
6. Naganobu K, Fujisawa Y, Ohde H, et al: Determination of the minimum anesthetic concentration and cardiovascular dose response for sevoflurane in chickens during controlled ventilation. Vet Surg 29:102–105, 2000.
7. Paul-Murphy J, Ludders JW: Avian analgesia. Vet Clin North Am Exotic Animal Pract 4:35–45, 2001.
8. Powell FL: Respiration. In Whittow GC (ed): Sturkies' Avian Physiology, 5th ed. San Diego, Academic Press, 2000, pp 233–264.
9. Quandt JE, Greenacre CB: Sevoflurane anesthesia in psittacines. J Zoo Wildl Med 30:308–309, 1999.
10. Schmitt PM, Gobel T, Trautvetter E: Evaluation of pulse oximetry as a monitoring method in avian anesthesia. J Avian Med Surg 12:91–99, 1998.

47. REPTILE ANESTHESIA AND ANALGESIA

Terrell G. Heaton-Jones, D.V.M., and Jeff C. H. Ko, D.V.M., M.S., D.A.C.V.A.

1. How does ambient temperature influence anesthesia in reptiles?

Unlike companion animals, reptiles are poikilothermic or ectothermic ("cold-blooded") vertebrates in which body temperature, metabolic rate, and immune function are directly influenced by external temperatures. Maintaining the reptile patient within the preferred optimal temperature zone (POTZ) for the species maximizes physiologic processes, immune function, drug metabolism, speed of induction, and speed of recovery. For example, the green iguana prefers daytime temperatures close to 100°F and nighttime temperatures above 80°F, which would require ambient temperatures for iguana anesthesia and recovery to be kept between 80 and 100°F.

2. Can hypothermia be used to produce anesthesia and analgesia in reptiles?

Hypothermia is not recommended as a method for anesthesia or analgesia in the reptile patient. Hypothermia only produces torpor in the reptile patient and sends it into a semihibernation state by slowing physiologic processes, biochemical reactions, and nerve impulse transmission. Nerve conduction studies in turtles have shown that "chilling down" the reptile does not abolish the nerve impulses but only slows the speed of conduction. Therefore, analgesia is absent while the animal appears unable to respond to any perceived pain stimuli.

3. Does hypothermia alter inhalant anesthesia in the reptile patient?

"Chilling down" an animal, whether or not fractious, does allow for ease of handling and endotracheal intubation. However, this method is not recommended as a form of restraint in reptiles because of its potential to deepen the level of anesthesia as well as prolong the recovery. This situation is likely to occur when a lipid-soluble gas inhalant (i.e., methoxyflurane) is used. Cooler temperatures reduce respiratory rates, prolong induction, and allow for increased amounts of inhalant gas to be "pumped" into the lung(s). This increased gas will collect in the air sacs and distribute systemically and be absorbed into fat stores. Consequently, rewarming the reptile during recovery from anesthesia increases the metabolic rate and systemic mobilization of the inhalant gas from the fat stores, potentially resulting in a deeper level of anesthesia as well as a prolonged recovery.

4. What reptile species are most commonly seen in the pet trade and are therefore likely to be treated by the veterinarian?

Reptiles are becoming very popular as pets, are increasing in monetary value, and are being bred in increasing numbers by private herpetologists and hobbyists. Among snake species, boids (boas and pythons) and colubrids (rat snakes, corn snakes, king snakes), are most commonly maintained as pets. Green iguanas, savannah monitors, and bearded dragons are the most populous lizard pet species, and various tortoise species (red-footed, Greek, Herman's, spur-thighed, and leopard tortoises) are maintained. Venomous species are maintained by many private herpetologists, but these should not be treated unless trained personnel are involved. Few people maintain crocodilians outside zoologic facilities. Other non-boid, non-colubrid species of snakes, tegu lizards, and aquatic turtles are also maintained in the private sector, but not in as large numbers. Consequently, the veterinarian must become knowledgeable with the species maintained, anatomic characteristics, and physiologic differences compared with mammals to successfully treat or anesthetize these animals.

5. What are some anatomic features in the respiratory system of reptiles that can affect anesthesia?

Unlike mammals, the glottis in reptiles is under voluntary muscular control of the glottis dilator muscle. Since most reptile species are capable of breath-holding, the glottis is usually kept tightly closed and intermittently opens during respiration. In snakes and lizards, the trachea is composed of incomplete C-shaped cartilaginous rings that allow partial collapse during feeding. In contrast, turtles and crocodilians have complete cartilaginous tracheal rings. Endotracheal intubation should be accomplished with a non-cuffed endotracheal tube, or a cuffed endotracheal tube inflated only sufficiently to form an effective seal when assisted or controlled ventilation is used. This is because the tracheal mucosa is easily damaged in these species.

Except for the crocodilians, whose lungs are complex and resemble mammalian lungs, the lungs of snakes, lizards, and turtles are simple sacular structures that contain hexagonal faviolae instead of alveolar pockets. Snakes and lizards have a caudal air sac that holds air once a breath is taken but is not involved in gas exchange. Consequently, the gas exchange surface is smaller in reptiles than in mammals, although the amount of air inspired is larger. The lung surface is also partly composed of smooth muscle, which helps to maintain the morphologic shape and prevents collapse if the coelomic cavity is penetrated (through trauma or surgically).

6. How do reptiles inspire and expire?

Reptiles do not possess a true diaphragm or a true thoracic cavity. They use one of two respiratory patterns: (1) inspire a single breath and breath-hold, or (2) inspire a series of breaths, expand the air sac, and breath-hold for a long period. The second method, an adaptation to staying under water for prolonged periods of time, can have profound influence on the time of anesthetic induction. Inspiration and expiration are both active processes requiring expansion of the coelomic cavity. Turtles have modified these processes because the lungs are placed dorsally to the viscera and attached to the upper, non-movable carapace. Internal viscera, attached to the caudoventral surface, is pushed forward (craniodorsal direction) to force air out during expiration. Pulling the viscera downward (caudoventral direction) expands the lungs and draws air in during inspiration. Turtles also utilize their front legs by extending them out of and retracting them into the shell increasing and decreasing the coelomic cavity size and therefore assisting respiration.

7. What are some cardiovascular anatomic differences between mammals and reptiles that affect anesthesia?

Crocodilians have a true four-chambered heart (two atria and two ventricles), similar to mammals. All other reptiles possess a three-chambered heart (two atria and one ventricle). The ventricle is subdivided into the cavum venosum, cavum pulmonale, and cavum arteriosum, which functionally divides the ventricle into three separate chambers and minimizes the mixture of oxygenated and deoxygenated blood. All reptiles have two aortae arising from the ventricle or ventricles. The aortae in crocodilians communicate through the foramen of Panizza and the caudal communicating artery posterior to the heart. The presence of the ventricular subdivisions and the two communicating aortae enables reptiles to redirect the flow of blood and shunt blood away from the lungs. This pulmonary bypass is an evolutionary adaptation to living in low O_2 and aquatic environments and occurs during the breath-holding periods. In these species, breath-holding and pulmonary shunting ability can result in greatly prolonged induction times if facemasks or chamber induction is used.

8. What other physiologic traits do reptiles possess that can affect anesthesia?

In addition to breath-holding and pulmonary shunting of blood, reptiles can also undergo anaerobic metabolism in low O_2 environments. This ability is especially well developed in aquatic species such as freshwater turtles (*Pseudemys* sp., *Trachemys* sp.). Green iguanas and freshwater turtles are capable of undergoing anaerobic metabolism for up to 4.5 and 27 hours, respectively, which is not practically feasible with facemask induction using inhalant anesthesia. Along with anaerobic metabolism, many reptile species can undergo bradycardia and blood pH fluctuations. Crocodilians have the ability to undergo wide fluctuations in their body pH ranging between 7.0 and 8.0, especially in response to preanesthetic manual restraint. Renal excretion is influenced by the renal portal system that directly drains venous blood from the tail and rear legs through the kidneys prior to return to the systemic circulation. Renal excretion of widely used injectable anesthetics such as ketamine may produce variable results when administered in the tail or rear legs. The administration of nephrotoxic drugs may have the potential of accumulating in the kidneys and inducing renal compromise.

9. What tests should be performed in a preanesthetic evaluation?

Ideally, the preanesthetic work-up for the reptile patient should include a thorough physical examination, accurate weight, blood work, hydration status, baseline electrocardiogram (ECG), and heart and lung radiographs. The physical examination should assess the eyes and nares for discharge that could indicate upper respiratory infection, the mouth and glottis for signs of infection or trauma that might impede endotracheal intubation, and the general body condition of the animal to assess nutritional and hydration status. Physiologically compromised animals present an increased anesthetic risk. An accurate weight is essential to determine the dosage of injectable anesthetic. Weights of large, aggressive, or venomous species are often "overestimated" resulting in anesthetic overdosing.

To rule out dehydration, anemia, infections, and renal and liver dysfunction, blood analysis should include a complete blood cell count (CBC) and chemistry panel to evaluate red blood cells, white blood cells, hematocrit, total proteins, uric acid, creatinine, and liver enzymes.

Other tests would include a baseline ECG, which may be obtained in the preanesthetized, awake animal. Alligator clips can be used in smaller reptile patients. In larger reptiles, however, the scales are usually too thick to use an alligator clip. Instead, surgical steel suture loops or a 27-gauge or 25-gauge metal hub needle inserted through the skin between the scales enables the alligator clips to be attached and the ECG recording to be made.

10. What does a reptile ECG look like and where should the leads be placed?

A reptile ECG should contain P, QRS, and T waves similar to a mammal ECG. Snake ECG patterns have an inverted QRS wave similar to an equine base-apex ECG in appearance, whereas lizards, turtles or tortoises, and crocodilians do not have an inverted QRS wave. The ECG should have variable speeds (slower speeds, ≤25 cm/sec) and sensitivities (increased sensitivities, 1 mV ≥1 cm) to account for the reptile's slower heart rate and greater electrical impedance. Heart location varies with the reptile species, and optimal lead placement will depend on the species being evaluated.

Species	Heart Location	ECG Lead Placement
Boa constrictor, pythons	Approximately cranial one-third of body length	Base-apex with one lead (RA) 10–12 ventral scale distance cranial and one lead (LA) 10–12 ventral scale distance caudal to the heart
Green iguana, chameleons	Between the front legs	Lead II—place the leads on the respective four legs or place the forelimb leads on the neck to enhance ECG
Savannah monitor, other monitors, tegu	Mid-body—approximately half the distance between the front and rear legs	Lead II—place the leads on the respective four legs
Tortoises—red-footed, Greek, Herman's, leopard, spur-thighed, etc.	Mid-body	Lead II—place the leads on the respective four legs

11. What are the advantages and disadvantages of using injectable anesthesia in reptiles?

Balanced anesthesia, a combination of injectable and inhalation anesthesia, is the best approach to use in the reptile patient. Preanesthetic sedation with injectable anesthetics is relatively easy to administer, avoids problems of prolonged induction periods associated with mask induction using inhalants alone, and "takes the edge off" aggressive species. Injectable agents can be delivered by a remote system such as a pole syringe or injectable dart (if the animal is sufficiently large) while maintaining safety of the personnel. The authors have used a pole syringe to anesthetize adult crocodilians prior to intubation and maintenance on inhalant anesthesia. Injectable preanesthetic drug administration should not be attempted in venomous species unless experienced personnel are handling the animals. In this instance, manipulating the venomous animal into a clear plastic tube of the appropriate size can facilitate safe handling and allow hand administration of an injectable anesthetic.

The greatest disadvantage of using injectable anesthetic agents for maintenance of anesthesia is inaccurate estimation of weight resulting in anesthetic overdose. Depending on the agent administered, cardiovascular depression, respiratory depression, prolonged recovery, and the inability for reversal are drawbacks associated with overdose using injectable anesthetics. We prefer to administer half of the calculated dose and then make a decision to administer half of the remainder of anesthetic. This titration method takes more time but avoids the problems associated with overdose.

12. What injectable anesthetic agents are recommended to use in reptiles?

Many injectable agents, opioids (etorphine), barbiturates (pentobarbital), skeletal muscle paralytic agents (succinylcholine, gallamine), dissociatives (ketamine, tiletamine), α_2-agonists (xylazine, detomidine, medetomidine), and steroidal compounds (alphaxalone-alphadolone), have been used to immobilize or anesthetize reptiles. However, many of these agents are unacceptable owing to variability of results, narrow margins of safety, and no antagonists for reversal in case of overdose. Injectable agents that have a wider safety margin, have specific antagonists for reversal (medetomidine and atipamezole), have a shorter metabolic half-life with minimal accumulation (propofol), produce consistent anesthesia, and can be combined in an anesthetic cocktail (medetomidine/ketamine) are available. These newer injectable agents can be used to maintain anesthesia if inhalant anesthetics are not easily accessible, such as in field situations. Examples of these newer injectable anesthetics are given in the table.

Name	Advantage	Disadvantage
Ketamine	Long history of use in many species Water-soluble, can be combined with many other agents, such as medetomidine Can be administered IV, IM, IO Inexpensive	Poorer analgesia Poor muscle relaxation No specific antagonist Prolonged recovery Renal excretion—unpredictable results may occur if administered in the tail or rear legs due to renal portal system
Tiletamine/Zolazepam Telazol	Easily administered IM Small injection volume with great potency (compared with ketamine alone) and more rapid onset of action	No specific antagonist Prolonged recovery May produce poor muscle relaxation
Medetomidine— Domitor	Easily administered IV, IM Can be combined with ketamine to lower the total dose of medetomidine or ketamine if used alone Analgesia provided Good muscle relaxation Specific antagonist available—atipamezole, which shortens the time of recovery	Bradycardia and bradypnea may occur but can be alleviated when used with ketamine Newer anesthetic drug that does not have a long history of use in many species of reptiles Relatively expensive
Propofol—Propoflo	Rapid induction period Short metabolic half-life with short recovery time Minimal cumulative effects seen with additional doses administered	Must be administered IV, IO to be effective Relatively expensive Short shelf life—prone to contamination once opened Potential to develop allergies due to egg-white base

13. Why should injectable anesthetics be administered in the front legs of turtles, lizards, and crocodilians and in the cranial half of the body in snakes?

This topic is still controversial. Reptiles possess a renal portal system in which venous blood is directed through the kidneys from the rear legs, tail, and caudal part of the trunk through the kidneys prior to entering the systemic circulation and returning to the heart. Renal excreted injectable anesthetics, administered in the rear legs in turtles, lizards, and crocodilians or in the caudal half of the body in snakes, must first pass through the kidneys and may be partially excreted before taking effect. If these drugs are nephrotoxic, the potential occurs for increased doses to directly affect the kidney and result in renal damage or even renal failure. Consequently, to avoid this first-pass effect through the kidneys, the authors recommend that injectable anesthetics be given in the cranial dorsal epaxial muscle in snakes and in the front legs in turtles, lizards, and crocodilians, if possible. Caution must be used with large, aggressive, or venomous species. The authors prefer administering injectable anesthetics and antagonists in the front legs in lizards, turtles, and crocodilians and in the cranial half in snakes to avoid complications associated with the renal portal system.

14. Can intraosseous drug administration be used in all reptiles?

Intraosseous administration of anesthetic drugs or fluids has been used successfully in a few species to administer fluids and maintain anesthesia without intubation or inhalant gases (propofol drips). This technique is effective in lizards (green iguanas and monitors) and select turtle species (sea turtles, some tortoises). The sites typically used are the long limb bones, distal end of the humerus in the front limbs (green iguanas, tortoises, sea turtles), distal end of the femur (green iguanas, monitors, other lizards), and proximal end of the tibia (green iguanas, monitors, other lizards) in the rear limbs. Some authors report using the bridge of the carapace/plastron in turtles as a potential intraosseous site, but we have not used this technique. Tortoises and crocodilians have heavily keratinized scales on their limbs requiring interscalar placement of the intraosseous cannulas. Large tortoises present a special problem by withdrawal of their limbs into the shell. Preanesthetic sedation to relax the patient and gain control of the limb becomes necessary in these species. Intraosseous administration is an invasive procedure and requires strict aseptic technique. This technique may prove useful in smaller animals ($\leq$1 meter long) with easier access and thinner bone cortices to penetrate but may be difficult in larger, heavily muscled individuals. This technique is not practical in snakes. More research needs to be conducted to evaluate the usefulness of intraosseous administration in reptiles.

15. What are advantages and disadvantages for using inhalant anesthesia in reptiles?

Some advantages of using inhalant anesthesia are (1) to provide a more precise control of the level of anesthesia compared with injectables, (2) easy adjustment of depth of anesthesia, (3) lack of accumulation with successive administrations, and (4) accurate weights are not needed especially if "masking down" a reptile patient. To achieve maximum precision, however, the reptile patient must be endotracheally intubated. Other advantages with using inhalant anesthesia include controlling respiratory rates and depth through intermittent positive pressure ventilation (IPPV) and providing the patient with supplemental oxygen. Assisted or controlled ventilation (IPPV, either manual or ventilator) is especially important when anesthetizing turtles during lengthy procedures in which the animal lies in dorsal recumbency and the visceral organs displace the dorsally located lungs against the carapace. Inhalant anesthetics can be reduced toward the end of a procedure to shorten the total anesthetic recovery time.

Some disadvantages with using inhalant anesthesia as the sole agent are the prolonged induction time associated with "masking down" a breath-holding species, the exposure of personnel to increased levels of waste gas, and personnel safety when aggressive or venomous species are being anesthetized (uncertainty about whether the animal is deeply anesthetized).

16. What factors affect inhalant anesthesia in reptiles?

Inhalant anesthesia in reptiles is influenced by ambient temperature, the reptile's body temperature, and other injectable anesthetics administered. Hypothermia, opioids, and other premedications lower the MAC of inhalant anesthetics, reducing the amount of gas required to maintain a surgical plane of anesthesia.

17. What inhalant anesthetics are recommended for use in reptiles?

Modern inhalant anesthetics such as halothane, isoflurane, or sevoflurane can be used with oxygen or oxygen-nitrous oxide mixture in reptiles. Combining the inhalant anesthetic with nitrous oxide reduces the amount of inhalant required for induction and maintenance. Nitrous oxide used as an anesthetic adjunct is rapidly absorbed into the systemic circulation, carrying the inhalant with it (second gas effect) and speeding the induction time. It is rapidly exhaled through the lungs, shortening the time for recovery.

Halothane and isoflurane are currently widely used for anesthesia maintenance in many animal species, including reptiles. Isoflurane is the inhalant anesthetic of choice because it has a lower blood/gas solubility compared with halothane, resulting in shorter induction and recovery periods. Additionally, prices of both inhalants are competitive. Sevoflurane, a new inhalant with lower blood/gas solubility than isoflurane, has been experimentally used in tortoises with good results. It has the potential to replace isoflurane in reptile anesthesia in the future.

18. Do analgesic drugs work in reptiles?

Reptile analgesia, whether used preemptively or during intraoperative, or postoperative periods, has traditionally received very little attention or research. No analgesics are licensed for veterinary use in reptiles. Analgesic drugs and dosages have usually been extrapolated from companion animals. However, reptiles do possess a well-developed central nervous system and feel pain when invasive procedures are applied. Research studies in a select number of reptile species (anole lizards, gopher tortoises, alligators, Nile crocodiles) with a select number of analgesics (morphine, meperidine, oxymorphone, and medetomidine) have revealed that these animals possess opiate receptors and do respond physiologically to noxious stimuli. Other analgesic drugs (flunixin, nalbuphine, pentazocine, buprenorphine, and lidocaine) have been reported in the literature for use in reptile species although the exact efficacy has not been evaluated. Topical 2% lidocaine has been applied to the glottis to desensitize this area and ease endotracheal intubation.

We have used butorphanol (0.1–0.2 mg/kg IM Q 48–72 hours) and morphine (0.5–1.5 mg/kg IM Q 48–72 hours) for postoperative pain relief in turtles and crocodilians. In addition to providing anesthesia, medetomidine has recently been shown to provide better analgesia in amphibians (leopard frogs and bullfrogs) compared with opioids. The authors have used medetomidine (40–160 μg/kg IM) in conjunction with opioids to provide anesthesia and analgesia during surgical procedures. However, if medetomidine is used as part of the anesthetic combination and then subsequently reversed, additional postoperative pain relief should be provided to ensure adequate analgesia, since reversing the anesthetic properties will also reverse the analgesic effects of medetomidine.

19. How are painful response and depth of anesthesia assessed in the reptile patient?

Pain assessment can be estimated using reflex responses to noxious stimuli during anesthesia, such as toe pinch withdrawal, righting reflex, corneal reflex, palpebral reflex, and cloacal pinch reflex. Loss of toe pinch withdrawal reflex in all four legs, palpebral (blink) reflex, head withdrawal reflex in turtles, and righting reflex in lizards, snakes, and crocodilians generally indicate that a surgical plane of anesthesia has been achieved. Corneal and cloacal reflexes are usually the last reflexes to be lost and can be used as an indicator of excessive anesthesia (too deep).

Snakes present a special challenge. These animals do not have legs or movable eyelids, so assessing limb withdrawal and palpebral and corneal reflexes is not possible. Tongue flick and withdrawal and tail pinch and cloacal pinch reflexes are used instead to estimate analgesia and anesthetic effects in the snake. Reflexes are lost in a head-to-tail direction and return in the opposite tail-to-head direction. The tongue flick reflex when the tongue is pulled out of the mouth (it remains extended and flaccid) is the first reflex to diminish and the last one to return during the anesthetic period. Once the tail and cloacal reflexes are diminished or absent, a surgical plane of anesthesia has been achieved.

20. Why use medetomidine or combinations with medetomidine in reptiles?

Medetomidine offers several advantages for use in reptiles. It provides profound sedation, muscle relaxation, and analgesia. A specific reversal drug, atipamezole, can be administered at the same injection volume as that of medetomidine used for reversal of medetomidine. However, clinical use of medetomidine alone (80–160 μg/kg) often produces variable results in reptiles. Consequently, it is often combined with other anesthetics such as ketamine, butorphanol, or midazolam to produce consistent results. The authors have successfully used medetomidine (80 μg/kg) and ketamine (5 mg/kg) combinations in several reptile species, including yellow rat snakes, Burmese python, green iguanas, gopher tortoises, Galapagos tortoise, Gila monsters, alligators, Nile crocodiles, and caimans. Medetomidine and ketamine can be used in a single intramuscular injection to immobilize or induce anesthesia in these species. If this dose of medetomidine and ketamine cannot induce a stage of anesthesia that would permit for endotracheal intubation, then butorphanol (0.2 mg/kg) with or without midazolam (0.2–0.4 mg/kg) can be added to deepen the anesthesia. Alternatively, an inhalant anesthetic with facemask can be used to deepen the anesthesia to achieve endotracheal intubation or surgical plane of anesthesia. At the end of the procedure, medetomidine can be reversed with atipamezole (at the same injection volume as that of medetomidine used), and the animal is readily awake within minutes of reversal.

21. Is intravenous fluid administration necessary in reptiles undergoing anesthesia?

Fluid therapy in reptiles is an area of anesthesia that has received very little interest or attention until recently. Evaluation of hydration status in the reptile patient can be very difficult because of the limited ability to assess skin turgor and mucous membrane moistness. An elevated hematocrit can be indicative of dehydration. All reptiles should have access to water ad libitum prior to anesthesia. Tropical and aquatic species (water turtles, boa constrictors, green iguanas, etc.) readily drink water and may be more prone to becoming dehydrated if kept away from a water source for prolonged periods of time such as during prolonged procedures and recoveries. Desert and arid species (some tortoises, desert iguanas, savannah monitors, etc.) will drink if provided with water but usually rely on obtaining water from food sources. They can metabolically conserve water through renal and cloacal reabsorption. Desert tortoises and giant tortoises use their bladder as a water storage organ for times of drought.

Intravenous fluid may be administered in some species such as green iguanas (midline abdominal vein) and large tortoises (dorsal tail vein). Intraosseous fluid administration has been successfully used in select species (green iguanas, tortoises, sea turtles). However, many species do not have easy venous or intraosseous access. The authors routinely administer fluids (orally, cloacally, or subcutaneously) to reptiles during or following anesthesia, especially if the anesthetic and recovery periods are prolonged and the patient must remain out of water. Although controversial and not recommended by some veterinarians, the lead author has given subcutaneous fluids (5–10 ml/kg) to crocodilians, monitors, and iguanas following surgery. Instead of creating one large subcutaneous bleb, multiple small blebs are made cranial to the rear legs and caudal to the ribs on both sides of the body. Multiple small blebs appear to enhance absorption. The scales in this area are usually not as heavily keratinized, the skin is loose, and subcutaneous blebs are easier to form.

22. What intravenous fluids can be given to the reptile patient?

Isotonic fluids are the fluids of choice. Lactated Ringer's solution and 0.9% saline have traditionally been administered to reptiles. Recently, lactated Ringer's solution administration has been questioned because of the long half-life of lactate in the plasma. Many reptiles, including green iguanas, water dragons, skinks, box turtles, water turtles, and crocodilians, undergo periods of anaerobic metabolism (during periods of hibernation or concentrated activity associated with struggling to avoid capture and resisting manual restraint) and produce lactic acid. Once lactate levels have increased, maintaining the reptile patient at suboptimal (too high or too low, not within the POTZ) temperatures decreases the rate of tissue oxygenation and lactate excretion, which allows for increased lactate levels to occur. Artificial increases in lactate associated with fluid therapy may exacerbate a lactic acidosis condition. Non–lactate-containing isotonic solutions, such as Normosol-R, may prove to be a better electrolyte solution replacement. We routinely administer Normosol-R to avoid potential lactic acidosis.

23. What anesthetic parameters should be monitored in the reptile patient?

According to the published position paper on monitoring by the American College of Veterinary Anesthesiologists, respiratory rates, heart rates and rhythms, blood pressures, and body temperatures should be monitored during anesthesia in all patients. Respiratory rates can be counted by observing the animal's chest excursion if the patient is not breath holding. IPPV is recommended to ensure adequate ventilation. Usually reptiles do not require high positive pressure to expand their lungs. Positive pressure at about 10–15 cm H_2O is more than adequate to maintain end-tidal CO_2 of 40 mm Hg. If the reptile patient is intubated, capnography (measurement of expired CO_2) can be used for monitoring of respiratory rate and ventilation efficiency. End-tidal CO_2 ($P_{ET}CO_2$) provides an indirect method to assess arterial CO_2 (P_ACO_2) and therefore assessing the ventilation efficiency and ventilator setting. The authors have used capnography in reptiles, but more research is needed to correlate this noninvasive method with arterial CO_2 levels, especially in turtle species that are capable of anaerobic metabolism.

24. How do you monitor heart rate?

Heart rates can be auscultated and accurately assessed with an esophageal stethoscope or Doppler ultrasonography if an electrocardiographic machine or pulse oximeter is not available. To assess heart rhythms, an ECG is essential. A combination of ECG with Doppler to assess heart rate, heart rhythm, and pulse quality (noise intensity) provides a reliable method of assessing both electrical and mechanical activity of the heart in the reptile. In snakes, lizards (green iguanas and monitors), and small crocodilians, the Doppler probe can be placed over the heart to detect the blood flow and therefore the pulse rate. Cardiac arrhythmias, including second-degree atrioventricular heart block and ventricular asystole, have been recorded during anesthetic periods using ECG in the reptile patient in our experience.

25. How do you monitor arterial oxygenation?

Arterial oxygenation can be measured using pulse oximetry. Pulse oximetry has been reported to be useful in evaluating arterial hemoglobin oxygen saturation (S_AO_2) during anesthesia in green iguanas. However, in the authors' experience, pulse oximeters have produced inconsistent results. Reptile scales contain too much keratine and are not highly vascular, preventing proper transmission and reflectance of the red and infrared lights. Rectal probes, used in the esophagus or the cloaca, did not produce consistent results, probably owing to the reduced vascular beds in reptiles (compared with mammals) and vasoconstriction during anesthesia. Furthermore, pulse oximeters used in small animals are programmed based on the hemoglobin dissociation curve of mammals and may not correlate properly with reptile's hemoglobin saturation. Pulse oximetry can only be used as a method to detect pulse rate and rhythm and only serve as a reference for the hemoglobin saturation in the reptile species.

26. How do you monitor blood pressure?

Using noninvasive blood pressure monitoring also has produced inconsistent results in the reptile. Reptiles have low systemic arterial blood pressures compared with domestic animals, heavily muscled legs, and deep-lying vessels that do not permit accurate and reliable blood pressures to be obtained by commercial noninvasive blood pressure monitors. Lack of superficial arteries prevent the use of direct percutaneous arterial blood pressure monitoring in these species.

27. How do you monitor body temperature?

Body temperatures in reptiles are dependent on ambient temperature (see questions 1, 2, and 3). Providing the POTZ during the anesthetic and recovery periods will (1) maximize drug absorption, distribution, and elimination; (2) minimize potential lactic acidosis; and (3) minimize the recovery period. It is important to monitor both the environmental and the reptile's temperatures simultaneously to provide POTZ in these species.

28. What anesthetic protocol is recommended for anesthetizing turtles?

Anesthesia in turtles involves using injectable anesthetics to relax the animal to get and keep the head out of the shell for endotracheal intubation. Many intramuscular combinations have been used in turtles and tortoises for sedation, but the authors like medetomidine (50–100 µg/kg IM) in combination with ketamine (5–10 mg/kg IM). Once the animal is sedate (the head and limbs can be easily extracted from the shell), the mouth can be propped open (with a syringe case) and endotracheal intubation can be performed. The glottis is located caudal to the fleshy tongue in tortoises, may be hard to visualize, and may be challenging to intubate, especially if the mouth cannot be opened widely. Topical lidocaine spray can be administered to desensitize the glottis and facilitate the intubation. Anesthesia is usually maintained with isoflurane (2–3%) in oxygen. Intubation is not practical in small turtles. If this is the case, a syringe case can be modified as a homemade facemask as a method for maintenance of anesthesia. [NOTE: Mask induction without prior sedation may be impractical if the turtle withdraws its head into the shell or may be prolonged if the turtle breath-holds and undergoes anaerobic metabolism.]

Once intubated, the patient will need to have either manual or mechanical assisted or controlled ventilation at 6–8 breaths per minute to ensure adequate ventilation and oxygenation. Advantages of this combination include (1) analgesia provided by medetomidine,(2) reduced dose of medetomidine since it works synergistically with ketamine, (3) reversibility of medetomidine by atipamezole which reduces the length of recovery, (4) reduced dose of ketamine, which acts synergistically with medetomidine, and (5) reduced incidences of apnea and bradycardia with reduced doses of either drug used alone. If medetomidine is used and reversed, supplemental analgesic should be administered. The patient is weaned off isoflurane toward the end of the procedure to shorten the recovery period. The authors have used this method and reversed the medetomidine while the animal is being maintained with isoflurane, which further shortens the recovery period.

29. What anesthetic do you recommend for anesthetizing lizards?

Again, medetomidine in combination with ketamine is a good combination that can be mixed into one syringe, and easily administered intramuscularly, and provides reliable sedation. Doses are the same as that used for turtles (medetomidine, 50–100 µg/kg IM; ketamine, 5–10 mg/kg IM). If analgesia is to be enhanced, butorphanol (0.2–0.4 mg/kg), morphine (0.5–1 mg/kg) or other types of opioid can be added as part of the combination. Medetomidine (80 µg/kg) and ketamine (5 mg/kg) can be used in a single intramuscular injection to immobilize or induce anesthesia in green iguanas. This combination is especially effective when dealing with aggressive male green iguanas. We wrap the iguana in a towel and administer the drugs intramuscularly in the front or rear leg. Lateral recumbency usually occurs in 8–10 minutes at which time the animal can be intubated. An alternative is a low dose of Telazol (tiletamine/zolazepam), which can be administered at 3–5 mg/kg IM. This is a low dose that will make an aggressive animal, such as large monitors, tractable. Additional supplemental analgesic, such as butorphanol or morphine, should be administered when medetomidine is reversed and opioid is not previously used as part of the combination.

Once the patient is sedate, the mouth can be opened and endotracheal intubation can be performed. Isoflurane (2–3%) maintenance is the inhalant of choice. Other alternative methods for maintaining anesthesia include intraosseous (5–10 mg/kg) or intravenous (5–10 mg/kg) administration of propofol. Although these are acceptable methods, propofol does cause respiratory and cardiovascular depression, requiring the administration of supplemental oxygen. Some authors advocate the use of mask induction with inhalant anesthesia alone, but we have found that using injectable pre-medications reduces the time for induction and the amount of waste gas exposure to personnel compared with the use of inhalant for induction.

30. What anesthetic protocols can be used for snakes?

Venomous species should be anesthetized only by experienced reptile specialists and zoo veterinarians. If venomous species are to be anesthetized, caution and extreme care should be taken to avoid accidents. The snake can be placed into a clear induction chamber or plastic tubing for induction with isoflurane 5% in oxygen until the righting reflexes are absent. Induction should be conducted in a secure, well ventilated room to prevent excessive build-up of waste gases and to prevent escape of the animal (if it is not fully anesthetized). If the snake is being held, experienced personnel should be handling the patient in a plastic tube to avoid being bitten. Once the snake is secured in a plastic tube, inhalant anesthetic can be used to fill the tube. Alternatively, an injectable anesthetic can be administered in the dorsal epaxial muscles.

Medetomidine (50–100 µg/kg IM) with ketamine (5–10 mg/kg IM) or Telazol (3–5 mg/kg IM) alone can be used to induce the animal prior to endotracheal intubation. Once anesthetized (loss of righting reflex), the mouth can be held opened using a soft rubber spatula to avoid damage to the recurved teeth. The glottis, located anterior, is readily visible and accessible and can be desensitized with topical 2% lidocaine prior to intubation. Isoflurane (2–3%) in oxygen is the inhalant anesthetic of choice. Manual or mechanical ventilation can be instituted at 6–8 breaths/min. Once the tail pinch reflex is lost, the patient has reached a surgical plane of anesthesia. Decreasing the level of anesthesia and inducing recovery can be estimated by return of the tail flick and progression of muscular contractions in a tail-to-head direction. Recovery is complete when the snake regains tongue flick control and its righting reflex. Atipamezole can be used for reversal of medetomidine. Telazol, on the other hand, cannot be reversed, and the recovery tends to be prolonged more than with the combination of medetomidine and ketamine.

BIBLIOGRAPHY

1. Bennett RA: A review of anesthesia and chemical restraint in reptiles. J Zoo Wildl Med 22:282–303,1991.
2. Frye FL (ed): Biomedical and Surgical Aspects of Captive Reptile Husbandry, vols 1 and 2. Melbourne, FL, Krieger Publishing, 1991.
3. Heard DJ (ed): Veterinary Clinics of North America: Exotic Animal Practice. Philadelphia, WB Saunders, 2001.
4. Mader DR: Reptile Medicine and Surgery. Philadelphia, WB Saunders, 1996.
5. Prezant RM, Jarchow JL: Lactated fluid use in reptiles: Is there a better solution?Proceedings of the 4th Annual Association of Reptile and Amphibian Veterinarians, Houston, 1997, pp 83–87.
6. Schaeffer DO: Anesthesia and analgesia in non-traditional laboratory animals. In Kohn DF, Wixson SK, White WJ, and Benson GJ (eds), Anesthesia and Analgesia in Laboratory Animals. San Diego, Academic Press, 1996, pp 337–378.
7. Schumacher J: Reptile anesthesia. In Thurmon JC, Tranquilli WJ, and Benson GJ (eds): Lumb and Jones' Veterinary Anesthesia, 3rd ed. Baltimore, Williams & Wilkins, 1996, pp 670–685.

48. ANESTHESIA OF URBAN WILDLIFE AND FARMED GAME

Nigel A. Caulkett, D.V.M., M.V.Sc., D.A.C.V.A.

1. What equipment is available to facilitate remote delivery of anesthetic agents?

A variety of techniques can be used to deliver anesthetic agents to free-ranging animals. Pole syringes can be used to deliver drugs up to about 2 meters. Lung-powered blow pipes are effective to about 10 meters. Blow pipes, powered with compressed air or CO_2, and CO_2 or air pistols can be used up to 15 or 20 meters. CO_2 rifles or cartridge rifles can be used to propel darts 30 meters and beyond.

2. What types of darts are available to facilitate drug delivery?

A variety of darts are available. Low-velocity darts (Dan-inject, Telinject) are generally manufactured from plastic, and injection of contents is powered by compressed gas. High-velocity darts are usually metal (Cap-Chur, Pneu-Dart), and injection of contents is powered by an explosive charge. Paxarms manufactures a high-velocity plastic dart that injects its contents using compressed air.

3. How do you choose appropriate equipment for a given situation?

The major factors to consider are the size of the animal and the range at which the drug can be delivered. Darts can produce significant injury or death if they are not used appropriately. The energy of impact is equal to the mass of the dart multiplied by the velocity squared. It is important to use the lightest possible dart, delivered at the lowest velocity possible, while maintaining an accurate trajectory. Rapid injection, from explosive-charge powered plungers, can also induce significant trauma. As a rule of thumb, metal darts should be reserved for large, well-muscled animals, when the dart must be delivered at a distance of greater than 20 meters. Low-velocity equipment should be used whenever possible.

4. How would you anesthetize a game-farmed white-tailed deer for physical examination and radiographs of the tarsus?

Several factors will enter into the choice of anesthetic agents for this procedure. The temperament of the individual is probably the biggest factor. A quiet female held in a dark room may require a very low dose of drug. A free-ranging male could require a higher dose, and an animal in rut may be very difficult to anesthetize. It is extremely important to work quietly around the animal, and, if possible, it helps to keep the animal in a darkened area prior to anesthesia. If the animal is stressed, its anesthetic requirements will be increased, particularly if α_2-agonists are used. Female white-tailed deer generally weigh 40–50 kg; mature male deer can weigh 60–90 kg.

Several drug combinations could be used in this situation; 6–10 µg/kg carfentanil plus 0.2 mg/kg of xylazine would be effective. The carfentanil should be antagonized with 0.6-1 mg/kg of naltrexone. Potent opioid narcotics should be used only by experienced personnel when adequate first aid facilities are available. Xylazine-ketamine could be used. If the deer is quiet and not stressed the xylazine can be administered at a dose of 2 mg/kg IM. Once the animal has become recumbent, 1–2 mg/kg can be administered intravenously via the jugular vein. Ketamine will need to be administered, at a dose of 0.5–1 mg/kg at 15- to 20-minute intervals. The advantage of this technique is that when the xylazine is antagonized, the deer will not experience rigidity or convulsive activity from residual ketamine. Xylazine can be antagonized with 0.1–0.2 mg/kg of yohimbine or 2–3 mg/kg of tolazoline. If the animal is free-ranging or stressed, xylazine-ketamine can be administered intramuscularly at a dose of 2 mg/kg of xylazine plus 4–6 mg/kg of ketamine. It is important not to antagonize the xylazine too early (< 30 minutes, unless in an emergency), as convulsive activity may result from residual intramuscular ketamine. Xylazine-Telazol is one of the most useful mixtures for immobilization of deer. Five hundred milligrams of Telazol powder is reconstituted with 2.5 ml of 100 mg/ml xylazine. The resulting solution has a volume of approximately 2.8 ml and contains approximately 90 mg/ml of xylazine and 180 mg/ml of Telazol. A quiet, confined white-tailed deer can be immobilized with 1 mg/kg of xylazine and 2 mg/kg of Telazol. In free-ranging or stressed animals, the dose should be increased to 1.5 mg/kg of xylazine plus 3 mg/kg of Telazol. Xylazine-Telazol anesthesia can be prolonged, or depth of anesthesia increased, with 1–2 mg/kg of ketamine at 10- to 15-minute intervals. The xylazine can be antagonized with yohimbine or tolazoline at the above dose, and recovery is usually smooth.

5. What kind of monitoring and supportive care should be used during the procedure?

The bare minimum should be to monitor pulse, respiratory rate, body temperature, and mucous membrane color every 5 minutes. Auricular and femoral arteries are good spots to palpate the pulse. Pulse oximetry is very useful during field anesthesia; it will give a continuous readout of heart rate and percent hemoglobin saturation. Supplemental inspired oxygen is indicated to treat hypoxemia, particularly if animals are also hyperthermic. Oxygen can be administered via a nasal canula, with the tip located at the level of the medial canthus of the eye. A flow rate of 6–8 L/min is usually adequate. Ophthalmic ointment should be used to help prevent corneal ulcers, and the animal should be kept in sternal recumbency whenever possible.

6. Are there any potential complications during anesthesia in deer?

Hypoxemia is a common complication of anesthesia, particularly when α_2-agonists are used. Saturations of 80–90% are common during anesthesia with α_2-agonist-based combinations. Hypoxemia is generally well tolerated, but can result in morbidity or mortality if hypoxemia is severe, or if it exists in combination with hyperthermia. Hyperthermia is a common complication of cervid anesthesia. Body temperatures over 41°C should be treated by actively cooling the deer. Body temperatures of more than 42°C are a medical emergency, and reversal of the anesthetic agents should be considered, combined with active cooling and supplemental inspired oxygen. Hyperthermia greatly increases oxygen demand and will result in complications rapidly if hypoxemia is also present. Supplemental inspired oxygen can be used to offset hypoxemia. Ruminal tympany can be a complication of anesthesia; although, in the author's experience, it is much less severe than in bovids. Fasting the animal for 24 hours prior to elective procedures, and maintenance in sternal recumbency will help to decrease the incidence and severity of ruminal tympany.

Capture myopathy can be seen during or following anesthesia of cervids. Capture myopathy may be acute, a shock-like syndrome, which may result in mortality during or immediately following anesthesia. It may be subacute, often manifested by severe muscle swelling, and myoglobinuria. This condition often results in mortality from renal failure or myocardial necrosis. The condition may be chronic. In cervids, this often presents as ruptured gastrocnemius muscles. In the author's experience, treatment of capture myopathy is usually unsuccessful, and it is extremely important to take steps to prevent capture myopathy. Avoid prolonged chases or stress prior to anesthesia. It is very important to keep stress levels to a minimum. Try to avoid anesthesia during the warm hours of the day. Always treat hyperthermia as a potentially serious complication, and administer supplemental inspired oxygen in the face of hyperthermia and hypoxemia. Try to avoid anesthetizing stags during the rut.

7. How would the anesthetic management differ if this were a free-ranging white-tailed deer in an urban environment?

The major difference with a free-ranging, wild white-tailed deer is that it would have a high level of background stress. Drug dosages should be increased to override the effects of the stress hormones. Either xylazine-Telazol or xylazine-ketamine could be used. Both combinations should be used at the high end of the dosage range given in question 4. Carfentanil-xylazine would produce an effective immobilization, but in an urban environment the risk of a lost dart may preclude its use.

A deer in this situation would be very prone to hyperthermia and capture myopathy. Chase times should be kept to a minimum to decrease the risk of these complications.

8. What would be the best site for dart placement?

The best site for dart placement would be the gluteal muscle mass or the semimembranosis-semitendonosis muscle mass. A large muscle mass is better able to tolerate dart-induced trauma, and drug absorption is optimized following injection into a large muscle mass with a good blood supply.

9. Would the anesthetic protocol be the same for a game-farmed wapiti (American elk)?

Most of the above would apply to wapiti, with a few differences. Wapiti require a relatively lower drug dosage than white-tailed deer. Xylazine can be administered at an intramuscular dose of 1 mg/kg, if the animal is calm. This can be followed by 1–2 mg/kg of ketamine IV for reliable immobilization. Xylazine-Telazol is usually effective at a dose of 1 mg/kg of xylazine plus 2 mg/kg of Telazol, or lower in very calm animals. Mature female wapiti weigh 200–300 kg; mature male wapiti weigh 300–450 kg.

10. What is the simplest way to block velvet antler, prior to surgical removal?

The simplest way to block velvet antler is to perform a ring block at the base of the antler pedicle. Lidocaine HCl (without epinephrine) is administered at a dose rate of 1 ml/cm of pedicle circumference. The block will produce surgical analgesia in 1–2 minutes and will last approximately 90 minutes.

11. What technique would be suitable for capture of a free-ranging moose?

Anesthesia of moose is very similar to anesthesia of other deer. All of the same precautions apply, and particular attention must be paid to the prevention of capture myopathy and hyperthermia. There are several drug choices for anesthesia of moose. A dose of 10 μg/kg of carfentanil plus 0.1 mg/kg of xylazine will produce reliable immobilization. The carfentanil should be antagonized with 100 mg of naltrexone/mg of carfentanil. If carfentanil is not available, or is inappropriate for the situation, 1 mg/kg of xylazine plus 2 mg/kg of Telazol will also provide reliable immobization. The xylazine can be antagonized with 1–2 mg/kg of tolazoline. A final option is 1 mg/kg of xylazine plus 4 mg/kg of ketamine. The major drawback of this technique is the volume of the drugs. If 100 mg/ml xylazine and 100 mg/ml ketamine were used, a volume of 30 ml could be required for a large moose. Mature moose weigh 400–600 kg.

12. What is a suitable anesthetic protocol for anesthesia of plains bison?

Bison can be extremely difficult to anesthetize. Anesthesia is much easier if the animal can be captured and restrained in a crush. Xylazine can be administered intravenously, into the tail vein at a dose of 0.3–0.5 mg/kg. This will often produce recumbency and should be followed by 2 mg/kg of ketamine IV. Anesthesia can be maintained with 1–2 mg/kg of ketamine, as needed. Five percent guaifenisin can also be administered via a jugular catheter. Guaifenisin should be used cautiously, and the animal should be monitored for signs of toxicity (extensor rigidity). If the bison is free-ranging, it can be immobilized with either 5–7 μg/kg of carfentanil plus 0.1–0.2 mg/kg of xylazine, or 1–1.5 mg/kg of xylazine plus 2–3 mg/kg of Telazol. Carfentanil should be antagonized with 0.5–0.7 mg/kg of naltrexone. The xylazine component of xylazine-Telazol should be antagonized with 2–3 mg/kg of tolazoline. It is important to use tolazoline or atipamezole, as yohimbine is not effective in bovids. The best sites for dart placement are the gluteal muscle mass and the semimembranosis, semitendonosis muscle mass. Xylazine-Telazol anesthesia can be prolonged, or depth of anesthesia increased, with 1-2 mg/kg of ketamine at 10- to 15-minute intervals. A mature female plains bison weighs approximately 500 kg. A large male bison can weigh 800–900 kg.

13. What kind of supportive care would you provide for the bison?

Care must be taken around the limbs, particularly if carfentanil-xylazine is used. It is not uncommon for animals to strike out with their hind limbs. The hind limbs may be tied up, to prevent injury. Kicking is usually indicative of light anesthesia or poor muscle relaxation, and the best treatment is intravenous xylazine at a dose of 0.05–0.1 mg/kg.

Bison are probably more prone to hypoxemia than cervids, and close monitoring of the percentage of hemoglobin saturation and supplemental inspired oxygen are recommended. Body temperature, heart rate, and respiratory rate should be monitored every 5 minutes. Bison are very prone to both ruminal tympany and regurgitation. Bison should be fasted for 24–48 hours prior to elective procedures and should be maintained in sternal recumbency when possible.

14. What are potential complications of bison anesthesia?

It has been stated that bison are prone to hyoxemia, ruminal tympany, and regurgitation. Bison are also very prone to hyperthermia and myopathy, particularly if they are captured after a prolonged chase; therefore, pursuit times should be kept to a minimum. Bison producers should be warned of this potential complication prior to any immobilization. Bison are prone to self-trauma during capture and it is not uncommon for herd mates to traumatize animals during the induction of anesthesia. It is important to antagonize the xylazine component of Xylazine-Telazol following immobilization. Tolazoline or atipamezole should be used, as yohimbine is not effective in bison.

15. You are assisting fish and wildlife officers with anesthesia of a black bear that has wandered into a populated area and may be injured. What precautions should you take in this situation?

Black bears are not usually aggressive but can become aggressive in some situations. It is important to work with trained people who have a good knowledge of bear behavior and can provide a firearm back-up and crowd control. If the bear is free-ranging, it is often best to attempt to "tree" the bear prior to drug delivery. Black bears will climb trees to escape from danger. Once the bear is treed, it is easier to dart the bear and there is less chance of a partially drugged bear injuring itself or personnel. Ideally the bear should be treed in an evergreen, such as a spruce or fir, as the branches tend to break the fall, once anesthesia is induced. Air mattresses or garbage bags filled with air can be used to help break the fall. Sometimes the bear will be induced to anesthesia and will not fall from the tree. In these situations the bear should be cautiously approached and lowered from the tree with ropes.

Once anesthesia is induced, bears should be cautiously approached. The person approaching should talk softly to the bear and watch for signs of head lifting and ear or eye movement. A pole syringe or long stick should be used for initial contact with the animal. Once it has been determined that the bear is anesthetized, it can be approached and the legs can be hobbled or a cable placed around the wrist and secured to a tree. Placement of a catheter in the jugular or medial saphenous vein will facilitate rapid venous access, if a top-up of anesthetic is required.

16. What anesthetic technique should be used on the bear?

Telazol is the drug of choice for black bear anesthesia. It will produce a safe, reliable immobilization, and has a high margin of safety. A dose of 5–6 mg/kg is sufficient for black bears. It will produce about 60 minutes of anesthesia. Full recovery can take 2–3 hours. The major advantage of Telazol is that recoveries are slow and predictable. Xylazine (2 mg/kg) plus ketamine (6 mg/kg) can be used if Telazol is not available. Xylazine-ketamine is not recommended for anesthesia of bears because sudden recoveries have been known to occur with this combination. If it is used, the bear should be worked on quickly and watched closely for signs of movement or nystagmus. There are some situations in which a "reversible" combination for anesthesia is useful. Sow bears with small cubs are one example. If a reversible combination is desired, 2 mg/kg of xylazine plus 3 mg/kg of Telazol will produce a rapid, reliable immobilization. The xylazine can be antagonized with 0.1–0.2 mg/kg of yohimbine, and recovery will occur more rapidly than with straight Telazol. Xylazine-Telazol can be administered in a much smaller volume than Telazol alone; plus, it produces a more rapid induction and will provide analgesia. It can be difficult to estimate the weight of bears. They often demonstrate piloerection that will make them look larger than they actually are. Bears demonstrate seasonal weight changes, with condition being poorest in the spring and best in the fall (opposite for polar bears). Adult black bears can weigh from 40–300 kg. Younger bears are commonly encountered in the course of wildlife management and generally weigh from 40–100 kg. It is generally wise to overestimate weight, as quick, reliable immobilization is required.

17. What is the preferred injection site for immobilizing drugs?

Bears have a large fat pad over their rump, particularly later in the fall. Drugs injected in this site will not be active. The neck and shoulders are the preferred location for drug administration. If only the hind end can be targeted, the dart should be placed into the semimebranosis/semitendonosis muscles.

18. What supportive care should be provided?

Bears act much like dogs during anesthesia. They are much less prone to complications than ruminants. Hyoxemia is rarely a problem with Telazol, but can be encountered with xylazine-Telazol or xylazine-ketamine. Supplemental inspired oxygen is usually not required, but oxygenation should be monitored closely. The bear should be maintained in sternal or lateral recumbency. Hyperthermia can occur, but with less frequency than in ruminants. Vomiting may occur and is most common during induction. If vomiting occurs, the mouth and pharynx should be carefully flushed and cleared of debris. Bears maintain jaw tone during light planes of anesthesia with Telazol and therefore caution is advised when examining the mouth.

Telazol–induced anesthesia can be difficult to monitor. Reliable signs of arousal include an increased activity of the tongue withdrawl and flexor withdrawl reflex and an increase in ear movement or head lifting. Anesthesia can be prolonged or depth of anesthesia increased by administration of 1–2 mg/kg of ketamine IV, or one-third of the intramuscular induction dose of Telazol. Head-lifting with xylazine-Telazol or with xylazine-ketamine indicates that the animal is very awake and potentially dangerous. Bears are frequently relocated via culvert traps. The bear should only be moved once it is awake, as bears can become compressed at the rear of the trap during movement and may lose their airway. If the bear is not recovered in a culvert trap, it should be watched from a safe distance until it can stand.

19. Would the procedure differ if the animal were a grizzly (brown) bear or a polar bear?

There is a much smaller chance of encountering these species in a populated area, but there are some populated areas where grizzly or polar bears may need to be immobilized for relocation. Both of these species are potentially more aggressive than black bears and must be dealt with very cautiously, by people who know their behavior. They will not tree, like black bears, and must be darted on the ground. Both of these species require a higher dose of Telazol than black bears, approximately 8 mg/kg. Xylazine-Telazol can be used at the same dose as in black bears. Grizzly bears weigh between 100–300 kg in the contiguous United States, the mountain parks of Canada, and the barren grounds. Bears along the northwest coast of Canada and Alaska can grow much larger, with weights up to 700 kg. Polar bears can reach up to 800 kg, and weights of 500 kg are not uncommon among male bears.

20. What can be used to facilitate the capture of feral dogs?

Chemical immobilization of feral dogs should be considered only after nonchemical techniques of capture have been attempted. One of the major considerations is the choice of appropriate remote delivery equipment. Low-velocity darting equipment and darts with contents ejected by compressed gas are the best choice for drug delivery. Metal darts with high-velocity injection can cause significant trauma to small muscle masses. Telazol is a good choice for immobilization of feral dogs, as it can be concentrated to a small volume, suitable for blow darts. Telazol has minimal adverse cardiopulmonary side effects, which contributes to its safety during field anesthesia. A dose of 5–6 mg/kg should be effective for immobilization. If Telazol is not available, 1 mg/kg of xylazine plus 4–6 mg/kg of ketamine or 20 μg/kg of medetomidine plus 2–4 mg/kg of ketamine can be used to facilitate capture of feral dogs. Equipment should be available to provide tracheal intubation, ventilation, and oxygenation under field conditions.

BIBLIOGRAPHY

1. Allan JL: Renarcotization following carfentanil immobilization of nondomestic ungulates. J Zoo Wildl Med 20:423–426, 1989.
2. Bush M: Remote drug delivery systems. J Zoo Wildl Med 23:159–180, 1992.
3. Caulkett NA: Anesthesia for North American cervids. Can Vet J. 38:389–390, 1997.
4. Caulkett NA, Cattet MRL, Cantwell S, et al: Anesthesia of Wood Bison with medetomidine-zolazepam/tiletamine and xylazine-zolazepam/tiletamine combinations. Can Vet J 41:49–54, 2000.
5. Haigh JC: Opiods in zoological medicine. J Zoo Wildl Med 21:391–413, 1990.
6. Haigh JC, Gates CC: Capture of wood bison (Bison bison athabascae) using carfentanil-based mixtures. J Wildl Dis 31:37–42, 1995.
7. Kock MD, Berger J: Chemical immobilization of free-ranging North American bison (Bison bison) in Badlands National Park, South Dakota. J Wildl Dis 23:625–633, 1987.
8. Kreeger TJ: Handbook of Wildlife Chemical Immobilization, 3rd printing with revisions. Fort Collins, Wildlife Pharmaceuticals, 1999.
9. Kreeger TJ, Del Giudice GD, Seal US, Karns PD: Immobilization of white-tailed deer with xylazine hydrochloride and ketamine hydrochloride and antagonism with tolazoline hydrochloride. J Wildl Dis 22:407–412, 1986.
10. Seal US, Schmitt SM, Peterson RD: Carfentanil and xylazine for immobilization of Moose (Alces alces) on Isle Royale. J Wildl Dis 21:48–51, 1985.
11. Wallace RS, Bush M, Montali RJ: Deaths from exertional myopathy at the national zoological park from 1975 to 1985. J Wildl Dis 23:454–462, 1987.

49. LABORATORY ANIMAL ANESTHESIA

Jennifer Fujimoto, D.V.M., D.A.C.V.A.

1. What is a laboratory animal?

A laboratory animal is any animal that is used for research purposes. This includes but is not limited to mice, rats, hamsters, gerbils, guinea pigs, rabbits, cats, dogs, ferrets, nonhuman primates, swine, goats, sheep, calves, reptiles, amphibians, birds, and fish. For the purposes of this chapter, only questions concerning rodents and rabbits will be asked.

2. Is preoperative fasting necessary in rodents and rabbits?

No, because vomiting during the induction of anesthesia does not occur in these species. All animals should be provided with water until approximately 60 minutes prior to the start of anesthesia.

3. What is a more effective anticholinergic for use in rabbits, atropine or glycopyrrolate?

Glycopyrrolate. Not only does it reduce salivary and bronchial secretions, but it is also more effective in protecting the heart from vagal inhibition. The effects of atropine may be unpredictable in rabbits, as many strains have high circulating levels of atropinase, which causes rapid enzymatic degradation of the drug.

4. Is it possible to intubate rodents?

Yes, but it requires skill and specialized equipment. Mice, hamsters, gerbils, and guinea pigs can be particularly challenging. Purpose-made laryngoscope blades or appropriately sized otoscope speculums can be used to visualize the vocal cords. It is also helpful to transilluminate the neck, as a spot of light can be observed in the oropharynx during each breath.

If a laryngoscope blade is used, the animal can be intubated with a suitably sized endotracheal tube with or without the use of a guide wire. If an otoscope speculum is used, the vocal cords are visualized and a guide wire (the guide wire from a Seldinger catheter is ideal, as it is flexible and has a soft blunt tip) is placed between them. The speculum is removed and an endotracheal tube is gently threaded over the wire into the trachea. The wire is removed and the endotracheal tube is secured. To facilitate passage of the guide wire from the side of the mouth, a slit can be cut the length of the speculum. As with larger animals, the tongue of rodents should be gently retracted prior to intubation. This can be accomplished with a cotton-tipped swab.

5. What can be done positionally to further facilitate the intubation of mice?

Mice can be suspended on a plexiglass board at approximately a 45-degree angle. They are held in this position by a rubber band, which attaches to the board and passes behind their front teeth. Once the mouse is intubated, it is removed from the board.

6. What unique anatomic features of guinea pigs makes intubation a challenge?

- Large tongue—only the rostral one third is mobile; the posterior two-thirds is fixed and has an elevated step or pad.
- Narrow buccal cavity due to cheek teeth.
- Soft palate is continuous with the base of the tongue. An opening, the palatal ostium, is the only communication between the oropharynx and the remainder of the pharynx. Modified laryngoscope blades or otoscope speculums must pass through the palatal ostium to visualize the vocal cords.

7. Why are rabbits considered difficult to intubate?

The oral cavity of rabbits is long and narrow and their mouths cannot be opened very wide, making visualization of their vocal cords difficult.

8. What different techniques can be used to intubate rabbits?

Rabbits can be intubated blindly or by visualization of the vocal cords with a laryngoscope or otoscope. An easy way to accomplish blind intubation in rabbits is to use a stethoscope from which the bell or diaphragm has been removed. An appropriately sized endotracheal tube is attached to the tubing and a small elliptical hole is made in the tubing, about 1 inch from the end. This hole allows the rabbit to breathe during the process of intubation. With the rabbit's head and neck gently extended, advance the lubricated tip of the endotracheal tube into the mouth, while listening to the breath sounds through the stethoscope. These sounds allow you to place the endotracheal tube just proximal to the glottis and, on inspiration, to gently advance the tube into the trachea. Proper placement usually results in a cough or visible fogging of the tube (or a mirror) during exhalation. If breath sounds disappear upon advancement of the endotracheal tube, it has probably been passed into the esophagus instead of the trachea.

When the vocal cords are visualized with a laryngoscope, the endotracheal tube can be passed directly into the trachea or threaded over a guide wire. If an otoscope and speculum are used, a guide wire must be initially passed into the trachea and an endotracheal tube threaded over it.

Rabbits can be intubated in either the prone or the supine position and, regardless of technique, should always have their head and neck extended and their tongue pulled forward. The endotracheal tube should never be advanced with force, as laryngeal trauma may result, with tissue swelling and bleeding. Lidocaine should be topically applied to the vocal cords to avoid laryngospasm.

9. Why should topical Cetacaine (benzocaine) not be used to anesthetize the larynx of rabbits?

Rabbits and other small mammals can develop methemoglobinemia when exposed to topical benzocaine (Cetacaine). Lidocaine should be used instead.

10. What size tubes can be used to cannulate the tracheas of rodents and rabbits?

- Mouse (25–35 g):
  - PE 90 tubing with the tip beveled at a 45-degree angle. The bevel should be rounded and on the convex side of the natural curve of the tubing.
  - 1.0 mm diameter tubing
- Rat (200–400 g):
  - 12 to 18 gauge plastic intravenous catheter
- Hamster (120 g):
  - 1.5 mm diameter tubing
- Guinea pig (400–1000 g)
  - 12 to 16 gauge plastic intravenous catheter
- Rabbit (1–3 kg):
  - 2 to 3 mm outside diameter tubing
- Rabbit (3–7 kg):
  - 3 to 6 mm outside diameter tubing

To avoid inadvertent intubation of a bronchus and to produce a seal with the larynx in rats, a small length (3 mm) of rubber tubing can be placed around the catheter approximately 0.5 to 1 cm from the tip.

11. What are the different routes of administering injectable anesthetics?

- Subcutaneous (SC):
  - Can be used in all animals, but the onset time of anesthesia is slow.
  - Common sites: in all animals, injections are usually made into the loose skin over the neck and upper back.
- Intramuscular (IM):
  - Can be used in all animals but may be difficult in rodents because of the smaller muscle mass that is available to inject into. Avoid injecting into or around the sciatic nerve.
  - Common sites: small rodents, hindlimb muscles; rabbits, hindlimb muscles or perilumbar muscles.

- Intravenous (IV)
  - Can be used in all animals but may be particularly difficult in mice.
  - The intravenous route is preferable when administering anesthetics because it is the most predictable route and it provides a rapid onset of effect. Drugs given intravenously can be titrated to produce a desired depth of anesthesia.
  - Common sites: mice and rats, lateral tail veins; guinea pigs, medial saphenous vein; rabbits, auricular vein located on the outer margin of each ear.
- Intraperitoneal (IP)
  - Most commonly used route in small rodents
  - As the entire dose is given at once, it is impossible to adjust the dose based on the individual animals' response. Over- or under-dosing can easily occur.
  - Inadvertent injection into organs or blood vessels is possible, and the animal consequently will not respond as expected to a given dose.

For all routes, always aspirate before injecting any drug.

12. Describe how to do an intraperitoneal injection.
- Appropriately restrain the animal manually.
- Tilt the head and body downward to move the abdominal contents toward the diaphragm.
- Insert the needle through the skin and the abdominal wall at a 30- to 45-degree angle, preferentially into the lower right quadrant of the animal's abdomen. Injection into this quadrant decreases the possibility of penetrating the cecum, stomach, or spleen.
- Gently aspirate before injecting the contents of the syringe into the peritoneal cavity. If intestinal contents are aspirated, discard the needle and syringe and start over. If blood is aspirated, reposition the needle and reaspirate.

13. What injectable anesthetics are commonly used in rodents and rabbits?
- Ketamine combinations (ketamine and a tranquilizer or an α_2-agonist)
- Pentobarbital

14. What kind of anesthetic is ketamine and why is it frequently combined with either a tranquilizer or α_2-agonist?

Ketamine is a dissociative anesthetic (there is dissociation between the thalamus and the limbic system of the brain) that produces a state of catalepsy, superficial analgesia, and profound amnesia. Ketamine alone produces immobility in most animals with a marked increase in skeletal muscle tone. When administered in combination with a tranquilizer (acepromazine, diazepam, or midazolam) or an α_2-agonist (xylazine or medetomidine), muscle relaxation is enhanced and the duration of anesthesia is prolonged. Ketamine combined with a tranquilizer produces good chemical restraint and/or a light plane of anesthesia. Ketamine combined with an α_2-agonist produces a surgical plane of anesthesia. Rabbits may self-mutilate if ketamine/xylazine is injected intramuscularly in close proximity to the sciatic nerve. Ketamine combinations may also cause localized tissue necrosis when given subcutaneously or intramuscularly.

15. What are the advantages and disadvantages of using α_2-agonists such as xylazine and medetomidine?

Advantages
- Potent sedatives
- In most animals produce mild to moderate analgesia
- Markedly potentiate the action of most anesthetic drugs
- Produce good muscle relaxation

Disadvantages
- Dose-dependent cardiovascular and respiratory depression
- Cause bradycardia
- Cause hyperglycemia and diuresis. This has been noted to occur in both mice and rats given a combination of ketamine/xylazine or ketamine/medetomidine.
- Recovery is prolonged

Medetomidine has effects similar to xylazine but because it is a more specific α_2-agonist, its side effects are fewer and not as pronounced.

16. Can α_2-agonists be reversed?

Yes. The effects of both xylazine and medetomidine can be reversed by either yohimbine or atipamezol. Yohimbine is a nonspecific antagonist, whereas atipamezole was specifically formulated to reverse the effects of medetomidine. However, atipamezole will work on xylazine-sedated animals and appears devoid of any undesirable side effects, unlike yohimbine.

17. What are the advantages and disadvantages of using pentobarbital for anesthesia?

Advantages
- Can be administered by either the intraperitoneal or the intravenous route
- Is a short-acting barbiturate that provides light anesthesia lasting anywhere from 15 to 60 minutes
- Relatively inexpensive
- A large amount of research data is available with pentobarbital as the anesthetic

Disadvantages
- Relatively narrow margin of safety between an effective and a lethal dose
- Dose-dependent respiratory and cardiovascular depression
- Excitement may be seen during the induction of anesthesia
- Not analgesic, and at subanesthetic concentrations may actually increase the awareness of pain
- Can cause significant hypothermia through interference with thermal regulation
- Given subcutaneously or intramuscularly can result in irritation or tissue necrosis at the site of injection due to the alkaline pH of the solution
- Prolonged recovery from anesthesia, especially if incremental boluses or a continuous infusion is used

18. What other factors influence the response of a mouse or rat to different anesthetic regimes?

- Strain: There are variable strain responses to any anesthetic and it is recommended that a pilot study be done whenever strains of animals or anesthetics are changed.
- Age: Neonatal animals are unable to adequately metabolize a wide range of drugs because of immature organ systems, whereas geriatric patients frequently have secondary health problems that can make routine anesthesia problematic.
- Sex: Male mice are more susceptible to the effects of intraperitoneal pentobarbital and sleep longer than females. Female rats, on the other hand, are less capable of metabolizing pentobarbital than males and may require a lower dose.
- Bedding: Soft wood bedding can induce liver microsomal enzymes, resulting in reduced sleep time after pentobarbital is given. This same effect may also be seen secondary to dirty bedding.
- Environmental temperature: In mice anesthetized with pentobarbital, sleep time was increased with decreasing environmental temperature.
- Nutritional status
- Time of day the anesthetic is given

19. What inhalant anesthetics are used to anesthetize laboratory animals?

- Ether (not common)
- Methoxyflurane (no longer commercially available in the United States)
- Halothane
- Isoflurane

20. Which inhalant anesthetics can be delivered relatively safely without the use of a vaporizer (open drop technique)?

Ether or methoxyflurane.

21. Why is it advisable to deliver halothane or isoflurane with a precision vaporizer?

Both halothane and isoflurane are potent inhalant anesthetics that can readily volatilize to lethal concentrations at room temperature. The use of a precision vaporizer allows for the delivery of controlled and safe concentrations of anesthetic to the animal.

22. Describe the open drop delivery of inhalant anesthetic.

A cotton ball or gauze sponge is saturated with either ether or methoxyflurane and placed in the bottom of a clear glass jar. A grid is placed over the cotton or gauze to prevent direct contact of the animal with the liquid anesthetic, as the anesthetic is irritating and can cause a contact dermatitis. Alternatively, the cotton or gauze can be fixed to the lid of the jar, eliminating the need for a grid. Once in the jar, the animal is closely observed. When it becomes recumbent, it is removed from the jar and anesthesia is maintained with a facemask. A suitable and inexpensive mask for rodents is a syringe case with a piece of cotton or gauze saturated with anesthetic placed in the bottom of the case. The depth of anesthesia can be controlled by the proximity of the animals nose to the source of the anesthetic.

23. Why is ether no longer commonly used as an anesthetic in laboratory animals?
- Newer and better inhalant anesthetics have been developed.
- Ether is flammable and potentially explosive. Special precautions must be taken when storing ether, and etherized carcasses must be placed in spark-proof refrigerators.

24. What are the advantages and disadvantages of using isoflurane?

Advantages
- Rapid induction and recovery
- Depth can be quickly altered
- Nonirritant, nonexplosive, and nonflammable
- Undergoes very little biotransformation; primary route of elimination is through exhalation
- Less of an effect on cerebral blood flow, especially with concomitant hyperventilation of the animal
- Does not sensitize the heart to circulating catecholamines

Disadvantages
- Dose-related cardiovascular and respiratory depression; causes peripheral vasodilation but has minimal direct depressant effects on the heart
- Pungent odor but does not seem to be a problem with most animals
- Requires delivery via a precision vaporizer

25. What other anesthetics are used in research?
- Propofol
- α-Chloralose
- Urethane
- Tribromoethanol
- Chloral hydrate
- Inactin

26. Which anesthetics should be used only in terminal research projects? Why?

α-Chloralose and urethane. Both α-chloralose and urethane produce long-lasting, light to surgical-level anesthesia with minimal cardiovascular or respiratory depression. (α-Chloralose produces light anesthesia and urethane surgical anesthesia). Urethane, however, is carcinogenic to both animals and people, and its use should be avoided if possible. Animals should not be allowed to recover from α-chloralose anesthesia because recovery is prolonged and is frequently associated with involuntary excitement.

27. Which anesthetic if incorrectly stored or prepared can be extremely irritating to the peritoneum when given intraperitoneally?

Tribromoethanol. If the stock solution of tribromoethanol is old or is not prepared and stored properly, the breakdown products of this anesthetic can cause abdominal adhesions, peritonitis, intestinal disorders, and death. Once formulated, tribromoethanol should be stored in a cool dark environment and used within a few weeks of preparation. It provides good surgical anesthesia in both mice and rats but should be used only once. Animals anesthetized a second time with tribromoethanol experience a high mortality rate.

28. What anesthetic, when given intraperitoneally to rats, can cause an adynamic ileus to develop?

Choral hydrate. This anesthetic when given intraperitoneally can lead to a high incidence of stasis and dilation of the bowel (adynamic ileus). Affected animals develop a distended abdomen and some may die. Using lower concentrations of chloral hydrate can decrease the incidence of the problem but cannot totally eliminate it. The development of adynamic ileus has also been reported to occur in guinea pigs after an intraperitoneal injection of chloral hydrate.

29. How can the development of hypothermia be minimized in rodents and rabbits undergoing anesthesia and surgery?

- Wrap the animal in saran wrap followed by an outer wrap of aluminum foil.
- Wrap the animal in bubble packing.
- Place the animal on a recirculating warm water blanket.
- Place the animal on a heat-activated gel pad.
- Lavage major body cavities with warm saline before closing.

Small animals are particularly susceptible to the development of hypothermia while under anesthesia, as they have a large surface area available for heat loss relative to their small body mass. Body temperature should be closely monitored.

30. Why is it important to minimize the development of hypothermia?

Hypothermia prolongs recovery from anesthesia and increases the incidence of anesthetic associated death, especially in small rodents.

31. How can the depth of anesthesia be assessed in rodents and rabbits?

- Observation of the pattern and rate of respiration.
- Palpebral reflex: This reflex is unreliable and difficult to assess in rodents. It may not be lost in the rabbit until dangerously deep levels of anesthesia have been attained.
- Pedal withdrawal reflex: In rodents, pinch the foot or tail and if the animal moves or experiences an increase in respiratory rate, anesthesia needs to be deepened before surgery is begun. In rabbits, pinch a toe and evaluate the animal's response to the stimulus.
- Ear pinch: At light levels of anesthesia, guinea pigs and rabbits may shake their heads or actually vocalize when their ears are pinched.
- Monitoring the rate and quality of the pulse, if the pulse is readily palpable.
- Monitoring the heart rate and blood pressure if applicable.

32. Describe different techniques to safely anesthetize neonatal mice and rats.

Hypothermia has long been popular for the anesthesia of neonatal rodents as it is relatively simple to accomplish and is inexpensive. However, it remains highly controversial because thorough investigations have not been done to indisputably establish its efficacy as an anesthetic in neonatal rodents.

At 9°C, neural conduction and synaptic transmission within the peripheral nervous system ceases. Similar effects appear to occur within the central nervous system. During profound hypothermia, it is unlikely that an animal is experiencing pain. Neonatal mice can be cooled to 1°C and can be safely maintained in a hypothermic state for up to 30 minutes. Reportedly, hypothermia can be used as an anesthetic in mice up to 6 or 7 days of age.

Induction of hypothermia usually takes 3 to 4 minutes after immersion in ice or ice water. Recovery is dependent on the duration of hypothermia but may take up to 1 hour. Maintenance of anesthesia requires that the animal be put on a bed of ice or a cooling pad. To decrease the incidence of distress (vocalizing and struggling) that can be associated with cooling, it is recommended that the pup be placed in a protective latex sleeve (the cut finger of a latex glove) prior to immersion. This provides partial insulation and also prevents the pup from coming into direct contact with the ice or cold water. During recovery, pups should be closely observed for possible discomfort, as humans describe the return of sensation as being painful.

The inhalant anesthetics offer distinct advantages for anesthetizing neonatal rodents. Induction and recovery are rapid, the pups are provided with oxygen, and the level of anesthesia can be easily individualized. However, the use of the inhalants requires proper equipment for agent delivery and adequate scavenging of the waste anesthetic gases. Methoxyflurane (no longer commercially available in the United States), halothane, and isoflurane have all been used safely and effectively in neonates.

The injectable anesthetics (pentobarbital, ketamine and ketamine combinations, urethane, and fentanyl combinations) have been used but with varying degrees of success. Neonatal animals have a decreased capacity to metabolize injectable anesthetics and their response to them is very different from their adult counterparts. Mortality, in general, is increased with the use of the injectable anesthetics even when reversal agents are administered.

BIBLIOGRAPHY

1. Brown RH, Walters DM, Greenberg RS, Mitzner W: A method of endotracheal intubation and pulmonary functional assessment for repeated studies in mice. J Appl Physiol 87(6):2362–2365, 1999.
2. Carraway JH, Gray LD: Blood collection and intravenous injection in the guinea pig via the medical saphenous vein. Lab Anim Sci 39:623–624, 1989.
3. Conlon KC, Corbally MT, Bading JR, Brennan MF: Atraumatic endotracheal intubation in small rabbits. Lab Anim Sci 40:221–222, 1990.
4. Danneman PJ, Mandrell TD: Evaluation of five agents/methods for anesthesia of neonatal rats. Lab Anim Sci 47:386–394, 1997.
5. Flecknell PA: Laboratory Animal Anesthesia, 2nd ed. San Diego, Harcourt Brace and Company, 1996.
6. Lovell DP: Variation in pentobarbitone sleeping time in mice 1: Strain and sex differences. Lab Anim 20:85–90, 1986.
7. Lovell DP: Variation in pentobarbitone sleeping time in mice 2: Variables affecting test results. Lab Anim 20:91–96, 1986.
8. Olson ME, Vizzutti D, Morck DW, Cox AK: The parasympatholytic effects of atropine sulfate and glycoprrolate in rats and rabbits. Can J Vet Res 57:254–258, 1993.
9. Papaioannou VE, Fox JG: Efficacy of tribromoethanol anesthesia in mice. Lab Anim Sci 43:189–192, 1993.
10. Phifer CB, Terry LM: Use of hypothermia for general anesthesia in preweanling rodents. Physiol Behav 38:887–890, 1986.
11. Sedgwick C, Jahn S: Techniques for endotracheal intubation and inhalation anesthesia for laboratory animals. Calif Vet 3:27–33, 1980.
12. Silverman J, Muir WWIII: Special topic overview: A review of laboratory animal anesthesia with chloral hydrate and chloralose. Lab Anim Sci 43:210–216, 1993.
13. Suckow MA, Danneman PJ, Brayton C: The Laboratory Mouse. Boca Raton, CRC Press LLC, 2001.
14. Timm KI, Jahn SE, Sedgwick CJ: The palatal ostium of the guinea pig. Lab Anim Sci 37: 801–802, 1987.
15. Waynforth HB, Flecknell PA: Experimental and Surgical Technique in the Rat, 2nd ed. San Diego, Harcourt Brace Jovanovich, 1992.

50. EUTHANASIA

Kurt A. Grimm, D.V.M., M.S., D.A.C.V.A., D.A.C.V.C.P.

1. What is euthanasia?

Etymology: Greek, easy death, from euthanatos, from eu- + thanatos (death): the act or practice of killing or permitting the death of hopelessly sick or injured individuals (domestic animals) in a relatively painless way for reasons of mercy.

The fundamental principal underlying euthanasia is the creation of an unconscious state before the termination of vital organ system function. This should be done with as little stress as possible to reduce the emotional distress of the animal and those witnessing or performing the procedure. If necessary, sedatives may be administered before the administration of the euthanasia agent to facilitate handling and reduce animal stress.

2. What agents can be used in dogs and cats to create unconsciousness?

All general anesthetic agents can be used to create unconsciousness. However, some are more acceptable for euthanasia based on the speed and ease with which they cause unconsciousness. Induction of anesthesia with an inhalant anesthetic generally requires a significant duration of restraint or confinement and may be stressful to the animal. Intramuscular administration will also require a significant time for absorption and peak effect to occur. When possible, intravenous administration of a hypnotic drug such as pentobarbital, thiopental, or propofol should be used.

3. What methods are acceptable for euthanasia of dogs and cats?

- Acceptable: barbiturates.
- Conditionally acceptable: inhalant anesthetics, CO, CO_2, N_2, Ar.

Conditionally acceptable methods should should be used only in unusual circumstances when barbiturates are unavailable. Special considerations apply to these methods and additional information or training should be sought before attempting these methods.

4. What methods are unacceptable for euthanasia of dogs and cats?

- **Exsanguination**—Because of the anxiety associated with extreme hypovolemia, exsanguination should be done only in stunned or anesthetized animals.
- **Air embolism**—Air embolism may be accompanied by convulsions, opisthotonos and vocalization. If used, it should be done only in anesthetized animals.
- **Drowning**—Drowning promotes escape behavior and is inhumane as a means of euthanasia.
- **Strychnine**—Strychnine causes violent convulsions and painful muscle contractions.
- **Nicotine, magnesium sulfate, potassium chloride, all curariform agents (neuromuscular blocking agents)**—When used alone, these drugs all cause respiratory or cardiac arrest before unconsciousness, so the animal may perceive pain or anxiety after it is immobilized.
- **Chloroform**—Chloroform is a known hepatotoxin and suspected carcinogen, and therefore hazardous to human beings.
- **Cyanide**—Cyanide poses an extreme danger to personnel and the manner of death is aesthetically objectionable.
- **Stunning**—Stunning may render an animal unconscious, but it is not a method of euthanasia. If used, it must be followed by a method to ensure death.

5. If drug combinations are used for euthanasia, is the order of administration important?

It is imperative that respiratory or cardiac arrests **not** precede unconsciousness. Neuromuscular junction blocking drugs such as succinylcholine or atracurium are not to be administered to assist in restraint or cause respiratory paralysis before unconsciousness is achieved. Likewise, administration of cardiotoxic substances such as potassium chloride and magnesium sulfate must not precede unconsciousness.

6. Can carbon monoxide be used for euthanasia of dogs and cats?

Carbon monoxide (CO) causes tissue hypoxia by incapacitating the major oxygen-carrying constituent of blood through occupation of oxygen-binding sites on hemoglobin. The loss of consciousness is believed to be relatively peaceful. This is because there is no hypoxia-driven chemoreceptor feedback, since dissolved oxygen in the plasma remains unchanged. Exposure of personnel to unscavenged CO results in unsafe workplace conditions and can result in toxicity. In summary, CO is not an acceptable method of euthanasia for cats and dogs when safer and faster methods are available.

7. I have heard of car exhaust being used as a source of carbon monoxide. Why isn't this acceptable?

Besides the above-mentioned concerns about the use of carbon monoxide, the use of internal combustion engines to produce carbon monoxide is unacceptable because of heat, noise, and difficulty in controlling the concentration.

8. How do argon, nitrogen, and other hypoxic gas mixtures cause death?

These agents dilute oxygen in the inspired gas until hypoxemia and hypoxia develop. These methods usually result in a short period of time before consciousness is lost during which the animal may be distressed. High inspired concentrations must be reached rapidly if these methods are to work humanely. These methods cannot be recommended when faster and less stressful methods are available.

9. If I must use hypoxic gases for animal euthanasia, are there special concerns for neonatal animals?

Neonatal animals have adapted to relatively hypoxic in utero conditions. Early in life, they may tolerate seemingly impossible periods of hypoxia, and death may be slow or not occur if proper conditions are not created.

10. Carbon dioxide is used during humane slaughter of swine. Why not for euthanasia?

At sufficiently high partial pressures, carbon dioxide (CO_2) is a rapid acting anesthetic and central nervous system (CNS) depressant. Some swine slaughter facilities use CO_2 to create unconsciousness before exsanguination. When done correctly, this method creates relatively rapid unconsciousness and eventual death. A compressed source of CO_2 must be used to ensure rapid production of high concentrations of inspired CO_2. Use of intravenous agents is preferred if they are available.

11. Is dry ice a good source of carbon dioxide?

Dry ice is not an acceptable source of CO_2 for euthanasia of dogs and cats. It may expose animals to uncomfortable temperatures, and gaseous CO_2 production may be difficult to control. Compressed gas sources are preferred.

12. Is an intravenous catheter necessary for euthanasia?

In some circumstances, the placement of an intravenous catheter may cause unnecessary stress to the animal and may result in additional expense. In many cases, however, the use of an indwelling intravenous catheter will prevent inadvertent perivascular injection and allow additional amounts of the agent to be administered under difficult circumstances. Catheters may prevent unnecessary distress to owners and staff and can be viewed as insurance against a "bad" euthanasia.

13. I have heard that α_2-agonists should not be used as sedatives because they slow the delivery of the barbiturate to the brain.

It is true that α_2-agonists, such as xylazine, decrease cardiac output. At modest doses, however, they redistribute the remaining cardiac output from peripheral tissues to the visceral organs including the brain, thereby maintaining brain blood flow. A slight increase in limb-brain circulation time following xylazine administration is often noted, but animals are typically heavily sedated and the few additional seconds seldom result in complications. The benefits of reduced stress, ease of handling, and decreased response to intravenous injection make the use of α_2-agonists beneficial in many cases.

14. What is T-61?

T-61 is a nonbarbiturate injectable euthanasia mixture containing embutramid (a hypnotic), mebezonium iodide (a neuromuscular junction blocker), and tetracaine hydrochloride (a local anesthetic). It was originally approved by the FDA–CVM for euthanasia by intracardiac, intraperitoneal, and intravenous injection to birds, cats, dogs, horses, laboratory animals, and mink. Since the product did not contain controlled substances, a DEA license was not required for purchase. However, concern over differences in the rates of absorption of the toxic and hypnotic components following injection by nonintravenous routes have led to withdrawal of the product in the United States. It is still available in Canada.

15. Are there alternatives to intravenous administration if peripheral veins are not accessible?

Intravenous access will usually result in the most rapid and smoothest loss of consciousness and death. However, in some instances, peripheral veins may not be accessible and alternative routes of administration are required. Intraperitoneal injection has been used in small animals and is an alternative only if intravenous access is not available. Intracardiac injection is associated with significant stress in many animals and is not acceptable. Premedication with sedatives with or without analgesic drugs will provide a more cooperative patient and smooth the loss of consciousness.

16. What is a good source for euthanasia information?

In 1993 the Animal Welfare Information Center of the United States Department of Agriculture distributed the Report of the AVMA Panel on Euthanasia on the Web at http://www.nal.usda.gov/awic/pubs/noawicpubs/avmaeuth.htm. It also appeared in print in the Journal of the American Veterinary Medical Association (1993;202:229–249). Another source is one of the many anesthesia texts such as *Lumb and Jones' Veterinary Anesthesia, 3rd edition*, which has a chapter dedicated to the subject.

17. How do I handle a staff member who objects to assisting with euthanasia?

Many people have a strong belief that the taking of life is wrong and will refuse to participate. Many others feel that euthanasia is a way to help end the suffering of an animal and view it as assisting nature by shortening the terminal stages of the dying process. Some veterinarians view it as a service to clients and choose to remain neutral on the issue. No matter what beliefs your staff have on euthanasia, participation should be voluntary and no one should be forced to participate in a procedure with which they are uncomfortable or unqualified to assist.

BIBLIOGRAPHY

1. Animal Welfare Information Center, United States Department of Agriculture National Agricultural Library: 1993 Report of the AVMA Panel on Euthanasia. J Am Vet Med Assoc 202:229–249. 1993.
2. Animal Welfare Information Center. http://www.nal.usda.gov/awic/pubs/noawicpubs/avmaeuth.htm
3. Euthanasia. In Thurmon JC, Tranquilli WJ, Benso, GJ (eds): Lumb and Jones' Veterinary Anesthesia, 3rd ed. Baltimore, Williams & Wilkins, 1996, pp 862–882.

VIII. Regional Anesthesia

51. DENTAL NERVE BLOCKS

Kurt A. Grimm, D.V.M., M.S., D.A.C.V.A., D.A.C.V.C.P.

1. If the animal is anesthetized during the dental procedure, why do I need to use nerve blocks?

When an animal is anesthetized with a general anesthetic, there will be no perception of pain. However, the transduction, transmission, and modulation (collectively called nociception) of noxious stimuli can continue. This will lead to increased anesthetic dose requirements, a greater requirement for postoperative analgesics, and potentially long-term nervous system changes resulting in allodynia and hyperalgesia. The use of dental blocks can reduce the amount of nociceptive processing and provide analgesia following recovery from general anesthesia.

2. What analgesic and anesthetic agents can be used for dental blocks?

Local anesthetics are administered to produce regional anesthesia for dental procedures. Lidocaine and bupivacaine appear to be most commonly used in companion animal practice. Local anesthetics are effective at inhibiting axon conduction and are therefore effective when deposited on the nerve near one of many easily palpated landmarks. Epinephrine may be added at 1:200,000 (1 mg/200 ml of local anesthetic) to reduce systemic uptake resulting in prolonged duration of effectiveness and reduced systemic toxicity.

3. What are toxic doses for lidocaine and bupivacaine?

Toxic doses will vary with route of administration, location of injection, rate of uptake, and individual differences in sensitivity. A good rule of thumb for infiltration of local anesthetics in the region of the head is 8–10 mg/kg of lidocaine and 2–3 mg/kg of bupivacaine for dogs. Toxic doses for cats may be $^3/_4$ to $^1/_2$ of those for dogs. By using diluted solutions, you can inject more volume to facilitate nerve conduction blockade at multiple sites and reduce the incidence of toxicity.

4. How much local anesthetic should I inject?

First, the toxic dose should be calculated and not exceeded. Next, the number of sites should be estimated and the desired dose (i.e., concentration multiplied by the volume) should be divided up between these sites. If the volume to be injected at each site is very small, then the local anesthetic can be diluted with saline to give the desired volume. In general, for dogs, $^1/_4$ to $^1/_2$ ml can be injected at the opening of the infraorbital, mental, and mandibular foramen. If the infraorbital canal is to be infiltrated, a slightly larger volume should be used to ensure the filling of the canal to provide adequate distribution. Cats generally will require less volume because of the smaller size of the anatomic structures.

5. What are the signs of local anesthetic toxicity?

Signs of toxicity will vary with the agent being used. Lidocaine will typically result in CNS excitation, leading to convulsions. Bupivacaine will also cause CNS excitation but will be followed by cardiac arrhythmias and myocardial depression at marginally higher doses.

6. What should I do if a patient seizes following a dental block?

While rare at recommended doses, seizures will usually indicate local anesthetic CNS toxicity. Seizures are often suppressed by general anesthetics and may not be appreciated if the blocks are performed at the beginning of the procedure. If seizures occur, treatment is intravenous administration of diazepam or another rapidly acting antiepileptic agent. A patent airway and adequacy of respiration should also be rapidly established. If bupivacaine was used, cardiac monitoring should include an electrocardiogram and blood pressure measurement. Unfortunately, there is no specific treatment for bupivacaine-induced myocardial toxicity, and treatment consists of treating the symptoms and reducing the exposure to the bupivacaine, if possible.

7. Which nerves innervate the upper dental arcade?

All innervation to the upper dental arcade is derived from the maxillary branch of the right and left trigeminal nerves. The maxillary nerve is neither superficial nor easily accessible. However, the infraorbital branch of the maxillary nerve gives rise to the innervating branches of the upper hemi-arcade and is easily located within the infraorbital canal. The caudal maxillary alveolar nerve, middle maxillary alveolar nerve, and rostral maxillary alveolar nerve provide sensation to the caudal, middle, and incisor teeth, respectively.

8. What are the anatomic landmarks I need to know to block the nerves of the upper teeth?

Local anesthetic is deposited at the infraorbital foramen if the rostral maxillary alveolar nerve is to be blocked, or at the deeper aspects of the infraorbital canal if the caudal, middle, and rostral maxillary alveolar nerves are to be blocked (see figure). The infraorbital foramen can usually be palpated inside the upper lip just above the second premolar tooth. The caudal opening of the infraorbital canal (the maxillary foramen) is usually at the level of the medial canthus of the eye, and needle insertion past this point may result in injury to deeper structures of the orbit.

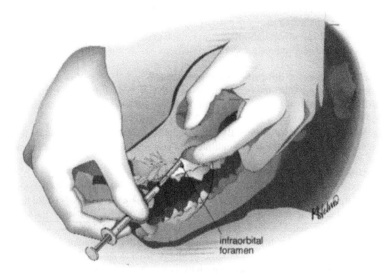

infraorbital
foramen

From Tranquilli WJ, Grimm KA, Lamont LA: Pain Management. Jackson, WY: Teton New Media, 2000, p. 49, with permission.

9. What nerves innervate the lower dental arcade?

The right and left mandibular nerves (also branches of the trigeminal nerve) innervate the lower dental arcade. At the rostralmost aspects, the mental nerve is a continuation of the mandibular nerve.

10. What are the landmarks for the nerve block locations of the lower jaw?

Unlike the maxillary nerve, the mandibular alveolar nerve is relatively accessible as it enters the mandibular foramen near the angle of the mandible. Anesthesia of the nerve at this point will block sensation to all lower teeth. If anesthesia of only the lower incisors and/or lower lip is required, the mental nerve (a continuation of the mandibular alveolar nerve) can be blocked. It may be blocked at the mental foramen located just below the lower second premolar tooth.

11. I have heard animals may mutilate themselves following dental blocks. Is this true?

These blocks are safe and effective in the majority of cases. There is some concern when blocks result in large areas of insensitivity around the lips and cheeks. Some animals may decide to chew on their facial features and should be closely observed for signs of self-mutilation. Fortunately, these episodes are very infrequent and most animals will not have any adverse effects following dental blocks. Tranquilization will often help animals that appear uneasy following loss of sensation to the face.

12. Is the addition of epinephrine to lidocaine contraindicated in patients anesthetized with halothane?

It is true that epinephrine increases the potential risk of cardiac arrhythmias during halothane anesthesia. However, epinephrine coadministered with lidocaine does not commonly lead to the development of serious ventricular arrhythmias. Isoflurane and sevoflurane do not appear to have the same arrhythmogenic interaction with epinephrine at doses commonly used for dental blocks.

13. How long does a nerve block last?

It is difficult to accurately predict the duration of nerve blocks. Proximity of local anesthetic placement to the nerve, agent used, type of nerve, concentration of the solution, local blood flow, intensity of the stimulus, and coadministration of epinephrine, sodium bicarbonate, and hyaluronidase will influence duration. Generally speaking, 60 to 90 minutes and 90 to 180 minutes of anesthesia should be expected from lidocaine and bupivacaine, respectively. Analgesia should be noticeable for a longer period of time.

14. What extra equipment is required for performing dental nerve blocks?

Anyone who can perform an intravenous or intramuscular injection has the necessary equipment. A tuberculin syringe, 22- to 25-gauge needle, and skin preparation supplies are all that are needed. Additional cost for the veterinarian is generally nominal per treatment. Knowledge and expertise in these techniques are what justifies the charges.

15. What are the contraindications to performing dental nerve blocks?

Absolute contraindications: Coagulopathies, infection at the site of injection, anatomic malformation at the site of injection that would result in uncertainty of needle placement.

Relative contraindications: Sensitivity to the local anesthetic being used.

16. Can systemic analgesics be administered before or after dental nerve blocks?

Absolutely. Preemptive administration of opioids, α_2-adrenergic agonists, nonsteroidal anti-inflammatory drugs, and other analgesic preparations will help to reduce the induction and maintenance doses of general anesthetics and enhance the intensity and duration of local nerve block–induced analgesia. If an animal displays pain-related behavior following a procedure, additional analgesics should not be withheld on the basis of local blocks having been performed. Block failure could result in inadequate analgesia and unneeded patient suffering if untreated. Behavior caused by pain should be differentiated from that caused by block-related anxiety. Anxiety may respond better to the administration of a sedative or tranquilizer such as acepromazine or medetomidine. Opioids may also provide sedation and analgesia and may be the drugs of choice when pain and anxiety cannot be differentiated.

17. Can I perform oral surgery with only dental nerve blocks and sedation?

While it may be possible to perform many general surgical procedures with local anesthesia and chemical or manual restraint, dental procedures are only safely done with general anesthesia.

General anesthesia will prevent voluntary or involuntary jaw movement, allow intubation with a cuffed endotracheal tube to prevent aspiration of blood and fluids, and, in most instances, is not associated with any greater risk to the patient than local anesthesia.

18. Can dental nerve blocks be performed on animals that are not sedated or anesthetized?
It may be tempting to perform dental nerve blocks on awake animals to provide additional postoperative analgesia. However, there is a greater chance of misguided needle placement and iatrogenic nerve injury if sudden movement occurs. Also, these blocks are performed in and around the mouth and there is the risk of defensive action by the animal that compromises the safety of the veterinarian.

BIBLIOGRAPHY

1. Hardie EM: Dental Blocks. In Predictable Pain Management: Symposium proceedings from the North American Veterinary Conference, Orlando, Florida, 1996, pp 45–47.
2. Lamont LA, Tranquilli WJ, Grimm KA: Physiology of Pain. Vet Clin North Am Small Anim Pract 30(4): 703–728, 2000.
3. Lemke KA, Dawson SD: Local and Regional Anesthesia. Vet Clin North Am Small Anim Pract 30(4): 839–857, 2000.
4. Skarda RT: Local and regional anesthetic and analgesic techniques: Dogs. In Thurmon JC, Tranquilli WJ, Benson GJ (eds): Lumb and Jones' Veterinary Anesthesia, 3rd ed. Baltimore, Williams & Wilkins, 1996.
5. Tranquilli WJ, Grimm KA, Lamont LA: Analgesic Techniques. In Tranquilli WJ, Grimm KA, Lamont LA (eds): Pain Management for the Small Animal Practitioner. Jackson, WY, Teton New Media, 2000, pp 32–72.

52. EPIDURAL ANESTHESIA

Kurt A. Grimm, D.V.M., M.S., D.A.C.V.A., D.A.C.V.C.P.

1. What are epidural, extradural, intrathecal, subarachnoid, and spinal anesthesia techniques?

The terms epidural and extradural anesthesia are used interchangeably. Both refer to the placement of an anesthetic solution upon (epi-) or outside (extra-) the dura mater. Intrathecal, subarachnoid, and spinal anesthesia are used synonymously by many veterinarians and refer to the placement of an anesthetic solution under the spinal arachnoid, but above the pia mater (within the subarachnoid space). The dura mater and arachnoid lie in close approximation and the small space in between is of little clinical importance. When the subarachnoid space is entered, cerebrospinal fluid (CSF) will usually drip from the hub of the spinal needle.

2. At what level does the subarachnoid space end in the dog and cat?

There are some interindividual and interspecies differences in the caudal extension of the spinal cord and subarachnoid space. The spinal cord usually ends at about L6 in the dog and the subarachnoid space will end approximately at the L7 region. In young animals and small-breed dogs, the subarachnoid space may extend into the sacral region. In the cat, both extend slightly caudal to their respective levels in the dog. The significance of this is that, in dogs, there is a minimal chance (approximately 5%) of obtaining CSF from an inadvertent subarachnoid puncture at the lumbosacral junction. However, there is a higher probability of subarachnoid puncture in cats. In either case, if subarachnoid penetration has occurred, the dose of anesthetic should be reduced by approximately 50%.

3. Will I damage the spinal cord by doing an epidural injection?

In dogs, the spinal cord tissue usually does not lie directly below the lumbosacral space, and the probability of direct spinal cord trauma is low. In 90% of dogs, the spinal cord terminates at the level of the 7th lumbar vertebral body. In cats, the spinal cord usually terminates more caudally, at the level of the sacrum. Still, when proper technique is used, the incidence of neurologic trauma is extremely low in cats.

4. Is the epidural space really an empty space?

Not at all! There is an extensive venous sinus network in addition to all of the semisolid epidural fat that surrounds and supports the spinal cord. Since the bony spinal canal has a fixed volume, when changes occur in the volume of the contents (such as decreased epidural fat in emaciated animals or increased blood volume during pregnancy), the volume available for drug solutions will change and cranial movement of drugs will vary.

5. What types of drugs can be administered in the epidural space?

Historically, local anesthetics have been the most widely used class of drugs for epidural anesthesia/analgesia. More recently, however, opioids, α_2-adrenergic agonists, and experimental classes of drug have been administered epidurally to enhance or produce anesthesia and/or analgesia.

6. What are the contraindications to epidural administration?

Absolute: Coagulopathies, septicemia, infection in the area of needle insertion, uncorrected hypotension (especially with local anesthetics), and lumbosacral pathologic lesion that would make needle placement difficult.

Relative: Bacteremia, neurologic disease that would be aggravated by epidural drug administration.

7. Why do I get blood back during an epidural needle placement?

Blood may come from a vessel that is punctured during insertion of the needle through the extraspinal muscle and connective tissue. More commonly, however, it is due to inadvertent entry of the needle into a venous sinus in the epidural space. Injection into the venous sinus is the same as intravenous injection elsewhere and is not recommended. Instead, the needle can be withdrawn and a new needle can be used to try again.

8. What signs can I use to be confident of correct needle placement?

The epidural space is at a slightly subatmospheric pressure. When it is entered for the first time, there is usually aspiration of any fluid in the hub of the spinal needle (hanging drop technique). Other signs of epidural needle placement are twitching of the tail and pelvic limb muscles as the needle touches the nerve roots, feeling a characteristic "pop" as the needle passes through the ligamentum flavum, loss of resistance to injection of a small volume of air, and a characteristic change in respiratory pattern during injection of a solution. The presence of CSF in the needle indicates inadvertent subarachnoid placement. It must be recognized and the dose reduced accordingly.

9. What effect does injection of air into the epidural space have?

Injection of a small volume of air (<1.0 ml) will generally not have any effect on the patient. It is absorbed from the epidural space and causes no adverse effects. Occasionally, injections of larger volumes of air have been blamed for "patchy" or inconsistent block in humans.

10. What is the mechanism of action of epidurally administered drugs?

No single mechanism is universally accepted. The most obvious (but not necessarily correct) mechanism is diffusion of the drug across the meninges to its site of action directly on the spinal cord. This mechanism may be more important for highly lipid-soluble agents such as fentanyl. Another mechanism is diffusion into the spinal nerve roots before or after they join and exit the intervertebral foramen. A third possible mechanism is the systemic uptake of the drugs by the venous sinus or by tissues outside the intervertebral foramen. This mechanism is unlikely to be important for local anesthetics but may be important for some opioids and α_2-adrenergic agonists.

11. What factors will decrease the dose of local anesthetic administration required?
- Pregnancy
- Obesity
- Old age (due to stenosis of intervertebral foramina)
- Increased concentration of solution
- Increased intra-abdominal pressure

12. Can preservative-containing solutions be placed in the epidural space?

There have been several reports of histologic changes occurring in the spinal cord following administration of preservative-containing solutions. It would appear that repeated administration would increase the exposure and result in a greater change. Therefore, it is commonly recommended that preservative-free solutions be used for epidural and spinal anesthesia and analgesia. However, clinical evidence suggests that single epidural administration of preservative-containing solutions does not result in observable changes on neurologic examination. The best advice is, if preservative-free solutions are available, they should be used.

13. What are the landmarks for lumbosacral epidural anesthesia?

The needle is inserted in line with the dorsal spinous processes of the lumbar and sacral vertebrae between L7 and S1. Commonly this is located just caudal to a line connecting the cranial edge of the wings of the ilia. Proper location can be double-checked by palpating the dorsal spinous process in the area. Remember the dorsal spinous processes of the lumbar vertebrae are separate and taller, whereas those of the sacrum are fused and shorter.

14. Which patient position is best, sternal or lateral recumbency?

Both are perfectly acceptable. Lateral recumbency is more amenable to positioning dogs with pelvic and hind limb fractures. However, the hanging-drop technique cannot be reliably used and needle placement is verified by "feel." Sternal recumbency may facilitate alignment of landmarks and is compatible with the hanging-drop technique. When performed by experienced veterinarians, both have similar success rates.

15. What is the hanging-drop technique?

The hanging-drop technique is a method of verification of epidural needle placement. Place the patient in sternal recumbency and insert the epidural needle through the skin. Next, remove the stylet and add anesthetic/analgesic solution to the hub of the needle until a meniscus is formed. Then slowly advance the needle until the needle is felt to enter the epidural space. The subatmospheric pressure in the epidural space should draw the fluid into the hub of the needle.

16. I am sure I injected into the epidural space but the block did not work. Why?

It is not uncommon to have one or more positive signs of correct needle placement, yet the block fails to work as expected. The explanation may be as simple as incorrect needle placement with misleading signs. Other explanations exist, however, and include leakage of solution out a nearby intervertebral foramen, inadvertent intravascular injection in a venous sinus, or direction of the solution away from the site of action by fibrous tissue or epidural fat.

17. What solutions are commonly used for epidural anesthesia and analgesia?

Anesthesia	*Analgesia*
2.0% lidocaine	2.0% lidocaine
0.5% bupivacaine	0.5% bupivacaine
	0.1% morphine (Astramorph)
	1.5% morphine
	0.1% medetomidine (Domitor)

18. Can epinephrine be combined with local anesthetics?

Epinephrine can be combined at 1:200,000 to prolong duration and slow absorption of the local anesthetic. A 1:200,000 mixture would be 1 mg of epinephrine for every 200 ml of local anesthetic.

19. Why do spinal needles have a stylet?

The stylet is there to occlude the end of the needle during puncture of the skin. Occasionally, a needle without a stylet will cut a plug as it passes through the skin and can carry it into the epidural space. This skin may serve as a nidus for infection and inflammation or, rarely, will continue to grow to form a tumor-like structure.

20. Am I really wimpy or are spinal needles really dull?

Spinal needles have a different bevel that is duller than that of hypodermic needles. The dullness allows the operator to have a better feel for the tissue layers and accentuates the "pop" as the needle penetrates the ligamentum flavum.

21. My boss won't let me do epidurals because it takes too long. How long does it take someone with experience?

As with all procedures, there is a learning curve. Speed will come with experience. Once experience is gained, epidural drug administration should only add 5 to 10 minutes to the procedure for most dogs. Some difficult dogs may require a longer effort, and the benefits should be weighed against the additional anesthesia time on a case-by-case basis. Very few veterinarians could spay a cat in less than 20 minutes their first time, but that didn't stop them from practicing and becoming proficient.

22. What supplies are required for epidural injection?

The only specialized piece of equipment is a spinal (epidural) needle. These are readily available and inexpensive. Most are disposable, and they are available in many types and sizes. A good general needle is a 22-gauge by 2- or 2.5-inch Quincke type. This will work for most mid-size and large dogs. Also required are a sterile syringe, sterile gloves, and supplies to clip and prepare the skin. Drugs are covered elsewhere, but new vials or single-dose vials should be used to reduce the risk of bacterial contamination; sterility is a must.

23. What side effects are commonly encountered?

The most noticeable side effect with local anesthetics is motor weakness immediately following recovery from anesthesia. This is usually a continuation of a desired effect during surgery. This typically resolves within a few hours but may take up to a day, depending on the drug and doses used. Other complications include urinary retention (local anesthetics and opioids), pruritus (opioids), nausea and vomiting (opioids and α_2-adrenergic agonists), respiratory depression (local anesthetics, opioids, α_2-adrenergic agonists), hypotension (local anesthetics and α_2-adrenergic agonists), and delayed hair growth over the needle insertion site. Another potential, albeit rare, complication is meningitis from a contaminated needle insertion.

BIBLIOGRAPHY

1. Hansen B: Epidural anesthesia and analgesia. In Predictable Pain Management: Symposium Proceedings from the North American Veterinary Conference, Orlando, Florida, 1996, pp 49–55.
2. Lamont LA, Tranquilli WJ, Grimm KA: Physiology of Pain. In Mathews, KA (ed): Veterinary Clinics of North America Small Animal Practice—Management of Pain. W.B. Saunders Company, Philadelphia, PA. 30:(4) 703–728, 2000.
3. Lemke KA, Dawson SD: Local and regional anesthesia. Vet Clin North Am Small Anim Pract. 30(4):839-857, 2000.
4. Skarda RT: Local and regional anesthetic and analgesic techniques: Dogs. In Thurmon JC, Tranquilli WJ, Benson GJ (eds): Lumb and Jones' Veterinary Anesthesia, 3rd ed. Baltimore, Williams & Wilkins, 1996.
5. Tranquilli WJ, Grimm KA, Lamont LA: Analgesic techniques. In Tranquilli WJ, Grimm KA, Lamont LA (eds): Pain Management for the Small Animal Practitioner. Jackson, WY, Teton New Media,2000, pp 32–72.

53. OTHER LOCAL ANESTHETIC TECHNIQUES

Kip A. Lemke, D.V.M., M.S., D.A.C.V.A.

1. Can local and regional anesthetic techniques be used in combination with analgesics and general anesthetics?

Yes, local and regional anesthetic techniques are often used in combination with analgesic and anesthetic drugs as part of a multimodal strategy to manage pain. Preoperatively and postoperatively, moderate to severe pain is usually easier to control if analgesics (e.g., opioids, α_2-agonists, anti-inflammatory drugs) are used in combination with local anesthetics.

2. When local and regional anesthetic techniques are used in combination with general anesthetics, should they be used before or after surgery?

The barrage of afferent input associated with surgical trauma alters nociceptive processing in the dorsal horn of the spinal cord, resulting in amplification and prolongation of postoperative pain. This alteration in spinal processing of nociceptive input is referred to as central sensitization. When local and regional anesthetic techniques are used before surgery, they have the unique ability to produce complete sensory blockade and prevent or preempt development of central sensitization. In addition to providing analgesia, intraoperative neural blockade improves muscle relaxation, attenuates autonomic and endocrine responses to surgery, and reduces anesthetic requirements.

3. Which local anesthetics are used in small animals?

Lidocaine is the most versatile and widely used local anesthetic in small animal practice. The drug is effective topically and can be used for local infiltration and intravenous regional anesthesia, as well as for peripheral and central (epidural, intrathecal) nerve blocks. Several formulations are available, including a 2% jelly, 10% spray, and 2% solution (20 mg/ml). When used for local and regional blocks, lidocaine has an onset time of 10–15 minutes and duration of action of 60–120 minutes.

Bupivacaine is a long-acting local anesthetic that is used to manage surgical and nonsurgical pain in small animals. The drug is not effective topically but can be used for local infiltration anesthesia and for peripheral and central nerve blocks. Several formulations are available including a 0.5% solution (5 mg/ml) with preservatives and one without. The potency—and toxicity—of bupivacaine is approximately four times that of lidocaine. When used for local and regional blocks, bupivacaine has an onset time of 20–30 minutes and duration of action of 240–360 minutes. Unlike lidocaine, administration of bupivacaine produces selective sensory blockade with limited motor blockade. Large doses of bupivacaine are selectively cardiotoxic, and accidental intravenous administration can cause ventricular arrhythmias (premature ventricular depolarizations, ventricular tachycardia, ventricular fibrillation).

4. How are specific nerves located?

Most local and regional anesthetic techniques are easy to perform if you review the anatomic location of the nerves, relevant landmarks, and major blood vessels before attempting the block. Some nerves can be located by identifying foramina from which they exit (e.g., infraorbital foramen), others can be palpated as they cross bony structures (e.g., fibular head), and still others can be located based on their relationship to distinct landmarks (e.g., lumbosacral space). Identification of peripheral nerves and precise placement of local anesthetic solution can also be accomplished with the use of an electronic nerve locator (see figure). One electrode is attached to the patient's skin and the other is attached to a coated, hollow needle with an exposed tip. The loca-

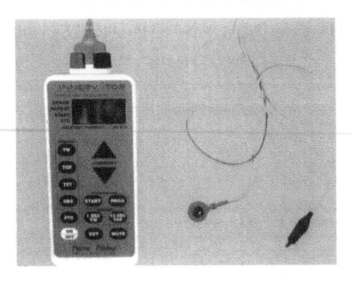

tor discharges at 1-second intervals while the needle is directed toward the nerve. As the needle approaches the nerve, a twitch response is observed and local anesthetic is administered through the hollow needle. Most local and regional anesthetic techniques do not require the use of a nerve locator; however, these devices can be very useful for blocks that are difficult to perform (e.g., brachial plexus block).

5. What peripheral techniques are used in dogs to block sensory innervation to the external ear?

Chronic otitis externa and otitis media are extremely painful conditions that often require medical and surgical intervention. The auriculotemporal and great auricular nerves provide sensory innervation to the external ear. Block the nerves with 1–2 ml of 2% lidocaine or 0.5% bupivacaine. Block the auriculotemporal nerve by injecting local anesthetic solution rostral to the vertical ear canal and caudal to the temporal component of the zygomatic arch. Block the great auricular nerve by injecting local anesthetic solution caudal to the vertical ear canal and ventral to the wing or the atlas.

6. What peripheral techniques are used in dogs to block sensory and motor innervation to the front limb?

Selective blockade of cervical and thoracic nerves (C_6, C_7, C_8, T_1) and their branches provides analgesia and muscle relaxation in dogs admitted for surgical procedures involving the front limb (see figure). Most nerves are blocked with 1–2 ml of 2% lidocaine or 0.5% bupivacaine. In small dogs, lower volumes are used to avoid toxicity.

The brachial plexus of the dog can be blocked proximally as the nerves exit the vertebral foramina (paravertebral brachial plexus block), or it can be blocked distally in the axillary space just above the level of the shoulder. The landmarks for the proximal technique are the transverse process of the sixth cervical vertebra and the head of the first rib. To perform this block, move the scapula caudally and palpate the transverse process and head or the rib. Next, block C_6 and C_7 by injecting local anesthetic dorsal to the cranial and caudal margins of the transverse process of the sixth cervical vertebra. Finally, block C_8 and T_1 by injecting local anesthetic dorsal to the cranial and caudal margins of the head of the first rib. Needles should be directed caudally when the paravertebral block is performed to avoid epidural or intrathecal injection. Additionally, the vertebral artery and branches of the costocervical artery run in close proximity to the nerves as they exit intervertebral foramina, and syringes should be aspirated before injection to avoid intravascular administration. Paralysis of the phrenic nerve can also occur, and this block should not be per-

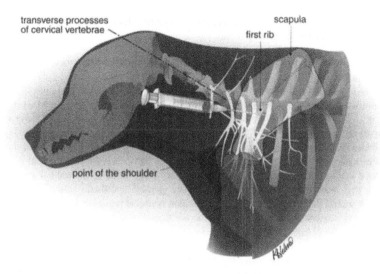

transverse processes
of cervical vertebrae

scapula

first rib

point of the shoulder

From Tranquilli WJ, Grimm KA, Lamont LA: Pain Management. Jackson, WY: Teton New Media, 2000, p. 41, with permission.

formed bilaterally or in animals with compromised pulmonary function. Unlike the distal technique, the paravertebral block has distinct landmarks, requires smaller amounts of local anesthetic solution, and produces anesthesia of the entire front limb distal to and including the shoulder.

Perform the distal block by injecting 5–10 ml of 2% lidocaine or 0.5% bupivacaine between the shoulder and the thoracic wall. Inject local anesthetic solution cranial to the first rib and caudal to the cranial border of the scapula. The axillary artery and vein are adjacent to the brachial plexus and syringes should be aspirated before injection to avoid intravascular administration. The block is used to provide analgesia and muscle relaxation for surgical procedures distal to and including the elbow.

Anesthesia of the front limb distal to the elbow joint is achieved by selective blockade of the radial, ulnar, median, and musculocutaneous nerves (RUMM block) in dogs. Block the radial nerve by injecting local anesthetic solution proximal to the lateral epicondyle of the humerus, between the biceps and triceps muscles. The ulnar, median, and musculocutaneous nerves are blocked by injecting local anesthetic solution proximal the medial epicondyle of the humerus, between the biceps and triceps muscles. In most dogs, these nerves can be palpated digitally. The brachial artery and vein are adjacent to the nerves on the medial side, and syringes should be aspirated before injection to avoid intravascular administration.

7. What peripheral techniques are used in cats to block sensory and motor innervation to the front limb?

The brachial plexus of the cat is blocked distally in the axillary space just above the level of the shoulder. Perform the block by injecting 1 ml of 2% lidocaine or 0.5% bupivacaine between the shoulder and the thoracic wall. Inject local anesthetic solution cranial to the first rib and caudal to the cranial border of the scapula. The axillary artery and vein are adjacent to the brachial plexus, and syringes should be aspirated before injection to avoid intravascular administration. The block is used to provide analgesia and muscle relaxation for surgical procedures distal to and including the elbow.

Selective blockade of the distal branches of the radial, ulnar, and median nerves provides analgesia in cats admitted for onchyectomy. Nerves are blocked with 0.2–0.3 ml of 2% lidocaine or 0.5% bupivacaine. Block distal branches of the radial nerve by injecting local anesthetic solution subcutaneously on the dorsomedial aspect of the carpus just proximal to the joint. Block distal branches of the median and ulnar nerves by injecting local anesthetic solution subcutaneously medial and lateral to the carpal pad.

8. What peripheral techniques are used in small animals to block sensory and motor innervation to the hind limb?

Selective blockade of lumbar and sacral nerves can provide analgesia and muscle relaxation in dogs admitted for surgical procedures involving the hind limb and perineum. Most nerves are blocked with 1–2 ml of 2% lidocaine or 0.5% bupivacaine. In small dogs and cats, lower volumes are used to avoid toxicity.

Anesthesia of the hind limb distal to the knee is achieved by selective blockade of the saphenous, common peroneal, and tibial nerves. The saphenous nerve runs through the femoral triangle on the medial surface of the thigh and provides sensory innervation to the medial surface of the thigh, stifle, and lower limb. Block the nerve injecting local anesthetic solution cranial to the femoral artery within the femoral triangle. The common peroneal nerve runs laterally over the head of the fibula and provides sensory innervation to the dorsal aspect of the lower limb. Block the nerve by injecting local anesthetic solution dorsal and caudal to the head of the fibula. The tibial nerve runs between the medial and lateral heads of the gastrocnemius and provides sensory innervation to the caudal aspect of the lower leg. Block the nerve by injection of local anesthetic solution between the medial and lateral heads of the gastrocnemius. The tibial nerve can also be blocked by injecting local anesthetic solution between the superficial and deep flexor tendons proximal to the hock. Syringes should be aspirated before injection to avoid intravascular administration.

BIBLIOGRAPHY

1. Dahl JB, Kehlet H: The value of preemptive analgesia in the treatment of postoperative pain. Br J Anaesth 70:434–439, 1993.
2. Kehlet H, Dahl JB: The value of multimodal or balanced analgesia in postoperative pain treatment. Anesth Analg 77:1048–1056, 1993.
3. Kehlet H: Multimodal approach to control postoperative pathophysiology and rehabilitation. Br J Anaesth 78:606–617, 1997.
4. Kissin I: Preemptive analgesia. Anesthesiology 93:1138–1143, 2000.
5. Lamont LA, Tranquilli WJ, Grimm KA: Physiology of pain. Vet Clin North Am Small Anim Pract 30:703–728, 2000.
6. Lemke KA, Dawson SD: Local and Regional Anesthesia. Vet Clin North Am Small Anim Pract 30:839–857, 2000.
7. McQuay HJ, Moore RA: Local anesthetics and epidurals. In Wall PD, Melzack R (ed): Textbook of Pain. New York, Churchill Livingstone, 1999, pp 1215–1231.
8. Skarda RT: Local and regional anesthetic and analgesic techniques. In Thurmon JC, Tranquilli WJ, Benson GJ (ed): Essentials of small animal anesthesia and analgesia. Philadelphia, Lippincott Williams & Wilkins, 1999, pp 203–224.
9. Torske KE, Dyson DH: Epidural anesthesia and analgesia.Vet Clin North Am Small Anim Pract 30:859–874, 2000.
10. Tranquilli WJ, Grimm KA, Lamont LA: Analgesic techniques. In Tranquilli WJ, Grimm KA, Lamont LA: Pain Management for the Small Animal Practitioner. Jackson, WY, Teton New Media, 2000, pp 31–72.
11. Woolf CJ, Chong MS: Preemptive analgesia: Treating postoperative pain by preventing the establishment of central sensitization. Anesth Analg 77:362–379, 1993.

IX. Pain Management for Small Animals

54. PHYSIOLOGY OF ACUTE PAIN

William J. Tranquilli, D.V.M., M.S., D.A.C.V.A.

1. What is the definition of *nociception*?

Nociception consists of the physiologic processes of (1) transduction of painful stimuli within the afferent nerve ending (nociceptor); (2) transmission of pain stimuli within sensory nerves to the dorsal horn of the spinal cord; and (3) modulation of painful stimuli within the spinal cord and supraspinal structures of the central nervous system (CNS) that finally result in the perception of pain.

2. What is nociceptive pain?

Nociceptive pain results from the activation of A-delta and C fiber sensory nerve endings (nociceptors) by mechanical, thermal, or chemical stimuli. This process can be sensitized by algogenic substances such that hyperalgesia results. This pain is often referred to as *physiologic pain* and subserves a protective function for the organism.

3. What is an algogenic substance?

Algogenic substances are endogenous chemical substrates that lower the threshold potential for activating nociceptors. Thus, nociceptors are said to be sensitized by these substances, which include but are not limited to histamine, serotonin, prostaglandins, kinins from plasma, and substance P from the afferent nerve terminals themselves.

4. How can pain be classified based on its neurophysiology?

Pain can be differentiated by basic mechanisms mediating its origin. Based on this method of classification, pain can be considered either nociceptive or non-nociceptive in origin. Nociceptive pain can then be divided into somatic or visceral and non-nociceptive into neuropathic or psychogenic pain (see Question 2).

5. Why is a pathophysiologic classification of pain preferred over an etiologic classification?

Etiologic classification refers to the primary disease process causing pain such as cancer pain, arthritic pain, burn pain, etc. Pathophysiologic classification describes both the neurologic basis and temporal pattern of pain, which is useful in selecting the correct therapeutic approach to alleviating pain.

6. What is meant by pain threshold?

Pain threshold refers to the minimal intensity at which a stimulus is perceived as painful. For a given stimulus, it is relatively constant for most individuals within a species.

7. What is meant by pain tolerance?

In contrast to pain threshold, pain tolerance may differ greatly among individuals with similar pain thresholds. Clinically, pain tolerance is more important than pain threshold and correlates with altered behavior patterns, more so than does pain threshold. It can be thought of as the level of pain an individual animal is willing to tolerate or endure. Thus, some animals are said to be quite stoic compared with others because of their apparent willingness to endure pain without outward changes in behavior.

8. What is the difference between an A-delta and a C sensory fiber?

A-delta fibers are small-diameter myelinated afferent fibers, whereas C fibers are very small unmyelinated nerves. The A-delta fibers conduct at velocities of 5 to 25 m/sec. C fibers transmit signals more slowly from polymodal nociceptors activated by thermal, chemical, and mechanical noxious stimuli. A-delta fibers react more selectively to specific noxious stimuli than do C fibers.

9. What is the relationship between afferent nerve size and its function?

Thin fibers conduct signals more slowly than larger diameter fibers and are less susceptible to electrical stimuli. This may be why transcutaneous electrical stimulation (TENS) is effective through its activation of larger diameter inhibitor fibers that can inhibit circuits in the spinal cord generated by small diameter nociceptive afferent nerves. Small fibers are more easily blocked by local anesthetics so differential blocks can be achieved (i.e., sensory nerve blockade, but not motor nerve blockade). Typically, sympathetic fibers are blocked first, followed by nociceptive afferent nerves, light mechanoreceptors, and then motor neurons.

10. What do "first" and "second" pain refer to?

This is the immediate and then delayed pain sensation one experiences after a noxious stimulus. This phenomenon is also described as "fast" and "slow" pain or "sharp" versus "dull, burning" pain. First pain is transmitted by the A-delta myelinated afferent fiber, whereas second pain results from stimuli passing through unmyelinated smaller C fibers.

11. Where does the first-order afferent neuron synapse with the second-order neuron?

The first-order neuron synapses with the second-order neuron within the dorsal horn of the spinal cord. Second-order neurons are the cells of origin of the ascending spinal sensory tracts, including many interneurons and projection neurons. Second-order neurons receive input not only from small-diameter nociceptive afferent nerves but also from large-diameter non-nociceptive afferent fibers.

12. What is central sensitization?

This occurs after dorsal horn neurons have received stimuli over a prolonged period and is thought to be mediated primarily through N-methyl-D-aspartate (NMDA) receptors within the dorsal horn of the spinal cord.

13. What neurotransmitters play a role in nociception at the level of the spinal cord?

Glutamate acts to depolarize second-order dorsal horn neurons via an influx of sodium and efflux of potassium. Substance P and calcitonin gene-related peptide, along with other neuropeptides, enhance passage of painful stimuli through the dorsal horn.

14. What neurotransmitters mediate descending inhibition within the spinal cord?

The two major inhibitory neurotransmitters are serotonin and norepinephrine. They enhance potassium conductance within neuronal cell membranes, hyperpolarizing and thus inhibiting neurons to future depolarizing events.

15. What neurotransmitters mediate local inhibitory interneuron activity within the dorsal horn of the spinal cord?

The majority of inhibitory interneurons release either glycine or gamma-aminobutyric acid (GABA). These substances inhibit the firing of dorsal horn nociceptive neurons both pre- and postsynaptically. Other interneurons contain enkephalins and dynorphins, which, when released, either increase potassium or block calcium conductance and thus nociceptive neurotransmitter release.

16. What receptors mediate inhibition of nociceptive pain within the dorsal horn of the spinal cord?

Several receptor populations mediate the antinociceptive effects of inhibitory neurotransmitters including presynaptic α_2, muscarinic, and opioid receptors and post-synaptic GABA and α_2-receptors.

17. What role does the NMDA receptor play in the production of pain?

NMDA receptors are activated by glutamate only following loss of a magnesium ion blockade. This blockade is relieved following glutamate activation of AMDA receptors that in turn depolarize neurons containing NMDA receptors. NMDA receptor activation induces a number of second messenger systems that can produce long-term biochemical and molecular changes in these neurons. The physiologic effects of these perturbations are (1) increased neuronal hyperexcitability, (2) decreased threshold, and (3) expanded receptive fields of nociresponsive neurons within the dorsal horn of the spinal cord. In the extreme, neurons may become spontaneously active. As such, the origin of pain is from the central nervous system itself (neuropathic pain). This state is referred to as "central hypersensitization."

18. What is the relationship between NMDA receptor activation and enhanced nociceptive syndromes?

NMDA-mediated (long-term or chronic) changes in dorsal horn neuronal processing may explain why pain can be either produced by non-noxious stimuli (allodynia) or exacerbated (hyperalgesia) following chronic nerve injuries (e.g., cervical disc disease) or barrages of painful stimuli to the spinal cord, such as might occur during prolonged surgical procedures.

BIBLIOGRAPHY

1. Carroll GL: Small Animal Pain Management. American Animal Hospital Association Press, 1998.
2. Flecknell P, Waterman-Pearson A: Pain Management in Animals. Philadelphia, WB Saunders, 2000.
3. Hellebrekers L: Animal Pain, Van Der Wees Publications, 2000.
4. Kanner R: Pain Management Secrets. Philadelphia, Hanley & Belfus, 1997.
5. Mathews K: Pain management. Ve. Clin North Am, 2000.
6. Thurmon JC, Tranquilli WJ, Benson GJ: Perioperative pain and distress. In Lumb and Jones' Veterinary Anesthesia, 3rd ed. Baltimore, Williams & Wilkins, 1996, pp 40–61.
7. Tranquilli WJ, Grimm KA, Lamont LA: Pain Management for the Small Animal Practitioner. Jackson, WY, Teton New Media,2000.
8. Yaksh TL, Lynch C III, Zapol, et al (eds): Anesthesia: Biological Foundations. Philadelphia, Lippincott-Raven, 1998.

55. RECOGNITION OF PAIN IN SMALL ANIMALS

Kurt A. Grimm, D.V.M., M.S., D.A.C.V.A., D.A.C.V.C.P.

1. What is involved in the "feeling" of pain?

The recognition of pain is a complex sensory process that is composed of four steps: transduction, transmission, modulation, and perception. The first three steps are collectively called nociception. The fourth is the individual processing of the nociceptive input by the cerebral cortex to formulate the sensory experience of pain. Pain perception depends on many confounding factors. Prior experience, current environment, and socialization are some of the factors that can alter the outward expression of pain. Without verbal descriptions of the pain experience, it is impossible to accurately measure an animal's "feeling" of pain with current technology.

2. What general types of assessment are used to recognize pain in animals?

Physiologic parameters, neuroendocrine values, and behavioral assessment have been used to attempt to recognize pain in animals.

3. What physiologic parameters can be useful for recognition of pain?

Heart rate, respiratory rate, and blood pressure are usually increased during the stress response to pain. While not specific for pain, these signs can often be correlated to the intensity of a noxious stimulus and presumably pain. These changes may also be present during periods of emotional or environmental stress in the absence of a noxious stimulus.

4. What is pain?

Pain is the unpleasant sensory or emotional experience (perception) following the application (or anticipated application) of a noxious stimulus. Pain can be experienced with or without accompanying physical signs of stress (e.g., tachycardia or hypertension).

5. What is stress?

Stress is the physiologic manifestation of bodily or mental tension resulting from factors that tend to alter an existent equilibrium, such as the application of a noxious stimulus, environmental changes, or pathologic processes.

6. What is distress?

Distress is the external expression through emotion or behavior of suffering. Distress is often recognized when an animal erupts in an outburst due to intolerable pain or stress. Current animal pain assessment schemes rely on signs of stress and distress to infer the presence of pain.

7. What is the difference between analgesia and hypoalgesia?

Many people use these terms interchangeably. By definition, however, analgesia is the absence of a response to noxious stimuli (i.e., complete absence of pain). Hypoalgesia is the decreased sensitivity to noxious stimuli (i.e., tolerance to pain). Clinically, the goal is often to make the patient's pain tolerable without causing excessive side effects that accompany higher doses of analgesic drugs required to provide analgesia. Hypoalgesia is often the correct terminology for the clinical treatment of pain.

8. What is a visual analog scale?

The visual analog scale (VAS) is a pain measurement tool developed for people. It is presented as a line of a fixed length (i.e., 100 mm), and the patient is asked to make a transecting line at the point that best represents his or her pain level. Adaptations of the VAS have been used in veterinary medicine. It should be remembered, however, that if the mark is made by anyone other than the person experiencing the noxious stimuli, the VAS represents the observer's *impression* of the intensity of pain being experienced by the patient.

9. What is a numerical rating scale?

The numerical rating scale has similar origins to the visual analog scale. It differs in that the scale is labeled from 0 to 10 or 0 to 5. These scales have been well studied in humans and appear to be valid assessors of human pain. Numerical rating scales have been adapted for use in veterinary medicine by incorporating descriptions of the numerical values. For example, a score of 0 may be associated with no vocalizing, whereas a score of 5 may correspond to severe agitation and vocalization that does not cease with human contact. These scales have been developed to reduce the reliance on the observer's impression of the animal's behavior. However, these systems are not specific for pain, are prone to inter- and intra-user variation, and, when used in veterinary medicine, suffer from the same problem as the VAS in that the rating is the observer's (not necessarily the animal's) impression of the animal's pain.

10. What does a behavioral assessment rating system tell the veterinarian?

Behavioral assessments range from rather simple methods incorporating a numerical rating scale to detailed time-consuming methods such as videotaping. These methods require the animal to display stereotypical behaviors that are associated with pain or the absence of pain. Videotaping an animal for a period of time ranging from a few minutes to a few days followed by quantification of the total time spent in each behavior provides an average behavioral assessment. Videotaping is not as clinically useful as other methods because there is a finite time required for gathering data before treatment decisions are made.

11. What exactly do neuroendocrine tests measure?

Neuroendocrine tests measure endogenous production of chemical mediators of the stress response. Norepinephrine, epinephrine, cortisol, and blood glucose are commonly measured. These tests are free of the observer bias that can confound numerical and visual scales when used for veterinary patients. However, these tests are invasive, require sample processing, are expensive, and have significant run times. These neurochemicals are not specific for pain but are indicators of the nonspecific stress response. It would be anticipated these values would be highly correlated with physiologic measurements for heart rate and blood pressure. The clinical usefulness of these tests is limited, and they are most applicable to research settings.

12. How do I assess the need for analgesic drug administration for perioperative acute pain in the clinic setting?

Most patients recovering from anesthesia following surgery will experience some degree of pain associated with tissue disruption. Many animals will not outwardly display signs of minor pain and will suffer quietly. Most patients will show signs of distress following major surgery for orthopedic or soft tissue procedures. Dysphoria due to anesthetic drug administration may also be marked and will confound the pain assessment.

A good starting place is observation of the patient from a distance. Note respiration rate and pattern as well as anxiety, vocalization, and body position. Next, approach the patient quietly and get a pulse rate while assessing the animal's reaction to human contact. Next, observe the animal's response to manipulation and palpation. Remember to palpate the nonpainful areas to have a control. Finally, remember what drugs have been given to the patient and correct your observations for their pharmacologic effects. For example, opioid agonists can induce dysphoria in some animals, and this may be mistaken as a vocalization due to pain. Use medical judgment to decide whether an intervention is required. Serial assessments will provide valuable baseline information and will enable detection of changes of the patient's status. Other assessment scales can be used to document or confirm the veterinarian's clinical impressions. When there is doubt as to the status of the animal, analgesic drugs should be administered if there are no medical contraindications.

13. What are some stereotypical behaviors of pain in dogs and cats?

A few of the stereotypical behaviors are vocalization, licking or chewing, restlessness, depression, aggression, trembling, and abnormal posture, gait, or movement. Cats tend to be withdrawn and do not vocalize to the same degree as dogs. It should be noted that tranquilizers such as acepromazine will often reduce these behavioral signs without significant analgesic effects.

14. Is it reasonable to anthropomorphize?

Yes. There are many similarities in the anatomy and the physiology of the mammalian nervous system that suggest that animals experience pain in much the same way as people. If a procedure would be painful to a human, it should be assumed it would be painful to an animal. Occasionally animals appear to be in less pain than humans are (e.g., in abdominal exploratory surgery) but it should be remembered there are individual and species differences in pain-related perception and behavior.

15. How is chronic pain assessed?

Functionality is a better measure of chronic pain than traditional behavioral and physiologic measurements. Symptoms such as decreased mobility, depression, reduced appetite, and weight loss are often associated with chronic pain states. Analgesic drug developments have outpaced the ability of veterinarians to assess need and efficacy for chronic pain treatment. Often the best measure of therapeutic efficacy is the owner's impression of the animal's functionality.

16. Why aren't behavioral and physiologic changes seen in animals with acute pain useful for those with chronic pain?

The classic behavioral and physiologic changes associated with acute perioperative pain serve no function if displayed chronically. Therefore, survival and homeostatic mechanisms tend to mask the intensity of pain when experienced chronically.

17. What is the Oxford Pain Chart?

The Oxford Pain Chart was developed as a subjective tracking device for chronic pain therapy in people. An adaptation can be used for veterinary patients. It should be noted the observations that are recorded are the owner's impressions of the animal's pain intensity.

BIBLIOGRAPHY

1. Johnston SA: Physiology, mechanisms, and identification of pain. In Predictable Pain Management: Symposium Proceedings from the North American Veterinary Conference, Orlando, Florida; January 14, 1996, pp 45–47.
2. Lamont LA, Tranquilli WJ, Grimm KA: Physiology of pain. Vet Clin North Am Small Anim Pract 30(4): 703–728, 2000.
3. Mathews KA: Pain assessment and general approach to management. Vet Clin North Am Small Anim Pract 30(4):729–756, 2000.
4. Tranquilli WJ, Grimm KA, Lamont LA: Managing chronic pain in dogs and cats. In Tranquilli WJ, Grimm KA, Lamont LA (eds.). Pain Management for the Small Animal Practitioner. Jackson, WY, Teton New Media, 2000, pp 104–114.

56. PRE-EMPTIVE ANALGESIA

Leigh A. Lamont, D.V.M.

1. What does the term *pre-emptive analgesia* mean?

Pre-emptive analgesia refers to the administration of analgesic interventions prior to the anticipated noxious insult (usually surgery) and throughout the perioperative period.

2. Since my patient is going to be anesthetized during surgery and unable to experience pain, what is the benefit of administering analgesics during this period?

Despite a number of other advantages, including reduced requirements of a basal anesthetic agent intraoperatively, the strategy behind pre-emptive analgesia focuses on inhibiting changes within the peripheral and central nervous systems that contribute to heightened pain postoperatively. It is important to remember that, even though a patient may be under general anesthesia and unable to perceive pain, nociceptive input to the nervous system continues throughout the surgical procedure, which may lead to a phenomenon known as *sensitization*.

3. How do surgical interventions cause sensitization of the nervous system?

It must be recognized that the nervous system does not function statically in response to noxious stimulation. On the contrary, peripheral tissue injury (such as with surgery) provokes dynamic changes in the responsiveness of the nervous system and alters how it processes noxious input. This phenomenon is called *sensitization* and affects both the peripheral and the central nervous systems. Peripheral sensitization is characterized by a reduction in the threshold of nociceptor afferent fibers, whereas central sensitization manifests as an activity-dependent increase in the excitability of neurons in the dorsal horn of the spinal cord. Together, these changes lead to post-injury pain hypersensitivity, which can be recognized clinically as an increase in the response to noxious stimuli and a decrease in the pain threshold, both at the site of injury and in surrounding tissues.

4. Is postoperative pain more difficult to manage once the nervous system has been sensitized?

Yes. Studies in both animal models and humans have demonstrated that once central sensitization has been established, traditional analgesic interventions become significantly less effective in treating pain, and higher doses of analgesic agents are required to achieve the desired effect. Simply put, pain is easier to prevent than it is to treat retroactively.

5. Does central nervous system sensitization predispose an individual to development of a chronic pain state?

Perhaps. Abnormal nervous system activity is a hallmark of chronic pain, which may persist long after the inciting stimulus has subsided. Although the exact mechanisms mediating chronic pain remain poorly understood and not all patients that experience post-injury pain go on to develop a chronic pain state, it is clear that sensitization can lead to nervous system memory, which may contribute to chronic pain.

6. What classes of drugs are appropriate for pre-emptive administration?

Traditional analgesic agents such as opioids, nonsteroidal anti-inflammatories, and local anesthetics form the foundation of most pre-emptive analgesic interventions. In addition, analgesic adjunctive agents such as α_2 adrenergic agonists (e.g., medetomidine), N-methyl-D-aspartate antagonists (ex. ketamine) and corticosteroids are also useful in a variety of situations.

7. How does pre-emptive administration of traditional analgesic agents inhibit or prevent the development of nervous system sensitization?

Opioids act centrally, and perhaps peripherally, to dampen afferent nociceptive transmission and modulate spinal pathways. Nonsteroidal anti-inflammatory agents reduce the activation and sensitization of nociceptors in the periphery, and recent evidence suggests that certain drugs in this class may have a central analgesic action as well. Local anesthetics block the transduction and transmission of nociceptive input to the dorsal horn of the spinal cord, thereby preventing postsynaptic sequelae.

8. How can opioids be incorporated into pre-emptive analgesic interventions?

Opioids can be administered systemically in the preanesthetic period or immediately post-induction intramuscularly, subcutaneously, or intravenously. An intravenous continuous infusion is a particularly effective means of delivery. Opioids are also beneficial when administered by the epidural, transdermal, or intra-articular route prior to surgical trespass. For more in-depth information on opioids, the reader is referred to Chapter 12.

9. Is it safe to administer nonsteroidal anti-inflammatory agents preoperatively?

Yes, in select patients. Although the risks associated with gastric ulceration, renal injury, and hemorrhage related to platelet dysfunction remain a legitimate concern with this class of agents, newer drugs with fewer adverse side effects are being marketed. In otherwise healthy animals, especially those undergoing elective or orthopedic procedures, the preoperative administration of a nonsteroidal anti-inflammatory agent will have significant benefits in the postoperative period. For additional information on nonsteroidal anti-inflammatories, the reader is referred to the article by Tranquilli et al.

10. How can local anesthetics be incorporated into a pre-emptive analgesic protocol?

Local anesthetics can be administered perineurally to produce a variety of regional blocks, including dental nerve blocks, intercostal nerve blocks, and brachial plexus blocks. They can also be administered epidurally, interpleurally, intra-articularly, infiltratively, and intravenously (for intravenous regional anesthesia). For more information on local anesthetics, see Chapters 17, 51, 52, 53.

11. Do combinations of analgesic agents offer any advantage?

Yes. This strategy is called balanced or multimodal analgesia. It involves the simultaneous administration of two or more of the analgesic drug classes or techniques mentioned above. Combination therapy has been shown to have additive or synergistic analgesic effects, and the dosages of individual drugs can typically be reduced. When used pre-emptively, multimodal analgesia helps to inhibit surgery-induced nervous system sensitization, minimize development of drug tolerance, suppress the neuroendocrine stress response to pain and injury, and shorten convalescence through improved tissue healing, maintenance of immune responses, and better patient mobility. For more information on multimodal analgesia, see Chapter 58.

12. What types of patients will benefit the most from pre-emptive analgesia?

Animals that are free from pain prior to surgery will benefit the most from pre-emptive analgesia. Such patients presumably have normal nervous systems that are functioning within expected physiologic limits to process nociceptive input. The goal of pre-emptive analgesia is to maintain this state postoperatively by preventing sensitization. Animals that present in pain prior to the surgical procedure may have already suffered varying degrees of nervous system sensitization and may be less responsive to this approach. In such cases, aggressive treatment is required, often with a variety of analgesic agents for an extended period of time.

13. Does pre-emptive analgesic administration mean that postoperative pain management is unnecessary?

No. Except for very minor procedures, it is unlikely that any pre-emptive analgesic intervention will completely obtund nervous system sensitization throughout the postoperative period.

This is because the inflammatory reaction to tissue damaged during surgery will persist even after the surgical procedure is completed, which may predispose to sensitization. Consequently, for invasive major surgeries, optimal pain management involves analgesic administration throughout the pre-, intra-, and postoperative periods.

14. My patients have always recovered quickly with no apparent detrimental effects following surgery. Why should I implement protocols addressing pre-emptive analgesia?

The ability of our patients to rapidly recover from major surgery and to mask signs of pain is truly remarkable. As veterinarians, we have committed ourselves to treating nonverbal patients who are unable to consent to the procedures we see fit to perform upon them. Consequently, we are obliged to provide them with analgesic treatment even if their outward behaviors do not demand it. The recognition that a given procedure may be painful to a human patient is enough reason to institute pre-emptive analgesic interventions as well as postoperative pain management strategies.

BIBLIOGRAPHY

1. Hansen B: Acute Pain management. Vet Clin North Am 30(4):899–916, 2000.
2. Lamont LA, Tranquilli WJ, Grimm KA: Physiology of pain. Vet Clin North Am 30(4):703–728, 2000.
3. Pascoe PJ: Perioperative pain management. Vet Clin North Am 30(4):917–932, 2000.
4. Tranquilli WJ, Grimm KA, Lamont LA: Pain management for the small animal practitioner. Jackson, WY, Teton NewMedia, 2000, pp 1–11.
5. Woolf CJ, Chong MS: Preemptive analgesia: Treating postoeprative pain by preventing the establishment of central sensitization. Anesth Analg 77:362–379, 1993.

57. POSTOPERATIVE ANALGESIC TECHNIQUES

Leigh A. Lamont, D.V.M.

1. Is postoperative pain undertreated in veterinary medicine?

Yes. A retrospective study from a veterinary teaching hospital spanning a 6-year period in the 1980s indicated that management of postoperative pain in companion animals was alarmingly inadequate. A more recent survey at another veterinary college demonstrated the continued reluctance of faculty, staff, house officers, and students to treat postoperative pain. Not surprisingly, these shortcomings are echoed in private practice, where various reports confirm that only 40 to 60% of veterinarians routinely administer any postoperative analgesic to their patients.

2. What are the reasons for undertreatment of postoperative pain in veterinary medicine?

In the past, a lack of understanding of the physiology and pathophysiology of pain and its effects on morbidity contributed to the problem. In fact, the undertreatment of pain in human patients has been recognized as a major issue only within the last 15 years, and attitudes that encourage patients to bear the pain rather than seek treatment have undoubtedly spilled over to veterinary medicine. Furthermore, there is the old adage that analgesics should not be used because the animal will be rendered pain-free and consequently may disrupt the surgical site. Unfortunately, this belief remains prevalent among many practitioners. Finally, the adverse effects of analgesic agents, notably the opioids, may have been overstated in the past. This, in combination with concerns about liability and record keeping, have made many veterinarians reluctant to take full advantage of this particular class of drugs.

3. What strategies are recommended to optimize treatment of pain postoperatively?

Effective postoperative pain management must be proactive. Efforts to prevent pain are, in general, more effectual than attempts to treat pain once it has already been established. This is the principle behind pre-emptive analgesia, which is discussed in more detail in the preceding chapter. By initiating treatment prior to the surgical insult and continuing it throughout the perioperative period, you can prevent sensitization of the nervous system, resulting in improved patient comfort and earlier return to function. Another strategy, known as multimodal analgesia, involves the administration of two or more analgesic drugs or techniques simultaneously. This approach allows multiple points along pain pathways to be targeted, and lower doses of each individual drug are required.

4. Which class of drugs is most commonly used to treat postoperative pain in companion animals?

Opioids appear to be the most efficacious class of drugs for the management of acute postoperative pain in companion animals. For mild to moderate pain, butorphanol and buprenorphine are commonly administered. For moderate to severe pain, morphine, oxymorphone, hydromorphone, and fentanyl are commonly employed. For more information on opioid pharmacology, see Chapter 12.

5. To provide optimal postoperative pain management, when should opioids be administered?

In almost all cases, incorporation of an opioid into an animal's preanesthetic medication is recommended. This accomplishes several goals: it provides a pre-emptive analgesic effect prior to surgery, it helps to calm the patient and alleviate stress (especially if combined with a sedative or tranquilizer), and it often decreases the doses of drugs required for induction and maintenance of anesthesia. Epidural administration of an opioid prior to surgery may also be indicated, depending on the type of surgical procedure to be performed. Alternatively, additional opioids may be administered systemically throughout the procedure, either as a constant rate infusion or as intermittent small boluses, to supplement analgesia during especially long, painful procedures. It is usually advisable to give a low dose of opioid near the end of the surgical procedure to ensure that the drug has time to reach its peak analgesic effect before the animal wakes up. This facilitates a smooth recovery and, if appropriate doses are given, does not excessively prolong the time to extubation. If intraoperative opioids have been administered throughout the surgical procedure, it may not be necessary to re-dose prior to recovery. Once the animal is extubated, a suitable opioid dosing regimen should be instituted to manage pain throughout the postoperative period.

6. For how long should opioids be administered postoperatively?

Clearly this will depend on the type of surgical procedure performed and the temperament and pain tolerance of the individual animal. In general, for procedures associated with mild to moderate pain, treatment over 12 to 24 hours with opioids is usually sufficient. However, just as in people, not all animals have the same pain tolerance, and a noxious insult that is only mildly uncomfortable to one animal may be extremely painful to another. For more invasive surgical procedures associated with moderate to severe pain, opioid treatment may be indicated well beyond the 24-hour mark. Remember that pain is an important contributor to morbidity and, if left untreated, can prolong hospital stays and significantly delay an animal's return to a normal level of activity.

7. What sort of postoperative opioid dosing regimen is most effective for pain management?

Unfortunately, the traditional approach was to wait for the animal to exhibit signs of pain (usually vocalization of some sort) before initiating treatment. This method is unacceptable for two reasons. First, it only attempts to treat pain after the fact, which we have already acknowledged is not the most effective strategy. Second, it assumes that veterinary caregivers can accurately and predictably identify animals in pain, which is an extremely difficult task. Instead, the best approach is to implement a fixed dosing interval for opioid administration. For example, after the initial dose at the time of recovery, morphine or oxymorphone is administered every 3 to 6 hours over the next 12 to 24 hours. The dose of drug, the dosing interval, the route of administration, and the duration of treatment are determined based on the patient's response to treatment during the recovery phase. The patient should be monitored during treatment for sensitivity upon manipulation of the surgical site, signs of respiratory depression, or excessive sedation.

8. In addition to intermittent bolus administration, what other approaches are available for delivery of opioids postoperatively?

A continuous intravenous infusion is an easy and inexpensive method for administration of opioid analgesics during the postoperative period. This approach maintains a constant plasma level of opioid, thereby eliminating the periods of waning analgesic effect that invariably occur with intermittent bolus administration. In addition, the dose can be more precisely titrated to achieve the desired analgesic effect without precipitating adverse side effects. Typically, a loading dose is given at the end of the surgical procedure to attain a therapeutic plasma level, and the infusion is immediately started. Attentive monitoring of physiologic parameters, including heart rate, respiratory rate, and mucous membrane color, is mandatory. The analgesic effect should be assessed by light manipulation of the surgical site and surrounding tissues. The infusion rate can then be adjusted if necessary to address the needs of each individual patient.

9. Which opioids are suitable for continuous intravenous infusions?

	Dogs	Cats
Morphine		
loading dose	0.3–0.5 mg/kg IV	0.08–0.1 mg/kg IV
infusion	0.1–0.3 mg/kg/hour IV	0.05–0.1 mg/kg/hour IV
Fentanyl		
loading dose	0.002–0.003 mg/kg IV	0.001–0.002 mg/kg IV
infusion	0.001–0.005 mg/kg/hour IV	0.001–0.005 mg/kg/hour IV

10. Do I need special equipment to set up an opioid continuous infusion?

Not necessarily. Obviously, an in-dwelling intravenous catheter is a prerequisite, and patients must be monitored to ensure catheter patency and an intact fluid delivery line. An automated fluid pump or, ideally, a syringe pump is a useful tool that facilitates precise delivery and decreases the likelihood of an overdose. However, if monitoring is vigilant, opioid infusions can safely be administered without special equipment, as long as the animal is closely supervised at all times. The simplest method is to add the calculated volume of opioid to a small bag of saline or lactated Ringer's solution and set the appropriate drip rate. This rate can then be dialed up or down to achieve the desired effect.

11. What if my patient has occasional painful periods while receiving an opioid continuous infusion?

This is referred to as "breakthrough pain." In some cases, the infusion may be sufficient to manage pain while the animal is resting and calm but may be inadequate if the patient is subjected to manipulation or additional noxious stimuli. If this is noted, one option is to increase the rate of the infusion by 20 to 30% and reassess in 30 minutes. Another possibility, if the periods of breakthrough pain are infrequent, is to leave the infusion rate where it is and administer small doses of supplemental opioid as necessary. If possible, it is best to administer these doses prior to initiation of potentially painful manipulations.

12. Can other analgesic agents be administered by a continuous infusion?

Although the opioids are the class of drugs most often administered as a continuous infusion, other analgesics may lend themselves to this approach. Ketamine, although not traditionally considered a good analgesic, is very useful in the management of certain types of pain and is best administered as a constant rate infusion, usually in combination with an opioid such as morphine or fentanyl. Lidocaine infusions may also be useful intra- or postoperatively and, in addition to providing systemic analgesia, may be beneficial in promoting normal gastrointestinal function. For more information on analgesic combinations, see Chapter 58.

13. Is a fentanyl patch a useful method for management of postoperative pain?

It can be. Fentanyl patches may provide a reasonable alternative to continuous intravenous opioid infusions, with the added bonus of convenience. Remember that it may take 12 to 24 hours after patch application before therapeutic plasma levels are reached, so patches should be applied the night before scheduled surgery if possible. Patch handling and placement are also important if transdermal absorption is to be predictable, and even so, a significant portion of patients probably never reach therapeutic plasma levels. Unlike intravenous opioid infusions, the patch cannot be modified to release more or less analgesic as required, so patients must be monitored closely for breakthrough pain and supplemental analgesics administered as needed. Just because a fentanyl patch was placed does not mean that the level of analgesia achieved is adequate.

14. What if an animal becomes dysphoric following opioid administration at recovery?

It is not unusual for some animals to experience a period of excitement or delirium at recovery. In most cases this phase is short-lived and, with gentle restraint and a soothing voice, many animals can be calmed and will revert to a resting state without pharmacologic intervention. Sometimes, however, this approach is not sufficient, and the next step is to attempt to discern between pain and dysphoria. Just because an opioid analgesic has already been administered at recovery does not eliminate the possibility that the animal is still in pain. If analgesia is deemed inadequate, an additional dose of an opioid, preferably one with a rapid onset of action, should be administered. If the animal is still agitated, there are a couple of options. First, a low dose of acepromazine or medetomidine can be administered to sedate the patient while retaining the analgesic benefits of the opioid. Second, if administration of additional doses of opioid has aggravated the signs of dysphoria, partial reversal can be accomplished with small incremental doses of intravenous butorphanol.

15. If my patient seems sedated postoperatively, does this mean the dose of opioid is too high?

Not necessarily. Major surgery is a stressful and exhausting ordeal and it is important for the animal to be able to get much needed sleep, especially during the first 12 hours postoperatively. The mild to moderate level of sedation that often accompanies opioid administration is actually desirable during this time frame. Ideally, the patient should rest comfortably but still show some response when stimulated either verbally or by gentle touch. As always, vital signs must be monitored regularly.

16. Are nonsteroidal anti-inflammatory drugs (NSAIDs) effective for the management of acute postoperative pain?

Yes. For major surgeries, NSAIDs play an important role in a multimodal pain management strategy, and for minor procedures, they often constitute a firstline approach for postoperative analgesia. With the availability of newer NSAIDs (including meloxicam, carprofen, ketoprofen, and etodolac) that are associated with fewer adverse effects, this class of drugs is no longer reserved only for the management of chronic pain.

17. To provide the most effective pain management, should an NSAID be administered pre-operatively or postoperatively?

From an analgesic standpoint, it is probable that an NSAID will be most efficacious if administered prior to surgery, according to the principles of pre-emptive analgesia. However, concerns about the risks of gastric ulceration, renal compromise, and antiplatelet effects exacerbated by general anesthesia and surgery have limited the preoperative use of these drugs in small animals. If reserved for young to middle-aged, otherwise healthy animals presenting for elective or orthopedic procedures, the benefits of preoperative administration of NSAIDs probably outweigh the risks.

18. Do I need to decrease the dose of opioid administered if I decide to administer an NSAID concurrently?

No, at least not initially. Although the combination of opioids and NSAIDs does produce additive or even synergistic analgesic effects in the postoperative period, there is no need to decrease the dose of opioid just because an NSAID is being administered concurrently. It is best to wait and tailor dosages based on the animal's response to treatment.

19. For how long should NSAIDs be administered postoperatively?

NSAIDs are commonly administered for anywhere from 24 hours to 3 to 7 days postoperatively, depending on the type of procedure performed and the individual patient. The availability of oral preparations means that NSAIDs can be dispensed to owners to administer at home once their pet has been discharged after surgery. Cats are usually restricted to 2 to 3 days of treatment.

20. Can local or regional anesthesia techniques be performed in the postoperative period?

Yes, although these techniques are most effective when administered before surgery. If the surgical procedure is particularly long, it may be beneficial to repeat a nerve block (for example, a brachial plexus block) at the end of surgery to extend its duration of effect. Certain techniques, such as intrapleural anesthesia/analgesia, are most easily accomplished at the end of the surgical procedure, and it may be feasible to repeat these techniques later in the postoperative period as needed.

21. What are the indications for placement of an epidural catheter?

Placement of an epidural catheter is indicated for the extended management of moderate to severe pain associated with major surgical interventions. The technique is also useful in other situations, including patients that have suffered significant trauma, patients with acute necrotizing pancreatitis, and patients with diffuse bacterial peritonitis.

22. What are the advantages and disadvantages of an epidural catheter over other analgesic techniques?

The tip of an epidural catheter can be placed precisely to achieve maximal effect at the desired location. For example, for forequarter amputations, the tip is positioned in the C6 to T1 region, for major abdominal procedures the tip should be at the thoracolumbar region, and for caudal surgeries the tip should be placed near the lumbosacral junction. This facilitates the delivery of small doses of analgesic agent to the target site. Unfortunately, the technique is more technically challenging than routine epidural drug administration and requires a special epidural catheter kit. Meticulous care of the catheter and strict aseptic technique are mandatory if complications are to be avoided.

23. What drugs can be infused through an epidural catheter?

Opioids and local anesthetics are the most commonly administered agents, although ketamine and α_2-agonists may also be useful adjuncts in some situations. Combinations of morphine or fentanyl with either lidocaine or bupivacaine are most often employed. A continuous epidural infusion is the optimal method of delivery; however, if a syringe pump is not available, intermittent injections can be made every 6 to 8 hours. Small volumes must be administered extremely slowly to avoid nausea and vomiting. For more information on epidural catheter placement, see the article by Pascoe.

24. For how long should an epidural catheter be left in place?

The longer the catheter is left in place, the greater the risk of complications resulting from infection. With meticulous care and vigilance, epidural catheters can be left in for 7 to 10 days if necessary. For major postoperative pain, 24 to 48 hours is often sufficient, and systemic opioids can be used to manage ongoing pain after this time. It is usually prudent to culture the tip of the catheter upon removal from the patient.

25. In addition to pharmacologic approaches, what other techniques can be used to make a patient more comfortable in the postoperative period?

Good surgical technique and efforts to minimize tissue trauma intraoperatively can improve patient comfort after surgery. In addition, the importance of good nursing care during the postoperative period cannot be overstated. Ensuring that the patient remain clean, dry, and comfortably bedded must be a priority. The application of support bandages, splints, or warm compresses may also be beneficial in certain instances. Finally, always remember that a soothing voice and a gentle touch can go a long way to calming an anxious animal in an unfamiliar setting, and even this simple human contact may alleviate pain and discomfort.

BIBLIOGRAPHY

1. Dobromylskyj P, Flecknell PA, Lascelles BD, et al: Management of postoperative and other acute pain. In Flecknell P, Waterman-Pearson A (eds): Pain Management in Animals. London, WB Saunders, 2000, pp 81–146.
2. Hansen B: Acute pain management. Vet Clin North Am 30(4):899–919, 2000.
3. Papich MG: Pharmacologic Considerations for Opiate Analgesic and Nonsteroidal Antiinflammatory Drugs. In Management of Pain, Vet Clin North Am 30(4):815–838, 2000.
4. Pascoe P: Perioperative pain management. Vet Clin North Am 30(4):917–932, 2000.
5. Tranquilli WJ, Grimm KA, Lamont LA: Pain Management for the Small Animal Practitioner. Jackson, WY, Teton New Media, 2000.

58. ANALGESIC COMBINATIONS

Leigh A. Lamont, D.V.M.

1. What does the term *multimodal analgesia* mean?

Multimodal, or *balanced*, *analgesia* refers to the simultaneous administration of drugs from two or more analgesic drug classes or application of two or more treatment modalities to achieve optimal pain management. In many ways, this is analogous to using several antineoplastic agents in a single patient in an attempt to inhibit tumor cell metabolism and replication through different mechanisms.

2. What classes of analgesic drugs are commonly used to target different points along the afferent pain pathway?

Three major classes of analgesic agents are currently used in veterinary medicine, and these are referred to as "traditional analgesics." First, nonsteroidal anti-inflammatory drugs can be used to inhibit transduction at peripheral nociceptors, while regional nerve blocks with local anesthetics are used to obtund nociceptive transmission to the central nervous system, and finally, opioids can be used to modulate processing of noxious input in the dorsal horn and in supraspinal structures. In addition to traditional analgesics, there are numerous other drugs, referred to as "analgesic adjuncts," that may be of use when incorporated into multimodal pain management strategies.

3. What are the benefits of combination analgesic therapy for pain management?

The rationale behind multimodal or combination analgesic therapy is that optimal analgesia can be achieved by additive or synergistic effects between analgesics with different mechanisms of action. Furthermore, lower doses of each individual agent can be administered, which results in fewer adverse side effects and delays the development of drug tolerance and diminished efficacy over time.

4. What types of pharmacodynamic interactions may be exploited by combination analgesic therapy?

Addition—Refers to the situation in which the administration of two analgesic drugs results in a response that is equal to the sum of the fractional doses. Additivity is strong support for the assumption that the drugs involved act via the same mechanism (i.e., usually the same receptor system).

Synergism—Refers to the circumstance in which the analgesic response achieved is greater than the sum of the fractional doses administered. Analgesic synergism is a primary goal of multimodal analgesic pain management strategies.

Potentiation—Refers to the enhancement of analgesic action of one drug by the administration of a second drug that has no inherent analgesic action of its own.

5. What is an analgesic adjunctive agent?

The term *analgesic adjunctive agent*, or *analgesic adjuvant*, refers to a diverse group of drugs, all of which have primary indications other than pain, but which may be analgesic in some painful conditions. Such drugs potentiate or enhance analgesia by interacting with a variety of receptors, or by altering nerve conduction processes implicated in pain-modulating systems and signal generation or transduction. In most cases, analgesic adjunctive agents are incorporated into a multimodal pain management strategy in conjunction with traditional analgesics, such as opioids and nonsteroidal anti-inflammatories. Although often reserved for chronic pain that is, or has become, refractory to other conventional treatment modalities, in some pain syndromes, therapy with an analgesic adjuvant may constitute a first-line approach.

6. List potential indications for analgesic adjunctive agents in veterinary medicine.

- Malignancy (e.g., osteosarcoma)
- Chronic inflammatory disorders (e.g., chronic otitis)
- Chronic orthopedic disorders (e.g., cervical disc disease)
- Chronic soft tissue injury (e.g., degloving injuries)
- Nervous tissue injury (e.g., phantom limb pain)

7. What factors must be considered prior to prescribing an analgesic adjunctive agent?

To select and administer an analgesic adjuvant properly, the veterinarian should be aware of the drug's clinical pharmacology. The following information is necessary: the drug's approved indication(s), potential unapproved indications (e.g., as an analgesic), common side effects and uncommon, but possibly serious, adverse effects, important pharmacokinetic features, and specific dosing guidelines for treating pain.

8. List analgesic adjunctive agents that may be useful in treating pain in companion animals.

- α_2-Adrenergic agonists: medetomidine, xylazine
- Antidepressants: amitriptyline, imipramine, paroxetine
- Topical preparations: EMLA cream, capsaicin
- NMDA receptor antagonists: ketamine
- Corticosteroids: prednisolone
- Antiarrhythmics: mexilitine, tocainide, lidocaine
- GABA agonists: diazepam, carbamazepine
- Anticonvulsants: gabapentin, phenytoin
- Neuroleptics: acepromazine

9. What is the mechanism of analgesic action of ketamine?

Ketamine has traditionally been viewed as a poor analgesic agent, and, although this is certainly the case when it comes to acute visceral pain, recent work has renewed interest in this old drug and revealed its potential as an analgesic adjuvant. Ketamine has historically been classified as a dissociative agent, and its labeled use is for chemical restraint and short-term anesthesia. We now know that it is an N-methyl-D-aspartate (NMDA) receptor antagonist in the central nervous system. By blocking the effects of the excitatory amino acid, glutamate, ketamine can reduce "wind-up" of dorsal horn neurons and diminish central sensitization. Evidence suggests that very low doses of ketamine may even be able to abolish hypersensitivity once it is already established. It is most often used in combination with opioids and seems particularly effective in managing pain of neuropathic origin.

10. What is the mechanism of analgesic action of α_2-adrenergic agonists?

Drugs such as medetomidine and xylazine bind to α_2-adrenoceptors located both pre- and post-synaptically in the dorsal horn of the spinal cord. This results in decreased release of a variety of neurotransmitters and neuropeptides (e.g., glutamate and substance P), as well as hyperpolarization of potassium channels. The net effect of these events is diminished ascending transmission of nociceptive input, which contributes to analgesia. For more information on α_2-adrenergic agonists, see Chapter 13.

11. What is the mechanism of analgesic action of intravenous lidocaine?

Local anesthetics are most commonly administered topically or regionally in relatively high concentrations directly in the vicinity of the nerve axon to induce conduction blockade and prevent nerve impulse propagation. For more information on local and regional analgesia, see Chapter 17 on the pharmacology of local anesthetics. Interestingly, the administration of lidocaine intravenously in very low doses has also been reported to have analgesic effects, especially in pain of neuropathic origin. The mechanism of this action remains unknown, but there are several possibilities. First, perhaps the sodium channels on injured axons may be more susceptible to conduction blockade induced by local anesthetics; consequently, low-dose intravenous administration may decrease peripheral transduction of the noxious stimulus and contribute to post-injury analgesia. Second, it is possible that the analgesic effect of intravenous lidocaine is not mediated by sodium channels at all, and other receptor systems, including NMDA, substance P, and acetylcholine receptors, have all been implicated as plausible targets. A sympatholytic effect may also contribute to analgesia in certain cases.

12. What does the term *neuroleptanalgesia* mean?

Neuroleptanalgesia refers to the unique state of hypnosis and analgesia produced by the combination of a neuroleptic drug and an analgesic drug. The only neuroleptic drug routinely used in veterinary medicine today is the phenothiazine acepromazine. It is important to remember that acepromazine has *no* inherent analgesic activity of its own; however, when combined with an opioid, acepromazine effectively prolongs and potentiates opioid-induced analgesia. The term *neuroleptanalgesia* is also used, in a more general sense, to describe the effect obtained when opioids are combined with other sedatives and tranquilizers, such as benzodiazepines and α_2-adrenergic agonists.

13. Are there any classes of analgesic drugs that should not be co-administered?

Yes, the combination of nonsteroidal anti-inflammatories and corticosteroids is contraindicated, as it may enhance the potential for serious gastrointestinal and/or renal toxicity. For more information on nonsteroidal anti-inflammatory agents, see the articles by Mathews, Papich, and Tranquilli et al.

14. List some common analgesic combinations that are useful in the preanesthetic period:
- Acepromazine + Opioid (e.g., morphine, oxymorphone, hydromorphone, fentanyl, meperidine, butorphanol, buprenorphine)
- α_2-Agonist (e.g., medetomidine, xylazine) + Opioid (as above)
- Benzodiazepine (e.g., diazepam, midazolam) + Opioid (as above)

15. List some common analgesic combinations that are useful intraoperatively or postoperatively:

Morphine 0.1–0.2 mg/kg/hour IV
or   +   **Ketamine** 0.5–1.5 mg/kg/hour IV
Fentanyl 0.001–0.004 mg/kg/hour IV

The opioid and ketamine are combined and administered as a continuous infusion. Nonsteroidal anti-inflammatory agents can also be administered with the above combination, and local and regional anesthetic techniques may also be indicated.

Morphine 0.1–0.2 mg/kg/hour IV
or   +   **Lidocaine** 1.0–3.0 mg/kg/hour IV
Fentanyl 0.001–0.004 mg/kg/hour IV

The opioid and lidocaine are combined and administered as a continuous infusion. If not contraindicated for other reasons, nonsteroidal anti-inflammatory agents can also be administered with these combinations.

BIBLIOGRAPHY

1. Kehlet H, Dahl JB: The value of "multimodal" or "balanced analgesia" in postoperative pain treatment. Anesth Analg 77:1048–1056, 1993.
2. Lamont LA, Tranquilli WJ, Mathews KA: Adjunctive analgesic therapy. Vet Clin North Am 30(4): 805–814, 2000.
3. Mathews KA: Nonsteroidal antiinflammatory anlagesics: Indications and contraindications for pain management in dogs and cats.Vet Clin North Am 30(4):783–804, 2000.
4. Papich MG: Pharmacologic considerations for opiate analgesic and nonsteroidal antiinflammatory drugs. Vet Clin North Am 30(4):815–838, 2000.
5. Tranquilli WJ, Grimm KA, Lamont LA: Pain Management for the Small Animal Practitioner. Jackson WY, Teton New Media, 2000.

59. PHYSIOLOGY OF CHRONIC PAIN

William Tranquilli, D.V.M., M.S., D.A.C.V.A.

1. What is the definition of *chronic pain*?

Chronic pain is generally thought of in terms of a prolonged time course of pain beyond that commonly experienced when somatic or visceral tissues are damaged. A number of disease entities are commonly associated with chronic pain syndromes, including cancer, arthritis, and a variety of neuropathies associated with abnormal peripheral (trigeminal neuralgia) or central (post-stroke pain) neuroprocessing.

2. What is neuropathic pain?

Neuropathic pain describes any acute or chronic pain syndrome sustained by aberrant somatosensory processing in either the peripheral or the central nervous system (CNS). In essence, pain originates from the nervous system itself rather than tissues that are innervated by afferent fibers and nociceptors.

3. How can chronic neuropathic pain be distinguished from other types of pain?

Pain type can be distinguished by inferred pathophysiology associated with pain. For example, the sustaining mechanisms of nociceptive somatic and visceral pain involves ongoing activation of pain-sensitive afferent somatic and visceral nerves that innervate these tissues and structures. *Psychogenic pain* refers to pain that has sustaining mechanisms related to psychological processes.

4. How does chronic inflammatory pain differ from chronic neuropathic pain?

Nociceptive pain mediates and is influenced by inflammatory changes, whereas neuropathic pain results from abnormal nerve function. Damage to peripheral tissues and injury to nerves typically produces persistent pain, hyperalgesia, and/or allodynia. Damage to cutaneous or deep (muscle, joint, viscera) tissue is associated with inflammation, whereas nerve damage leads to pathologic peripheral nerve changes, including neural degeneration, neuroma formation, and spontaneous neural discharge. Evidence suggests that although chronic nociceptive pain and neuropathic pain have separate origins and mechanisms of action, they both alter central neuroprocessing and, in turn, are influenced by psychogenic activity.

5. What is the most common cause of pain in cancer patients?

Either tumor involvement of pain sensitive tissue or organs or complications of therapy can cause pain in cancer patients. The most common type of cancer pain is bone metastasis, which can induce severe nociceptive pain.

6. Do NSAIDS have direct effects upon tumors?

Yes, NSAIDS produce their analgesic effects in cancer patients partially through their effects on the margins of tumors and the inflammation that exists at this site. Metastases of some tumor types require prostaglandins E_2 for growth, and NSAIDs inhibit prostaglandin production.

7. What is meant by *central sensitization*?

Central sensitization involves functional and structural changes in the CNS pathways that mediate nociception. Changes occur as a consequence of specific mechanisms that are only now being elucidated. Recent studies have documented the role of glutamate and *N*-methyl-D-aspartate (NMDA) receptors in producing sensitization of dorsal horn neurons. These changes underscore the plasticity of the central connections modulating nociception and pain processing within the CNS.

8. What are some of the changes induced by sustained aberrant neuroprocessing accompanying a variety of chronic pain syndromes?

Functional changes include lowered pain threshold, exaggerated activation, ectopic discharge, enlarged receptive fields, and loss of normal inhibitory processes. Structural changes include transsynaptic degeneration, transganglionic degeneration, and collateral sprouting.

9. What is phantom pain?

This term is applied to pain following amputation of a body part. The specific mechanisms that cause phantom pain are unknown. It may be conceptualized as "somatosensory memory" that does not reside in a specific location of the CNS but may involve complex interactions of neural networks in the brain and, as such, can be initiated by seemingly unrelated stimuli to the amputated structure.

10. How can you distinguish between neuropathic pain and nociceptive pain?

In nonverbal patients (young children, animals), this distinction is exceedingly difficult. Human patients describe neuropathic pain as burning, electric-like, or lancinating. Examination often reveals allodynia (pain on light touch), hyperalgesia (increased perception of pain), hyperesthesia (increased perception of non-noxious stimulus) or hyperpathia (exaggerated pain response). Veterinarians must infer these changes based on their knowledge and perceived changes in response patterns or behavior in the animal being examined.

11. What classes of analgesic agents can be used to treat chronic pain syndromes unresponsive to traditional analgesics?

Several classes of drugs considered *adjuvant* analgesics might be used. These include antidepressants, anticonvulsants, gamma-aminobutyric acid (GABA) agonists, oral local anesthetics, NMDA receptor antagonist (e.g., ketamine or dextromethorphan), and valproic acid. In addition, multipurpose agents such as the α_2-agonists, neuroleptics and corticosteroids may be helpful. As suggested by the term *adjuvant*, these analgesics are often coadministered with traditional analgesics to enhance efficacy and prolong analgesic activity.

12. What mechanisms mediate analgesia achieved with antidepressant drugs?

The analgesic action of antidepressants occurs more quickly and at a much lower dose than that necessary to treat depression. It is thought that antidepressants block re-uptake of monoaminergic neurotransmitters (e.g., serotonin and norepinephrine). Increased levels of these neurotransmitters may enhance pain inhibition within the spinal cord and higher centers.

13. Where does modulation of painful stimuli occur within the spinal cord?

Modulation occurs via endogenous systems that either inhibit or facilitate passage of pain stimuli through dorsal horn cells within the spinal cord and higher CNS centers.

14. What type of receptors located within the dorsal horn of the spinal cord facilitate pain transmission?

Substance P activates NK-1 type receptors to facilitate acute pain transmission while glutamate activates NMDA receptors. Prostaglandin receptors may also be activated by local release of prostaglandins within the dorsal horn.

15. What receptors inhibit pain transmission within the dorsal horn of the spinal cord?

Spinal receptors that are primarily inhibitory include the muscarinic, GABA, somatostatin, opioid, α_2, and adenosine receptors.

16. During a protracted period of surgery, does general anesthesia with an inhalant anesthetic prevent the development of central sensitization?

No. There is no evidence that clinical concentrations of inhalant anesthetics sufficiently dampen the neuroprocessing responsible for sensitization of pain pathways at the level of the spinal cord and above within the CNS.

BIBLIOGRAPHY

1. Tranquilli WJ, Grimm KA, Lamont LA: Pain Management for the Small Animal Practitioner. Jackson, WY, Teton New Media, 2000.

60. MANAGEMENT OF CHRONIC PAIN

Leigh A. Lamont, D.V.M.

1. Is chronic pain more difficult to treat than acute pain?

Yes. In chronic pain states, the nervous system itself becomes the focus of pathology. Abnormal activity in the peripheral and/or central nervous system results in misinterpretation of afferent input, which may be sustained long after the inciting noxious stimulus has subsided. Normal endogenous hypoalgesic mechanisms become less effective and, consequently, chronic pain is seldom permanently alleviated by administration of traditional analgesics.

2. Is chronic pain more difficult to recognize than acute pain?

Yes. Chronic pain is often insidious in onset, with the intensity of the pain gradually increasing over time. This, in combination with the remarkable ability of our patients to mask signs of pain or discomfort, makes recognizing chronic pain a challenge. Furthermore, the pain intensity assessment scales that are currently used in veterinary patients for acute pain are of little value for chronic pain recognition. Owners are probably the best equipped to perceive subtle changes in their animal's behavior, which may reflect pain.

3. Is implementing a pain management strategy a substitute for a thorough work-up?

No, absolutely not. Animals presenting with vague signs, such as decreased activity level, altered mood, and diminished appetite, should undergo a complete diagnostic evaluation with the goal of obtaining a correct medical diagnosis. Pain may be a symptom of a serious underlying condition and, if left untreated, may cause the patient permanent injury or even death. If a patient has been diagnosed with a terminal disease or is experiencing intractable pain secondary to an undiagnosable condition, attempts should be made to improve quality of life with analgesics while minimizing adverse reactions.

4. What is the Oxford Pain Chart?

Please fill in this chart each evening. Record an estimation of your pet's pain intensity and the amount of pain relief. If your pet had any side-effects, please note them in the side-effects box.

	Date							
Pain Intensity How bad was your pet's pain today?	Severe Moderate Mild None							
Pain Relief How much pain relief has the medication given your pet today?	Complete Good Moderate Slight None							
Side-effects Has the treatment upset your pet in any way?								
How effective was the treatment this week?	Poor ☐ Fair ☐ Good ☐ Very Good ☐ Excellent ☐							

Name _____ Treatment Week _____

From Tranquilli WJ, Grimm KA, Lamont LA: Pain Management. Jackson, WY: Teton New Media, 2000, p. 109, with permission.

This is a tool that can be used in assessing chronic pain in pets. The chart has been adapted from human medicine and is designed for owners to track the intensity of their animal's pain and response to treatment.

5. What are common conditions that may lead to development of a chronic pain state?
Conditions such as cancer (e.g., osteosarcoma), chronic inflammatory disease (e.g., chronic otitis), chronic orthopedic disease (e.g., osteoarthritis), chronic soft tissue injury (ex. degloving injuries), and nervous tissue injury (e.g., cervical intervertebral disc disease) are all common causes of chronic pain in dogs and cats.

6. When implementing an "at home" treatment program for chronic pain, what factors must be considered?
The treatment schedule, method of administration, and associated side effects must be amenable to both the owner and the patient, otherwise compliance will be poor. If long-term treatment is deemed appropriate, it may be prudent to collect baseline hematologic and biochemical data followed by periodic re-checks to monitor for adverse side effects associated with analgesic treatment. What works for one patient may not work for another, so if a particular approach is ineffective, alternative treatments should be explored. Remember that in some cases drug tolerance may develop, so chronic pain management strategies need to be flexible and evolve over time. Finally, many drug protocols for management of chronic pain are extra-label or off-label uses, so there is a degree of liability incurred by the practitioner, and this should be communicated to the owner prior to initiating treatment.

7. What drug delivery methods are most appropriate for managing chronic pain?
The oral route of administration is most common, and most owners and patients are comfortable with this technique. Owners can also be trained to administer medications by subcutaneous injection if necessary. Novel techniques are becoming increasingly available such as the fentanyl patch for transdermal opioid delivery, topical capsaicin ointment for management of neuropathic pain, and a variety of topical pleuronic gel formulations ranging from ketamine to ketoprofen.

8. What is the World Health Organization ladder for cancer pain management and is it applicable to managing chronic pain in dogs and cats?
The World Health Organization (WHO) has proposed a guideline for the treatment of chronic cancer pain in humans. The principles behind this simplified approach can be applied to chronic pain management in companion animals. See figure.

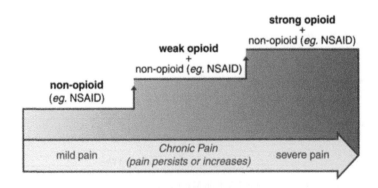

From Tranquilli WJ, Grimm KA, Lamont LA: Pain Management. Jackson, WY: Teton New Media, 2000, p. 110, with permission.

9. Are there studies documenting the analgesic efficacy of the drugs used to treat chronic pain in dogs and cats?

No, there are currently no systematic reviews of analgesic drugs and techniques used to treat chronic pain clinically in dogs and cats. Consequently, recommendations are based on treatment strategies used in human medicine, anecdotal reports in veterinary patients, and extrapolation from what we know about managing acute surgical pain in companion animals.

10. What drugs are commonly used to manage chronic pain in companion animals?

Initially, therapy with drugs classified as traditional or conventional analgesics should be instituted. Usually, oral nonsteroidal anti-inflammatory drugs (NSAIDs) are prescribed first and oral opioids are added if, or when, NSAIDs alone become ineffective. The most commonly administered NSAIDs are carprofen, etodolac, meloxicam, ketoprofen, and aspirin. Butor-phanol, codeine, and morphine are the most commonly used oral opioids. Transdermal fentanyl (in the form of the fentanyl patch) is another popular alternative. If the pain persists or increases in severity despite combination treatment with NSAIDs and opioids, or if the side effects associated with treatment become intolerable, therapy with analgesic adjuvant drugs should be initiated.

11. Are analgesic adjunctive agents potentially useful in the management of chronic pain?

Yes. Analgesic adjunctive agents are addressed in more detail in the chapter entitled "Analgesic Combinations." This diverse group of drugs, ranging from antidepressants to anticonvulsants to antiarrhythmics, has proven particularly useful in managing a variety of chronic pain syndromes in human patients. Since the focus of chronic pain is the nervous system itself, these drugs act at a variety of specific receptor systems to modulate signal generation or transmission. The analgesic effects seen in patients suffering from chronic pain are presumably a byproduct of these activities, although a common theme that adequately describes the mechanism of all such analgesic drugs is yet to be determined.

12. List some representative analgesic adjunctive agents with doses for dogs and cats.

	DOG	CAT
Amitriptyline • tricyclic antidepressant • duration of effect is 6–12 hrs	1.0 mg/kg PO	0.5–1.0 mg/kg PO
Mexiletene • oral antiarrhythmic • duration of effect is 6–12 hrs	10-20 mg/kg PO	5–10 mg/kg PO
Gabapentin • anticonvulsant • duration of effect is 8–12 hrs	2.5–5.0 mg/kg PO	2.5–5.0 mg/kg PO
Ketamine • N-methyl-D-aspartate receptor antagonist • duration of effect is 4–6 hrs	0.1–1.0 mg/kg IM, SC, PO	0.1–1.0 mg/kg IM, SC, PO
EMLA Cream • topical local anesthetic		
Capsaicin Cream • active ingredient in hot peppers		

13. What other techniques are potentially useful in managing chronic pain?

Veterinarians have an increasing variety of nonpharmacologic options available for the treatment of chronic pain. Acupuncture can be particularly effective in certain chronic pain syndromes and is discussed in more detail in chapter 67. Trancutaneous electrical nerve stimulation (TENS), trancutaneous acupoint electrical stimulation (TAES) and percutaneous electrical nerve stimulation (PENS) have been used as adjuvants to treat numerous types of chronic pain in human patients and may prove useful in veterinary patients as well. Other upcoming possibilities include magnetic field induction, iontophoretic delivery of local anesthetics and neurolysis.

BIBLIOGRAPHY

1. Brearley JC, Brearley MJ: Chronic pain in animals. In Flecknell P, Waterman-Pearson A (eds): Pain Management in Animals. London, WB Saunders, 2000, pp 147–160.
2. Lamont LA, Tranquilli WJ, Mathews KA: Adjunctive analgesic therapy. Vet Clin North Am 30(4): 805–814, 2000.
3. Lester P, Gaynor JS: Management of Cancer Pain. Vet Clin North Am 30(4):951–966, 2000.
4. McLaughlin R: Management of chronic osteoarthritic pain. Vet Clin North Am 30(4):933–950, 2000.
5. Tranquilli WJ, Grimm KA, Lamont LA: Pain Management for the Small Animal Practitioner. Jackson, WY, Teton NewMedia, 2000.

61. ACUPUNCTURE ANALGESIA

Stephen A. Greene, D.V.M., M.S., D.A.C.V.A.

1. What is acupuncture?

Acupuncture is the placement of needles through the skin at specific anatomical sites to produce an analgesic or therapeutic benefit. Stimulation of acupuncture points is believed to "re-balance" the flow of energy through channels or "meridians" within the body. According to traditional Chinese medical theory, imbalance in energy flow is the fundamental underlying cause of pain and pathologic conditions.

2. What is the mechanism of acupuncture analgesia?

Stimulation of nerve endings by acupuncture needles sends afferent traffic to the spinal cord. At the level of the spinal cord, descending pathways inhibitory to pain may be activated, or further transmission along ascending pathways to the brain may occur. Brain responses may include release of endorphins and enkephalins. These substances can have central nervous system (CNS) analgesic effects, or they may enter the systemic circulation for transport to the local area of pain where they bind to receptors. In addition, brain activity can be initiated to stimulate descending spinal pathways that are inhibitory to pain transmission. Finally, local disruption of blood vessels by the acupuncture needle may lead to release of neurotransmitters, complement activators, and other chemical mediators that modulate pain transmission.

3. In traditional Chinese medicine, what is the underlying imbalance associated with joint pain?

According to theory of traditional Chinese medicine, joint pain may be caused by stagnation of energy ("chi") flow. Imbalance in the energy flow through a specific joint may occur because of various influences that upset the balance of energy within an individual. Thus, the goal in treating pain is to treat the underlying cause of the stagnation and energy flow imbalance. This may be accomplished using acupuncture points that are close in proximity to the painful joint as well as points that are distant yet functionally related (in Chinese medical theory) to the local region afflicted.

4. What pharmacologic agents interfere with acupuncture analgesia?

Agents that are likely to interfere with acupuncture analgesia include drugs that decrease serotonin (e.g., cinanserin), naloxone, drugs that block acetylcholine production (e.g., hemicholine), α-agonists (e.g., clonidine), propranolol, aminophyline, and paracetamol. Depending on the stimulus, neurotransmitters such as norepinephrine can be either inhibitory or promoters of acupuncture analgesia. Exogenous steroids (e.g., dexamethasone) may also inhibit acupuncture analgesia.

5. For what conditions does acupuncture analgesia seem appropriate in animals?

In veterinary practice, animals are frequently treated with acupuncture for chronic pain conditions associated with joints. Osteoarthritis is a common condition for which pet owners seek alternatives to pharmacologic analgesic therapy to preserve the desirable personality, energy level, or liver function of their animals. Chronic pain conditions are likely not cured by acupuncture and may require continuously repeated treatments. Pain arising from other causes and location can also be treated by acupuncture. Acute pain associated with surgery is not readily managed by acupuncture alone. Postoperative pain control using acupuncture as an adjunct to pharmacologic analgesics may allow use of lower doses or less frequent dosing regimens.

6. How is surgical anesthesia produced by acupuncture?

Surgical analgesia in human volunteers has been demonstrated by experienced Chinese acupuncturists. People who are specifically suited to this type of analgesic technique are selected for demonstration purposes. Similarly, animals with behavior traits amenable to conscious immobilization have undergone successful surgical procedures using acupuncture analgesia. In contemporary accounts, electroacupuncture has been used to provide surgical analgesia rather than simple needle acupuncture. Selection of acupuncture points is determined by the location of the surgical site and the general condition of the patient. Acupuncture for surgical analgesia requires a long preparatory time before the patient is ready. At this time, pharmacologically induced analgesia or anesthesia is more efficient and reliable for most surgical procedures in animals.

7. What is electroacupuncture?

Electroacupuncture is the application of electrical stimuli to acupuncture points. The electrical stimuli may be delivered transcutaneously or via acupuncture needles. Electrostimulation of acupuncture points can produce more controllable and higher intensity stimulation than manual needle stimulation. Physiologic changes induced by electroacupuncture include cardiovascular effects, altered gastrointestinal motility, and analgesia. Some indications for electroacupuncture are chronic pain, induction of surgical anesthesia, and paralysis. Electroacupuncture should not be used in animals that are pregnant or in animals with shock, hypotension, epilepsy, or cardiac dysrhythmias.

8. How does electroacupuncture differ from transcutaneous electrical nerve stimulation (TENS)?

For treatment of painful conditions, electroacupuncture is used, with low-frequency, high-intensity stimulation (1–5 Hz and 15–50 mA). This type of stimulation can produce general anesthesia and is associated with liberation of endorphins. When used over a period of several treatment days, effects of electroacupuncture tend to be cumulative.

TENS is usually a high-frequency, low-intensity stimulation (> 70 Hz and < 10 mA) and activates large-diameter sensory nerve fibers. The analgesia from TENS is rapid in onset, not cumulative with repeated treatment, and mediated by serotonin, norepinephrine, and dynorphins rather than endorphins. TENS is delivered transcutaneously via broad electrodes applied to the skin surface.

BIBLIOGRAPHY

1. Altman S: Techniques and instrumentation. In Schoen AM (ed): Veterinary Acupuncture, 2nd ed. St. Louis, Mosby, 2001, pp 95–111.
2. Chapman CR, Gunn CC: Acupuncture. In Bonica JJ (ed): The Management of Pain, 2nd ed. Philadelphia, Lea & Febiger, 1990, pp 1805–1821.
3. Cheng E, Pomeranz B, Yue G: Dexamethasone partially reduces and 2% saline treatment abolishes electroacupuncture analgesia: These findings implicate pituitary endorphins. Life Sci 24:1481–1486, 1979.
4. Gaynor JS: Acupuncture for management of pain. Vet Clin North Am Small Anim Prac 30:875–881, 2000.
5. Kendall DE: A scientific model for acupuncture: Part 1. Am J Acupuncture 17:251–268, 1989.
6. Kendall DE: A scientific model for acupuncture: Part 2. Am J Acupuncture 17:343–360, 1989.
7. Melzack R, Wall PD: Pain mechanisms: A new theory. Science 150:971, 1965.
8. Price DD et al: A psychophysical analysis of acupuncture analgesia. Pain 19:27–32, 1984.
9. Sjölund BH, Eriksson M, Loeser JD: Transcutaneous and implanted electric stimulation of peripheral nerves. . In: Bonica JJ (ed), The Management of Pain, 2nd ed. Philadelphia, Lea & Febiger, 1990, pp 1852–1861.
10. Steiss JE: The neurophysiologic basis of acupuncture. In: Schoen AM (ed): Veterinary Acupuncture, 2nd ed. St. Louis, Mosby, 2001, pp 27–46.

INDEX

Entries in **boldface** type signify complete chapters.

Printed and bound by CPI Group (UK) Ltd, Croydon, CR0 4YY

03/10/2024

01040848-0011